CANCER
the full menu

Rolf Gordon

DULWICH HEALTH
130 GIPSY HILL, LONDON SE19 1PL

DEDICATED to my darling wife Lena, our very active son Mads, my vibrant sister Brita and my exciting sister-in-law Adda, who may not have died of cancer if I had known all the information in this book at the time they were diagnosed.

ACKNOWLEDGEMENT I am grateful for the encouragement, advice and help given to me by doctors, health practitioners and numerous people including many cancer patients from all over the world. I would also like to thank all my staff and friends for their criticism, inspiration and help in producing this book from my longhand scripts.

Book also by Rolf Gordon 'Are You Sleeping In A Safe Place?'

Published by Dulwich Health Limited, 130 Gipsy Hill, London, SE19 1PL
Tel: +44 (0)20 8670 5883   Fax: +44 (0)20 8766 6616

ISBN 978 0 951 4017 0 6

PREFACE

'CANCER - the full menu' is written not just for the approximately two million people in the UK who have had cancer diagnosed and for their family and close friends, but for everyone to help prevent them getting cancer in the first place. Don't forget that one in three people will die of cancer. Even though this book is, in my opinion, one of the most comprehensive written on the subject of cancer, it is not necessary for you to read it from cover to cover. You can very quickly read what is relevant to your problem.

When you are first told by your doctor that you have cancer, you are in shock and will most likely remember very little of what you were told. Here you can quickly read about diagnosis and the latest orthodox treatments available. So when you next talk with your doctor and medical team, you can concentrate on finding out more about your individual case and concerns.

You can then read about the 'BIG FOUR', which must be dealt with quickly to ensure that your treatment results in you being given the 'all clear' as soon as possible and reduce the likelihood of your cancer returning. Take a look through the index - you may well find the help and advice you need in just one or two chapters.

Please note that I have no medical qualifications, but have gathered my information from many doctors, cancer specialists, health practitioners and thousands of cancer patients I have been involved with over the last 24 years. I therefore recommend you contact your doctor first if you are worried and take your doctor's advice.

I alone take responsibility for any errors or misinterpretations of text and illustrations which have all been drawn freehand by me.

"This is the most comprehensive and informative book written on cancer. I strongly recommend it to anybody, whether or not they have cancer".
Dr Patrick Kingsley M.B., B.S., M.R.C.S., L.R.C.P., F.A.A.E.M., D.A., D.Obst., R.C.O.G. who has dealt with thousands of cancer patients during 30 years in practice.

"This book is essential reading for anyone wishing to understand and compare immuno-supportive and immuno-suppressive approaches to cancer management. It is clearly written, scholarly and informative".
Dr Stephen Bourne M.B., M.R.C.G.P., Dip. Homotox (Hons)

"I was very impressed with your book. It has been written from the heart and without ego".
High Court Judge, Michael H.D.

CONTENTS

CANCER - the full menu
Cancer Cesspit

42% of you may have to be rescued from the cancer cesspit by the modern orthodox medical profession involving powerful drugs, highly skilled surgeons and very accurate radiotherapy (all described in great detail in over 25 chapters on individual cancers).

Having been treated, you are then thrown back into the cesspit often for the cancer to return, when even more powerful treatment has to be carried out, nearly always with very severe side-effects. This is all because doctors are unlikely to know why you got cancer in the first place. You certainly do not get cancer by chance. 1 in 2 men and 1 in 3 women die of cancer.

I make no excuses for using the strong words 'cancer cesspit' after having been with my darling wife Lena, my vibrant sister Brita and our fantastic son Mads while they were dying of cancer. Our son was 26 when he died. Has anybody got more appropriate words?

Hundreds of times I have heard cancer patients in their thirties and forties say: "I eat a healthy diet, am slim, do not smoke, drink very little alcohol, exercise on a regular basis and have no history of cancer in my family. I have done all the things the cancer research charities say I should do to prevent getting cancer - so why did I get cancer?"

Every 2 minutes someone is diagnosed with cancer in the UK, (over 270,000 per year). If cancer continues to increase at today's rate, it will soon be the main cause of death. Already one in three women and one in two men will develop cancer at some point during their life time. Once diagnosed, cancer is fatal in 47% of young women and 37% of young men.

I have been involved with well over 5,000 people who have been diagnosed with cancer over the last 24 years. **All** had problems with THE BIG FOUR, which are not generally checked for by doctors. The most harmful of THE BIG FOUR is **Geopathic Stress** - which luckily the majority of you are not most of the time. It was proved to the complete satisfaction of all doctors at a cancer conference in Berlin about 80 years ago that, **one is unlikely to develop cancer unless one has slept or stayed for long periods in places of Geopathic Stress.** Thousands of medical doctors and therapists now confirm Geopathic Stress must be cleared before any cancer treatment can be 100% successful. Many eminent doctors who specialise in cancer, have associated cancer directly with Geopathic Stress in tens of thousands of cases (see my book 'Are You Sleeping In A Safe Place'?).

Even if you have a certain gene, which in cases of breast cancer gives you a higher risk, this is unlikely to have an effect on you unless you are Geopathic Stressed. Most childhood cancers are caused by the mother having slept in a Geopathic Stress place during pregnancy and the child then sleeping in a Geopathic Stress place afterwards.

Unfortunately, most doctors still completely dismiss Geopathic Stress and say it has not been scientifically proven. In fact, it has far more scientific evidence than many pharmaceutical drugs and the only 'side-effect' by moving your bed into a Geopathic Stress free place is you will most likely sleep and feel better!

Geopathic Stress is one of the main causes of depression, which makes any physical illness even worse and more difficult to recover from. Most people who get cancer have very acidic blood and are high in micro-parasites (who love Geopathic Stress). They are also low in certain vital enzymes, vitamins, minerals and trace elements due to a poor absorption rate caused by Geopathic Stress, subsequently resulting in malnutrition.

The above results in a weakened immune system, the main cause of your cancer. Also many people die of other illnesses after cancer treatment, like pneumonia, septicaemia, heart attack etc. due to an impaired immune system, which has been further damaged by the cancer treatment. It is one statistic which is not published, but combined with cancer is no doubt the major cause of death today. We all create hundreds of pre-cancerous cells every day, but they are normally destroyed by our strong immune system.

Very little orthodox treatment can boost your immune system, so to be on the safe side and prevent getting cancer again - often in a different place - you must incorporate complementary remedies.

Unfortunately, Britain is at the bottom of the cancer survival league in Europe, apart from some former Eastern Block countries such as Estonia, Poland and Slovenia[1]. This is often due to general practitioners failing to spot cancer symptoms (insist on a second opinion if you have any suspicions), finding it hard to access a cancer specialist and the average long waiting time to be diagnosed and for the orthodox treatment to start. Also very successful treatments carried out widely for many years in the USA and other Western countries are only available in a few UK hospitals [2]. It is, therefore, even more important that complementary remedies are considered as they can sometimes delay the spread of the cancer and often reduce tumours, so they are easier to treat by orthodox means. This can also ensure you are not among the more than 50% who, on average, do not survive cancer for more than five years.

The wonderful thing about complementary remedies is that you often get amazing results and even if they do not work, you seldom suffer any bad side-effects. The only warning is some therapists may charge you a large fee for little results, and there are certain herbs that you should not take before an operation (see details under operation in Part Two), as they may increase your blood flow.

The irony is, many doctors say "do not try complementary remedies, they might do you harm", when tens of thousands of people in the UK die of orthodox medicine every year.

It has now been revealed, that 40% more men die of cancer than women, excluding breast and prostate cancer. The three main reasons are:

Firstly - Men are usually more reluctant to visit their GP, so their cancer is diagnosed at a later stage, making successful treatment less likely. Five out of six men's jobs are full time, compared with only half of women's jobs and GP surgeries are generally closed when full-time workers might want to visit their doctor.

Secondly - Of the thousands of people who have come to me for advice on cancer, about three out of four are women, who contact me both on behalf of themselves or their husband/partner etc. When given vital recommendations, the answer is often 'he will only believe in what his doctor tells him'. In only a few cases is it the other way round i.e. the woman is the one who does not believe in life saving complementary remedies.

Thirdly - Cancer experts blame the NHS for being in favour of saving women victims.

Do try to incorporate simple preventative measures described in the following chapters to ensure you are unlikely to get cancer again or do not get cancer in the first place.

[1] Britain spends twice as much per head of population on medical care as countries which are higher on the survival league table such as Portugal.
[2] Such as Photo Dynamic Laser Treatment and Cyberknife radiotherapy.

Here is a typical case of combining orthodox treatment with complementary remedies

Malcolm, from Kent, was very grateful that the remedies and treatment I suggested, which he carried out himself, reduced the size of the very rare bone cancer in his lower right leg by some 80%. Instead of the initial recommended leg amputation above his knee, a small operation was carried out to remove the dead cancer cells. He also had secondary cancer in his lungs, which again reduced by a massive amount thereby enabling a small operation to remove the remaining cancer (see copy of letter from Malcolm under bone cancer).

Geopathic Stress is caused by the earth's good vibrations, which rise up through the earth and are distorted by weak electromagnetic fields created mainly by subterranean running water, but often strengthened by certain mineral concentrations, fault lines and underground cavities. The distorted vibrations become abnormally high and harmful to living organisms.

Unfortunately, Geopathic Stress has become many times stronger during the last few years due to 'solar weather ' - the effect of the sun's rays have become much more damaging because of the weaker ozone layer, thereby increasing the Geopathic Stress vibrations. This is one of the main causes of the steady increase in cancer cases and other illnesses.

Even after investing TEN TIMES as much now on cancer research and treatment (about £200 billion world-wide per year) as 20 years ago, the death rate from cancer has DOUBLED (in the USA from 300,000 to 600,000 per year). During the same period Geopathic Stress has become about three times stronger.

Cases, where cancer patients have benefited by eliminating the Geopathic Stress

Often people with a brain tumour, who have taken my advice, have told me days after moving their bed into a safe place, they wake up without a headache and feel much better for the first time in a long while.

Bill had leukaemia when he was born. He was still being treated, when he was four years old. I told his mother how to move Bill's bed into a Geopathic Stress-free place. A few months later Bill's mother rang me to say their doctor had just told her, "It is a miracle. Bill no longer has leukaemia." This good result cost nothing.

Beverley had just had a brain tumour operation. The doctor told Bob, her husband, she only had days to live. Bob could feel his wife's hospital bed was in a very strong Geopathic Stress place. He managed to get his wife's bed moved across the ward into a Geopathic Stress-free place. Beverley was discharged from hospital within two weeks!

John, with lung cancer, said "I slept so much better immediately after moving my bed into a good place" and his skin colour became remarkably healthy-looking overnight.

16 year old Peter was diagnosed with Hodgkin's disease and diabetes. Chemotherapy was recommended, but refused by Peter's parents, as Peter's mother, a nurse, had seen the terrible side-effects of chemotherapy. They signed a disclaimer and Peter was discharged from hospital. Having heard about Geopathic Stress, they found Peter's bed was very Geopathically Stressed and therefore moved it into a safe place. This is almost 20 years ago and Peter is now not only in excellent health, but also is no longer diabetic.

12 year old Edward had a non-operable tumour as big as a melon in his abdomen. His bed was found to be very Geopathic Stressed and was therefore moved into a safe place. Soon, his tumour shrunk to the size of a lemon and eventually vanished altogether. It was confirmed he no longer had cancer. Doctors agreed the chemotherapy Edward was having at the time would not have made his tumour vanish.
(Chemotherapy is not very effective on large tumours).
His doctors said it was 'spontaneous remission'. Edward soon became a strong member of his school's rugby team.

Thomas was diagnosed with testicular cancer when he was 25 years old. He refused orthodox treatment including chemotherapy. Thomas discovered he was sleeping in a Geopathic Stress place and immediately moved his bed into a good place. This is over 15 years ago and Thomas is now very healthy and completely free of cancer.

Jette had surgery to remove cancerous tumours on both her ovaries, followed by intensive chemotherapy treatment. Her doctor told her without hesitation, that her type of cancer most often came back and was then terminal. Jette's bed was found to be very Geopathic Stressed. She had slept there for 18 years and always had cold feet and sweated profusely each night. As soon as Jette's bed was moved into a Geopathic Stress-free place, Jette's feet immediately became warm during the night and she was no longer sweating. It is almost seven years since Jette had cancer. She is now back in a full time job, a healthy person, full of life with sparkling eyes much to the delight of her husband and children.

Linda went through a very tough chemotherapy, radiotherapy and bone marrow treatment for leukaemia at the age of 15. This resulted in her being clear of cancer. She went home and for the first few months she slept in her mother's cosy bed and her health improved from week to week. Linda then went back to her own bed and a hospital check-up soon afterwards showed the leukaemia might have recurred and her doctors were very worried. When one of Linda's mother's work colleagues heard about Linda's problems, she agreed to check Linda's bed and found it very Geopathic Stressed. Linda's bed was immediately moved into a safe place and tests soon showed Linda's cancer had gone. It is now 20 years ago since Linda escaped cancer and is now a very healthy woman in her thirties, but she will always ensure she sleeps in a good place.

There are many more successful cases described in the chapters dealing with the individual types of cancer.

Gradually many doctors and nurses now realise orthodox and complementary remedies must work in tandem to obtain the best results. But why do most doctors still not believe in anything other than orthodox treatment? Let me give you an example:

Hundreds of thousands of people have safely eliminated gall bladder stones in days, (all soft and many as large as nails) without pain, using a combination of apple juice, olive oil and lemon juice. The success rate is over 95%. Yet surgeons carry out hundreds of thousands of major painful operations a year to remove gall bladders or carry out keyhole surgery, which is not always successful. There is sometimes a lengthy recovery time and you cannot eat normally for a long time - if ever - afterwards. Often people have continuous pain waiting over a year for an operation, which can cost over £4,000. So, if doctors do not believe in this simple remedy, which can relieve sufferers of so much discomfort quickly and save the nation millions each year, why should doctors believe in anything not orthodox? I have personal experience that the gall bladder flush works 100%. (See Part Nine for full details of the gall bladder flush).

I will explain later how you can check for Geopathic Stress very quickly and easily with a simple home-made device made in minutes and costing nothing. There are other simple methods of checking including the muscle test (kinesiology) which can also check which remedies or therapies are best for you. Do not forget you are unique, so what is good for other people, may not be suitable for you. These tests are already used by millions of people all over the world.

Cancer - the full menu

It is vital you know 'the full menu' to ensure the most successful outcome. Many oncologists (cancer specialists) do not discuss 'the full menu' if the ideal treatment is not available at their hospital. As mentioned before, the amazing Photo Dynamic treatment and Cyberknife radiotherapy are only available at one or two UK hospitals. So get a second opinion, as you can now be treated at a hospital of your choice. Also most doctors are unlikely to recommend important complementary remedies to give you the best chance to ensure your cancer does not come back.

Quick and easy read

Each type of cancer has a separate chapter including children's and animal cancers and can be read on its own. All is written in an easy-to-read language with great detail about symptoms, research, individual cancers, diagnosis, latest orthodox treatment and how to ensure a high success rate. You would be lucky to find all this information within hundreds of hours on the internet or in books - in my opinion this is one of the most comprehensive book written on cancer, yet what you are interested in can be read very quickly.

There are also chapters on chemotherapy, radiotherapy, surgery, lasers, nutrition, some very powerful and very successful complementary therapies not even mentioned by cancer charities, how your immune system works, why we in Britain are thousands of times more likely to get breast cancer and prostate cancer than in China etc. I also explain how to kill micro parasites present in all cancer patients, which most doctors do not understand and have no remedy for and why in all cancer cases the liver is weak, so it cannot produce enough Co-enzyme Q10 which is the sparking plug for all our cells and vital for the body's metabolism. Also how chemists have recently managed to extract highly reactive compounds from a well known herb, which has been shown to have a very beneficial effect on cancer patients, destroy micro parasites, boost the immune system and deal with pneumonia, septicaemia and even eliminate MRSA and E-Coli in most cases. There are also chapters on hospitals, financial help, insurance and vaccinations when travelling abroad and how to help friends with cancer etc. (See contents for full list of chapters).

Is it imperative you incorporate proven, simple and powerful changes to ensure you live a full natural life without cancer coming back or developing it in the first place. Remember the term 'survival' used by doctors, only means cancer has not come back within 5 years.

THE BIG FOUR are fully explained and how to deal with them.

Change before you have to.

Take charge of your own health.

Over 90% of children and 75% of adults will sleep much better if they move their beds out of Geopathic Stress (babies, who are continuously crying at night, will nearly always start to sleep peacefully). Most animals in the wild and domestic animals in the open will seek to sleep in Geopathic Stress free place. Nearly all trees and plants will thrive better when they grow in Geopathic Stress free places.

CHARLOTTE

Charlotte was a very pleasant, smiling, happy child who interacted well with others up until approximately 2 years ago when she was moved into her present bedroom.

All round she began to go downhill. With time she became very morose and uninterested in interacting with others. Her appetite became very poor; she pushed food around her plate or refused to eat. She was very pale and was always listless, continuously complaining of tiredness. She spent her time lying on a couch with her thumb in her mouth and her teddy over her face. She also had a problem with bed wetting. Worst of all her temper tantrums were so bad they had to be seen to be believed. Her mother found her very difficult, in addition to the temper tantrums she wouldn't do as she was told.

"We decided to ask Rolf Gordon to check her room for Geopathic Stress". A strong Geopathic Stress line was found to be running the length of her bedroom and through two other rooms. The line ran lengthways down the middle of her bed. Her bed was moved away from the Geopathic Stress line and almost immediately she started to improve. Bed wetting went down to once a week and within a few weeks had stopped altogether. Her colour improved, she had pink cheeks instead of pale and washed-out. She became much livelier and started interacting better with others, spending more time playing happily with her brother. Her behaviour otherwise improved considerably with only a normal child's transient reaction if told off by parents. Her appetite increased, she started asking for second helpings. At school her reading ability suddenly went up, almost as if something had suddenly clicked.

"Thanks to the discovery by Rolf Gordon that my granddaughter was sleeping in a Geopathically Stressed area and consequently moving her bed, Charlotte now aged 5 years, is a much more pleasant, happy and healthier child. The improvement is quite amazing".

**Linda M, Northern Ireland
(Charlotte's grandmother)**

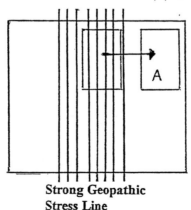

**Charlotte's bed
moved to A**

**Strong Geopathic
Stress Line**

Do you need more proof how harmful Geopathic Stress is?

PART ONE

The BIG FOUR

> The BIG FOUR have been known for years and must first of all be dealt with. I have found them a problem in all the over 5,000 cancer cases I have been involved with during the last 24 years. They are the main reason why your immune system has become weak, which is the major problem in all cancer cases. No medical drug will prevent this.

ONE

Geopathic Stress As this is one of the prime reasons you got cancer in the first place, you must deal with this immediately, not only to strengthen your immune system, but also so you can get over any harsh orthodox treatments quicker and make sure they work better for you. So you have to ensure that you sleep and sit in a Geopathic Stress-free place.

TWO

Micro Parasites Dr Helda Clark found after more than ten years of research that, in most cancer cases, there was a large presence of micro parasites. One of the quickest and most successful methods of killing all types of micro parasites without any side-effects, is to take 100% stabilised allicin derived by a patented process from garlic. It is also a very strong immune booster before and after any cancer treatment.

THREE

Q10 (Co-enzyme) This is the enzyme in every cell in your body which gives them 90% of their energy. This is why the largest amount of Q10 is in your heart. Q10 is developed in the liver from food. Your liver is often weak if you have cancer, so it cannot produce enough Q10. You normally die if you have 30% or less of normal amounts of Q10 in your body. Many cancer patients I have checked out only have 60% on a scale where 100% is normal.

FOUR

Acid-Alkaline Balance of your blood. Nurses confirm that nearly all patients in hospital cancer wards have very acidic blood. This causes vital alkaline minerals to be used up in your body in an attempt to neutralise your blood balance. High acidic levels also decrease your oxygen levels and your body cells will start to die.

76% of people who die of cancer are over 65 This is caused by elderly people having stayed longer in Geopathic Stress places, their bodies not producing enough Q10 and the fact that they are likely to eat more acidic food. They have also been damaged longer by free radicals and are generally lower in vital nutrients. They delay going to their doctor as they feel cancer symptoms are normal signs of getting older. Finally, they do less exercise, which among other things prevents their lymph system detoxifying their body adequately.

Most people who get cancer suffer from malnutrition even if they have been on a healthy diet. Read in PART FOUR why and how to correct this with essential supplements. Also learn why dairy products and artificial sweeteners may cause cancer.

The BIG FOUR has also been found to affect most people with other serious illnesses including multiple sclerosis, Alzheimer's disease, dementia, upper respiratory infection, motor neurone disease, Lyme and Lupus disease etc.

GEOPATHIC STRESS

> It was proved almost 80 years ago that **one is unlikely to develop cancer unless one has slept or stayed for long periods in places of Geopathic Stress.**

In 1929 Gustav von Pohl, a German scientist, proved the above to the satisfaction of the Central Committee for Cancer Research in Berlin.[1] Dr Hans MD checked the beds of 5,346 people who had died of cancer and found they had all slept in very Geopathic Stress (GS) places. The world renowned cancer specialist, Dr Hans Nieper stated "92% of all my cancer patients are GS".[1] It is estimated more than 4,000 medical doctors, on the continent of Europe, arranged to have the beds (of patients who suffer from cancer and other serious illnesses) checked out for GS.

Professor Otto Berman carried out a double-blind test on almost one thousand people to prove the harmful effect GS has on the human body.[1]

What is Geopathic Stress

Geopathic Stress is the earth's vibrations which rise up through the earth and are distorted by weak electromagnetic fields created by subterranean running water, certain mineral concentrations, fault lines and underground cavities. The distorted vibrations become abnormally high and harmful to living organisms.

GS has become much stronger over the last few years due to the sun penetrating the weaker ozone layer more easily and increasing the strength of the GS, thereby causing even more cancer cases each year (double over the last 20 years in the USA).

How Do I Know If I Am Geopathic Stressed?

If you cannot shake off an illness, depression or feel below par, ask yourself:

1. Did my health problem begin shortly after moving into my home or place of work?
2. Do I feel better when I am away from home or my place of work?
3. Do any of my family feel uneasy about the 'atmosphere' at home?
4. Did the previous occupants suffer from any serious or long-term illness?
5. Does the illness seem to be worse during autumn or spring or wet stormy weather (when underground water may be flowing at higher velocity thereby causing more Geopathic Stress)?
6. Were there any nearby disturbances, which may have caused underground water veins to flow into different channels under my house prior to my illness (landslides, building and road work, working quarries and mines etc.)?
7. Does my home or any part of it feel unnaturally cold or damp?

Geopathic Stress and Sleep

Sleeping in a GS place is particularly stressful, as a large area of your body is exposed to the GS. Also most people sleep during the night, when GS is stronger. During sleep, your

---

[1] See full details in my book 'Are You Sleeping In A Safe Place'.

brain is supposed to rest half the time and is busy healing your body the other half. However, if you are GS during sleep, your brain has to spend all of its time working due to the strain of GS and you wake up tired.

The 1 sq. metre (10 sq.ft.) you sleep on and therefore spend about one third of your life on, must be free from Geopathic Stress.

Read later, (under Nutrition), how GS can cause you to absorb as little as 50% of the vital minerals, vitamins and trace elements from your food.

Answer to Sceptics

Many feel the effect of GS is purely psychological and due to suggestion, but then you cannot influence the behaviour of animals, plants and babies.

Most animals will try to sleep in a good place and will become ill if forced to live in a GS home, stable, etc.
Most types of trees will have stunted growth and not bear fruit in GS places.
You will often find indoor plants will not thrive in a GS place in a home.

Cancer

I have found in all cases of cancer, tumours first developed when two or more GS lines crossed, or there was one very strong GS line. In cases of cancer of the blood or lymph system, GS lines often covered the whole bed.

Here are just a few of the thousands of cancer cases I have checked out.

| Brain Tumour | Cervical Cancer | Tumour in RH lung | Prostate Cancer | RH Breast Cancer |

Hospitals

Most hospital nurses will tell you some beds have a 'reputation' where patients, who occupy them, seem to have more difficulty in recovering or where the death rate is higher. The beds are GS.

Checking for Geopathic Stress

Most people can check for themselves if there is Geopathic Stress in their home but there is no scientific instrument yet which is sensitive and selective enough. There are also recognised methods of detecting GS in people, like the VEGA Test and Kinesiology. (See Part Nine).

Other problems caused by Geopathic Stress

- M.E., asthma, P.M.S., cot death, heart problems, bipolar disorder and depression.
- Long-term physical and mental illnesses where treatment does not seem to work.
- Children who are hyperactive - have learning difficulties - are difficult to control.
- Children born with defects.
- Long-term stress in relationships/at work.
- Miscarriage, premature birth, not being able to conceive and difficult pregnancies.
- Allergies to food and drink.
- Child abuse.
- Road rage.

More Successful Surgery

You are much more relaxed if you are not Geopathically Stressed. Research carried out by the University of Texas has shown that patients who were relaxed before cancer surgery, had a more active immune system 48 hours afterwards which improved healing. The patients also had greater activity of their natural killer T-cells (see page 247), which help protect the body from inflammation and infection. Natural killer T-cells also detach and destroy rogue cancer cells. Many surgeons in Germany will not carry out major surgery on patients who are Geopathically Stressed.

Swine Flu

All the people who have died of swine flu were Geopathic Stressed, even the ones who had no 'underlying health matters'.

Mental Illness

Making a patient Geopathic Stress free, showing the patient kindness and understanding and sharing their feelings are much more effective than any antidepressant medical drug.

MICRO PARASITES

It is claimed micro parasites are present in most people who get cancer. So to eliminate cancer it is very important you kill these micro parasites. This can in most cases be successfully done with a powerful 100% stabilised allicin extract.

Diseases caused by micro parasites have now reached epidemic proportions and one of the most under diagnosed and under appreciated health threats in the world. Not only do doctors not, as a general rule, check for micro parasites as you need a dark field microscope of which there are very few in the UK, but medical drugs are not very successful in killing them all.

You can check if you have micro parasites by using the Muscle Test (see page 269) or a health practitioner can check you out on a VEGATEST (See page 276).

AlliTech is nature's very powerful way of destroying micro parasites. It is also a successful antibiotic, anti-viral, anti-fungal immune booster. AlliTech is a patented product containing 100% stabilised Allisure®. Allicin is created from the two compounds Allinase and Alliin, which are kept completely separate inside garlic, until the bulb is attacked by microbes in the soil.

Dr Hulda Regehr Clark Ph.D. in her book 'The Cure For All Cancer' describes how she, over ten years ago, discovered the true cause of cancer. She claims the cause of every type of cancer, whether it be leukaemia or breast cancer, is the fluke parasite.

How can the human intestinal fluke cause cancer? This parasite typically lives in the intestine, where it might do little harm, causing colitis, Crohn's disease or irritable bowel syndrome, or perhaps nothing at all, but if it invades a different organ like the uterus, kidneys or liver, it does a great deal of harm.

If it establishes itself in the liver, Clark claims it causes cancer. She also claimed cancer starts in the liver. Clark further claims the great increase in propyl alcohol entering into our bodies, assists the growth of micro parasites.

Flukes and Propyl Alcohol

Dr Clark maintains that something special happens to people who have propyl alcohol in their bodies preventing the liver from trapping and killing those tiny flukes' parasites which are actually allowed to make their home in the liver and other tissues.

It is as if the immune system has no power to kill them. The flukes begin to multiply in people with propyl alcohol in their bodies! The *micracidiae* (hatchlings) start to make little balls inside themselves, called *radiae*, but each *radiae* is alive! It pops itself out of the *micracidiae* and begins to reproduce itself. Each *radiae* can each make forty more *radiae* right inside your body – in your cervix or lungs, whenever you cancer is growing! These *radiae* are swept along in your blood, landing in whatever tissue lets them in. Smoker's lungs, breast with benign lumps, prostate glands full of heavy metals are examples of tissues that give the *radiae* their landing permits.

Geopathic Stress

Micro parasites love Geopathic Stress, so it is no coincidence that cancer nearly always develops in the region of your body where Geopathic Stress is strongest when you are asleep. During sleep your body has time to strengthen your immune system, except if it has to spend time fighting the Geopathic Stress.

Clearly you need to do four things:

1. Ensure you do not sleep or sit in a Geopathic Stressed place.
2. Kill the parasite and all its stages and boost your immune system.
3. Stop letting propyl alcohol into your body.

It is not only fluke parasites you have to destroy, but the many other microbes your body can harbour, which cause all sorts of illnesses. However, getting rid of all these microbes would be impossible using conventional medicines that can only kill one or two types of microbes at a time. Many medicines can make you quite ill and can cause extreme nausea, vomiting, make you itch all over and some are very toxic. Imagine taking ten such drugs to kill a dozen types of microbes.

100% stabilised allicin extract from garlic is nature's very powerful method of killing all types of microbes. In cancer cases, it is recommended you start off taking up to 25 ml per day of the liquid. After two weeks, you can reduce it to 10-15 ml per day. Some find it best to mix it with fruit juice, milk or smoothies. Allicin extract is also a powerful natural antibiotic, anti-viral, anti-fungal, anti-inflammatory and immune booster (see details in PART FOUR).

You are always picking up parasites. Parasites are everywhere outdoors. You also get them from other people, your family, your home, your pets and uncooked meat. After we are infected with it this way, we can give it to each other through blood, saliva, semen, breast milk etc. The only thing which should touch our mouth is food, drinks and kisses!

Parasites Gone, Propyl Alcohol Next

Now that you have killed the intestinal fluke, what next? Stop getting propyl alcohol into your body. Propyl alcohol is the antiseptic commonly used in cosmetics, anti-perspirants, shampoos, hair sprays, mousse, body lotions, shaving supplies and rubbing alcohol.

If in doubt check with dowsing or the muscle test (see Part Nine). Check the ingredients for 'proponal' or 'isoproponal' on the label. Also propyl compounds like propomide, propacetamid, propyl gallate or calcium propionate can be converted by the body to propyl alcohol. Do not use anything that has 'prop' in the list of ingredients. Don't give your discarded products to anybody. Throw them out.

Dispensing of Dead Parasites

It is most important to clear your body not only of the dead parasites and their eggs, but also the waste products and toxins they have produced. This is best done with an oxygen enriched capsule producing, like OxyTech, several bowel movements a day. Using natural detoxing footpads are also a good way of detoxifying your body.

Keep Yourself Clean

Wash your hands regularly and in particular when you come home; also wash your feet if you've been outside with bare feet. Use liquid soap from containers, as parasites etc can live on bars of soap. Change your shoes at the outside door, when you come home. You can unknowingly pick up parasites under your shoes from bird droppings, animal excreta etc. Wear non-slip 'flip-flops' (rubber slippers/sandals) when visiting swimming pools. Around eight thousand infectious moulds, parasites etc lurk in each $10cm^2$ area of pool changing rooms.

Sterilising Food & Cleaning Materials etc

It is also important you clean fruit and vegetables such as lettuce, tomatoes, apples, pears etc. A very powerful sterilising liquid can be made up by putting water into a 'spray container' (a thoroughly cleansed 500ml empty spray bottle will be fine) with three drops of Super Strength Oil of Oregano or ten drops of Regular Oil of Oregano. This solution can also sterilise kitchen and bathroom cloths, sponges, brushes etc. Fruit vinegar can also be used. Place the kitchen cloths etc (no metal) wet in your microwave for one minute or in your freezer for over six hours. Wash at over 60° C in a washing machine. Germ-a-Clenz is a 100% natural germicidal spray made from wild oregano to protect you in the home, workplace or hospital from the dangers of airborne and surface bacteria, mould, parasites and fungal spores. It can also be sprayed on fruit etc.

Water and Ozonated Water

Drink plenty of water which stimulates your immune system (see Part Four), helps increase the body's white blood cells and flushes out dead parasites and accumulated toxins. Even better is ozonated water, which helps destroy micro-parasites, bacteria, viruses, fungi and revitalises your body. You can make one glass of ozonated water in one minute with a small apparatus from Commercial Science. [1]

Exercise

Exercise helps move your lymph round your body, thereby transporting your toxins and dead parasites to your liver and kidneys for filtration and elimination. Try and get three 40 minute walks a week. A very quick and efficient way to exercise is on a Rebounder. Two minutes on a Rebounder will double your white blood cell count, which produces most of the cells in your immune system, which fight your parasites (see Part Five).

Other illnesses

Parasites and other microbes are present in most cases of minor and major illnesses such as AIDS, Alzheimer's, hepatitis, Lupus, Lyme disease, MRSA, Multiple Sclerosis, Parkinson's disease, TB etc.

P.S. Chemotherapy is a very effective way to kill parasites BUT it also destroys 30% of your immune system!!!

[1] Made in England by Commercial Science, 11 Hyland Close, Crawley, West Sussex, RH10 6RX

CO-ENZYME Q10

> **The body's content of Q10 has been low in all the thousands of cancer cases I have been involved with. Q10 is the sparking plug for all your cells, creating the substance ATP (Adenosin Tri-phosphate) which is your cells' most important source of energy for all your biological functions, such as physical and mental activity and those dozens of energy-needing systems like digestion and organ activities.**

Your liver converts the lower Co-Enzyme Qs from your food into Q10, which can be absorbed by your body. Only animals can utilise the lower Qs. Your liver needs Q10 to operate 100%. Unfortunately Geopathic Stress creates a vicious circle. Your liver becomes weak, so it cannot produce enough Q10 which it needs to function normally, so it can produce enough Q10.

Also if we have cancer and/or get older, our liver becomes less efficient due to lack of Q10. Our body contains 45% less Q10 at 80 than at birth. An adult body contains only 2,000 mg of Q10. Death may occur somewhere between 25%-35% of normal. Many people with cancer have at the time of diagnosis, a content below 60% causing a weak immune system, which cannot destroy cancer cells.

The largest amount of Q10 is found in your heart to give it energy. That is why Q10 has shown over many years to be very effective in treating heart problems. Healthy people in their 90's have been found to have a high quantity of Q10, whereas people with dementia and Alzheimer's disease are very low in Q10. Extra Q10 has shown to prevent periodontal diseases, which affect the tissues in the gums that support your teeth.

It is vital to take extra Q10 if you are taking statins for lowering cholesterol, as you are depleting your body of Q10 because they share the same biosynthetic pathway in your liver. There are no known interactions or contra-indications with Q10, so it is vital you take Q10 if you have cancer especially when you are in hospital having treatment, all the time.

Scientific evidence There have been hundreds of scientific papers published over the last 40 years to show the beneficial effect of Q10.

Recommended daily dose if you have cancer.
<u>Children</u> 30-100 mg   <u>Adult</u> 100-400 mg

Scientific tests show Q10 in oil, in soft gelatine capsules, is the easiest for your body to absorb. As Q10 gives you more energy, do not take capsules in the evening, otherwise they may keep you awake.

Successful Trials

Remission of Breast Cancer in 'High risk' Patients supplemented with Co-enzyme Q10
Trials were carried out in Denmark by Dr Knud Lockwood, Sven Moesgaard, Takeshi, Hanioka and Karl Folkers in which 32 typical breast cancer patients between 31 and 81

years of age classified as 'high risk' or secondary cancer were treated over 11 years from 1990 to 2001 with Q10.

Main observations:
1. Only two of the patients died of cancer during this period. Normally, one would have expected half of the women to have died over this period.
2. None of the patients showed signs of further distance metastasis.
3. Quality of life improved (increase in weight and reduced use of pain-killers).
4. Many of the patients showed total remission.

The patients were initially treated according to the routine procedure in Denmark i.e. surgery, chemotherapy, radiotherapy and in some cases, Tamoxifen.

All the patients were taking about 400 mg of Q10 daily.

One 59 year old woman had, for one year before the trial, taken 90 mg of Q10 per day. This had 'stabilised' her 1.5 to 2 cm tumour. After 3 months on 390 mg of Q10 per day, the tumour was no longer present and all necessary examinations confirmed this. This indicated that Q10 was dominant in the complete regression over and above any benefit from nutritional supplements also taken.

One doctor, who had treated about 7,000 breast cancer patients over 35 years, said she had never seen a spontaneous comparable regression of a 1.5 to 2 cm breast cancer tumour before.

ACID-ALKALINE BALANCE re CANCER
Also important information for people who do not have cancer

> **The acid alkaline balance of your blood must be dealt with to prevent you getting cancer, or if you have cancer. Nurses, who had worked for some time on a hospital cancer wards, informed me that all cancer patients there had very acidic blood, especially if they have had chemotherapy. If you have anxiety and worries, it can also lower your acid alkaline balance.**

The single most important measurement of your health is the pH of your blood and tissues - how acidic or alkaline it is. Different areas of your body have different ideal pH levels, but your blood pH is the most telling of all. Your body will go to great lengths to preserve it.

The acid/alkaline balance (also called acid/base balance) is measured on a pH (potential hydrogen's) scale from 1 (very acidic) to 7.4 (neutral) to 10 (very alkaline). 7.4 to 7.5 are slightly alkaline and are associated with good health. Cancer cells give off lactic acid in anaerobic fermentation of food which generates a lower pH and thereby further compromises the cell's ability to fight off the cancer. In other words, cancer likes an acid environment.

Just as your body temperature is rigidly regulated, your blood must be kept in a very narrow pH range - mildly acidic or alkaline. Your body will go to great lengths to preserve it including wreaking havoc on other tissues or systems. Your correct pH is more important than blood pressure, cholesterol count, blood sugar, hormone levels, calorie count etc.

How to encourage a healthy pH

- Try to eat 70-80% alkaline food such as wholegrain products, fresh vegetables and other plant food. Fresh fruit is alkaline, but turns acidic when made into juice or cooked. In particular the acidity level of courgettes, peppers, onions and aubergines increase when roasted. Milk and lean meat such as chicken, fish and turkey is only slightly acidic.
- Tomatoes and oranges are very acidic. Lemons and vinegar transform into alkaline in your body.
- Deep breathing exercise and drink plenty of water.
- Try to eat only 20-30% acid forming food such as meat, sugar, cheese, butter, processed and refined food, yeast products, fermented food, grain, artificial sweeteners, fizzy drinks, coffee and alcoholic drinks. (Ardent vegetarians may have an abnormally high pH and may need to eat some acidic food to bring their pH down to a normal healthy level).
- Raw foods are more alkaline, while cooked food is more acidic.
- Drink alkaline juices made up mostly of green vegetables and grasses. (Go easy on fruit juices as they contain large amounts of sugars). To get used to the more subtle sweeteners found in greens, you may want to add some beetroot and carrots. These vegetables are sweet because they have higher levels of sugars, so keep them to 20% or less of your juices. (Peppers are not so high in sugars, so you can use them freely).
- Bicarbonate of Soda (without aluminium) is very effective in bringing up your pH. Several months supply will cost less than £1.00 from your local supermarket. For 7 to 10 days, take one to two teaspoonful a day in a small cup of water first thing in the morning half an hour before any food. If your pH is very low, take two teaspoonful first thing in the morning for 7 days, then one teaspoonful for another 7 days. Later take one teaspoonful once or twice a week. This may also prevent you getting colds and flu.
- By taking Bicarbonate of Soda first thing in the morning, it passes through your empty stomach quickly into your small intestines, where it is absorbed into your blood. Taking Bicarbonate of Soda half an hour before food enables your stomach to become acidic again so it can digest your food.
- If you are anxious or worried, one or two half teaspoonfuls a day can be very effective.
- To test if you need Bicarbonate of Soda, take 2-3 teaspoonfuls first thing in the morning in a small cup of water. If you belch within 5 minutes you have enough and your pH should be OK.

Why very acidic blood is bad for you

Acids and alkaline are opposites and when they meet in certain ratios, they cancel each other out creating a neutral pH. It takes about twenty times as much alkaline to neutralise any given amount of acid, so it is easier to maintain than to regain a balance.

Sodium, potassium, calcium and magnesium react with acids to create a much less detrimental substance, which can then be eliminated by the body. These alkaline minerals are kept in reserve in a healthy body to meet an emergency, but if there are insufficient amounts in the diet or in reserve, the body has to absorb them from elsewhere, like calcium from your bones or magnesium from your muscles.

If pH tissue deviates too far to the acid side, oxygen levels decrease and your body cells will start to die. Cancer cannot survive in oxygen.

To ensure your body has enough reserve of the above, particularly when your health is under par, add the following to a healthy diet:

Magnesium - take 350-700 mg supplements per day. Magnesium helps to hold potassium in your cells.

Sodium - two teaspoonfuls a day of Bicarbonate of Soda several times a week.

<u>Potassium</u> - Seaweed.

<u>Calcium</u> - best form of calcium supplements are calcium amino acid chelate or citrate, which is twice as well absorbed as calcium carbonate. Pulverised clean eggshells are very good.

<u>Vitamin D</u> - this helps your body absorb calcium and magnesium from your food and supplements. Take 20-40 mcg per day.

Why Geopathic Stress causes acidic blood

During sleep your brain does your body's "housekeeping" looking after your organs, creating new cells etc. Unfortunately, due the brain having to struggle with Geopathic Stress, it decides to delay the proper operation of your digestion system, so you no longer absorb the correct amount of minerals, vitamins and trace elements from your food, thereby creating more acidic blood.

How to measure your pH balance

You can measure the pH balance in your saliva or urine with pH litmus test strips from your chemist or the internet. For testing your urine, collect fresh urine in a container first thing in the morning, after you have fasted overnight. Tear off a test strip with dry fingers. Dip the test strip into the urine for 2 seconds. Pull it out and shake off surplus liquid. The test strip changes colour depending on the pH value at the moistened patch. Compare the colour with the colour scale on the container.

A blood pH test is the most reliable, as taken from blood samples taken at your doctor's clinic or hospital after fasting overnight. However, they cannot be done on a daily basis as you might experiment with different diets and take, for example, Bicarbonate of Soda.

Bicarbonate of Soda

According to Dr Tullio Simoncini, the famous oncologist in Rome, Italy, Bicarbonate of Soda hits cancer cells with a shock wave of alkalinity, which allows much more oxygen into the cells than cancer can tolerate. Cancer cells cannot survive in the presence of high levels of oxygen. Bicarbonate of Soda is effective in treating poisoning or overdoses from many chemicals and pharmaceutical drugs by negating the cardiotoxic and neurotoxic effect. The safe oral use of Bicarbonate of Soda should be taken very seriously no matter what other treatment is used. It will also mean that you do not have to alter your diet too drastically, particularly if you are underweight and have little appetite due to cancer and rely on your favourite food.

Remember what I say *"you must feed your soul"*.

P.S. If you cannot tolerate Bicarbonate of Soda, squeeze juice from half a lemon into a glass and fill up with luke warm water. Add a sweetener like honey or sugar if necessary. Drink first thing in the morning, half an hour before breakfast. This is almost as good as taking Bicarbonate of Soda, as it will also help your blood become more alkaline, because lemon turns alkaline in your body.

PART TWO

CONVENTIONAL (ORTHODOX) TREATMENT

Very few oncologists (cancer specialists) will discuss <u>the full menu</u> of conventional cancer treatments, mainly because some treatments may not be available at their hospital (see below).(')
It is vital you take into account the BIG FOUR and other recommendations to ensure a successful outcome, by making you stronger before conventional treatments and so you can survive afterwards from many very aggressive conventional treatments.

The following pages will give you details of the main conventional cancer treatments which can be used alone, or in combination, so you can refer to them before or after seeing your oncologist.

Being told you have cancer is such a shock that you will probably only remember 10% of what your cancer specialist tells you, so it is vital you take a relative or friend along who can take notes of what you are being told. Most doctors will allow you to use a tape recorder, so you can listen to it when you come home. Take the 'Questions to ask your Consultant' with you.

SUMMARY
- **Questions to ask your Consultant about your Treatment**
- **Giving your consent**
- **Conventional Treatment**
    Surgery - operating the cancer tumour away
    Radiotherapy - involves penetrating radiation or radiation seeds
    Chemotherapy - the use of chemical substances
    Laser - high energy light beams
    Hyperthermia - heat therapy
    Hormonal - the use of hormones
    Biological - boosting the body's own defences against cancer
    Bone Marrow Transplant

(') If the best treatment for you is not available, you may decide to see an oncologist at a hospital where they can carry out such treatment like the very successful, non invasive and quick PhotoDynamic Treatment (see under Laser Treatment) or keyhole surgery which leaves hardly any operation scars and you can come home from hospital sooner. The Habib Resection Device is used by some surgeons during operations on the liver, so very little blood is lost (see under Liver Cancer).

Questions to ask your Consultant about your Treatment

Tell the consultant at the outset if you wish to be told the whole truth. Feel free to ask any questions you wish.

- Ask to have your cancer explained.
- What treatment or combined treatments are recommended?
- How successful do you expect the treatments to be?
- Are there any side-effects and what can be done to relieve them?
- Any alternative treatments?
- Can I have a second opinion regarding treatment?
- If I agree to the treatment, when can it be carried out, how long will it take and if it entails a hospital stay, how long?
- Are any complementary therapy and supplements recommended? Don't expect the consultant to appreciate the BIG FOUR.
- If there is anything you do not fully understand, ask the consultant to explain.
- If you find you have more questions to ask after the consultation, can you have another meeting or can you make a phone call to the consultant?

Remember, you are in overall charge of the situation, not the consultant.

Giving your Consent

No treatment can be given without you signing a consent form, so make sure you fully understand:

- The type and length of treatment you are advised to have.
- The advantages and disadvantages of the cancer treatment.
- Whether there is any alternative treatment available.
- Any significant risks and side-effects.

Do not let yourself be rushed or bullied into signing the consent form.

DIAGNOSES - CONVENTIONAL (ORTHODOX)

In order for your doctor to confirm you have cancer, where, and what type, it is necessary to carry out a series of diagnostic tests. The results can then be discussed with you by an oncologist (cancer specialist) and/or a multi disciplinary team of doctors and nurses, to establish the best treatment.

The earlier cancer is detected; hopefully a less aggressive conventional treatment is needed with a much better chance of a full recovery. You should have a diagnosis as soon as you are aware something new has happened to your body for example:

- Unusual bleeding or discharge.
- Change in bowel or bladder habits.
- Indigestion or difficulty in swallowing.
- Nagging cough or hoarseness.
- Thickening or lump in breast or elsewhere.
- A sore that does not heal.
- Obvious change in a wart or mole.

The kind of test will depend upon the problem you have, what kind of cancer is suspected and the degree to which it might have spread.

Many cancer tests can be interpreted in different ways by individual doctors. Medicine is not an exact science.
Don't be surprised if you get varying opinions from different types of specialists. Surgeons, oncologists who specialise in radiotherapy or chemotherapy etc. look at cancer and its treatment from different viewpoints. As mentioned above, it is best to discuss any suggested treatment with a multi-disciplinary team of doctors and nurses, or at least get a second opinion if you are only seeing one doctor.

Don't forget to take a friend along to record details, as you may well remember very little yourself afterwards.

Positive and negative
Positive usually means that something has been found. In most cases it is something that is not normally supposed to be there.
Negative means that nothing was found as a result of the test.

SUMMARY
- **Physical Examination and medical history**
- **Laboratory Tests - blood, tumour markers and urine**
- **Endoscope - inserting lighted instrument**
- **Cytology - study of cells under a microscope**
- **Imaging Techniques - ultrasound, MRI, CT, PET and X-ray**
- **Biopsy - microscope examination of tissue**

Physical Examination and Medical History

Write down and take with you a list of any symptoms and when they started. Also an outline of your illnesses through your life, even though most people's details are on their doctor's computer.

If your doctor feels you have a problem after a physical examination, he/she will book you an appointment with a consultant. (see under individual cancers, which physical examination is carried out).

Laboratory Tests

Complete blood count is carried out to check the number of red cells, white cells and platelets in a sample of your blood. A check will also be done on the portion of blood value made up of red blood cells and your blood's oxygen carrying capacity, along with the red blood cells indices (size and haemoglobin concentration of red blood cells) and white blood differential (percentage of each type of white blood cells).

Tumour markers

See under individual cancers how tumour markers can indicate the aggressiveness of any cancer.

Urine Test

A test of your urine sample is often done by your doctor using a special chemical strip that reacts with substances in your urine and changes colour. A more detailed analysis under a microscope may be done in a laboratory.

Faecal occult blood (FOB) test

This test detects tiny amounts of blood in your faeces (stools) which you cannot normally see and which can sometimes be caused by bowel cancer or polyps.

Endoscopy

Endoscopes are instruments which are inserted into your body's orifices to examine you internally. See details under individual cancers such as neck, oesophagus, lungs, stomach, prostate, bladder, bowel, vagina etc.

Cytology (exfoliation cytology)

This is the process of examining isolated cells, obtained from cervical smears (Pap smear test) to determine whether or not they are cancerous.

Imaging Techniques

Ultrasound

This is a very safe way of examining the inside of the body by very high 'sound' frequency of about three to ten million cycles per second (Hz). Our ears only hear sound between about 12 and 20,000 Hz.

Ultrasound is mainly used for fluid-filled organs such as the gall bladder, bladder and soft organs such as liver, pancreas and kidneys. It cannot easily pass through body parts surrounded by bone, such as the brain and spinal cord.

Transvaginal ultrasound

By placing a transducer in the vagina, an ultrasound image of the pelvic structure can provide valuable information about the lining of the womb.

CT Scan (computerised tomography)

This uses a rotating X-ray beam to scan the body from several angles.

MRI Scan (Magnetic Resonance Imaging)

This scan creates a cross section of selected parts of the body by using magnetic fields.

Isotope Bone Scan

This is a test which shows up any abnormal areas of bone. A very small amount of a mildly radioactive substance is injected into a vein, usually in the arm. Two to three hours later, a scan is taken of the whole body. As abnormal bone absorbs more of the radioactive substance than normal bone, any abnormal areas show up on the scan as highlighted areas (sometimes known as hot spots).

Bone Density Test (BMD)

BMD is an X-ray scan that measures bone mass.

PET (Positron emission tomography)

Images are in 3D. Most malignant tumours use a lot of glucose and will 'light up' on a PET scan. PET scans can be used in conjunction with CT and MRI scans, to show that 'something is taking up space'. PET is more accurate than CT and MRI scans and is now commonly used to scan for staging of lung cancer and melanoma and detecting secondary cancer cells which have spread to lymph nodes (metastases).

X-ray

This is the oldest form of diagnosis and involves passing a small dose of ionizing radiation through specific areas of the body onto a film.

Mammogram

This is a type of X-ray to check for tumours in the breast. It is not a very accurate test as only 20-30% of tumours detected prove to be cancerous after a biopsy has been taken.

Standard mammogram is not very safe as it produces radiation doses 1000 times greater than an ordinary X-ray.

Digital Mammography is much less invasive and better at detecting tumours in young women who have dense breasts. Images can be manipulated and magnified immediately, highlighting tiny and subtle tumours, reducing the need for recall. See further details under breast cancer.

Biopsy

This is a process of taking a specimen by a cutting needle or open operation from tissues of tumours or lymph nodes, for examination under a microscope to see if they are cancerous. See further details under breast and prostate cancer.

Tests carried out to detect brain cancer:

Lumbar puncture

This test may be performed to get a sample of *cerebrospinal fluid* (CSF) which is the fluid around the brain and the spinal cord. A needle is pushed through the skin of your back, between the bones of your spine to collect a sample of the CSF. This may be slightly painful, but only lasts a few minutes.

Myelogram

These checks for any spread of brain cancer to the spinal cord. A fluid, which shows on X-ray, is injected into the CSF to show an outline of the spinal cord.

Angiogram

A dye is injected to show up the blood vessels in the brain through a series of X-rays. The dye is injected through a thin flexible tube (catheter) into an artery in the groin, arm or neck.

SURGERY

Surgery is the oldest approach to cancer treatment and involves cutting away the cancer tumour or certain organs affected by cancer. Surgery is also used in diagnosis (biopsy), reconstruction (such as after breast cancer surgery) and for reducing the effect of blockages, discomfort or other complications.

Apart from using a surgical knife (scalpel), other types of surgery can be carried out, such as lasers (using high energy light beams) and cryotherapy (removing tumours using freezing probes). Surgery can also be used in conjunction with the other therapies described in this chapter.

SUMMARY
- **Diagnosis (biopsy)**
- **Before your operation**
- **Staging**
- **Secondary Treatment**
- **Reconstruction**
- **After your operation**
- **Long term complications**
  - **Nerve damage**
  - **Lymphoedema**

Diagnosis (biopsy)
This procedure entails removing a small piece of tissue to confirm the diagnosis of cancer and find out what cancer it is. The sample is examined in the laboratory. (See more details under breast and prostate cancer).

Before your operation
In addition to the questions you have asked your consultant about your treatment, you need to ask your surgeon who is to carry out the operation:
- Please explain in simple terms, what you plan to do. Show me what part of my body is involved and tell me how extensive the surgery will be. Is it possible to do keyhole surgery, photodynamic or cryosurgery?
- What sort of scan will I have?
- Is this surgery dangerous? What are the risks and what are the benefits?
- Will I have to stay in hospital after the operation? If so, how long?
- How long will the operation take?
- How long will it take to recover?
- How disfiguring will the operation be?
- Will the operation be disabling? Temporarily? Permanently?
- Will I have drains, catheters or intravenous lines after the surgery?
- Will I need a blood transfusion? Can I bank my own blood?

Make sure you discuss with your surgeon, not only any medication you are taking, but also any herbal remedies or supplements, to avoid a potentially dangerous reaction during or immediately after surgery. The following in particular you should stop taking before surgery:

Echinacea Possible risk: allergic reaction; impairs immune suppressive drugs; could slow wound healing. Advise: stop taking it as far in advance of surgery as possible.

Garlic Possible risk: bleeding, especially when combined with other drugs that inhibit clotting. Advise: stop several days before surgery. See 100% stabilised allicin later under 'after your surgery'.

Ginkgo Possible risk: bleeding, especially when combined with other drugs that 'thin' the blood. Advise: stop taking it at least 36 hours before surgery.

Ginseng Possible risk: lowers blood sugar levels; increases the risk of bleeding; interferes with warfarin. Advise: stop taking at least seven days before surgery.

St. John's Wort Possible risk: alters metabolism when taken at the same time as drugs such as steroids, warfarin and cyclosporine. Advise: stop taking it at least five days before surgery.

But do take the Bach Flower **Rescue Remedy** before surgery to calm you down.

Staging

Oncologists use staging to work out the size of the cancer tumour and whether it has spread (metastasised), to other parts of the body. Staging can be done at the same time as surgery when removing the cancer. See staging under certain individual cancers.

Surgery

The main type of surgery is to remove the tumour and nearby tissues and lymph nodes, which might contain cancer cells, preferably by keyhole surgery which leaves a smaller scar and involves a shorter stay in hospital.

Other types of surgery are:

Laser - including Photodynamic - (see under laser).

Cryosurgery - using cold liquid gas to destroy a tumour by freezing (see under prostate cancer).

Robotic surgery

A growing number of robotic devices in UK hospitals are performing minimally invasive surgery at extraordinary levels of accuracy, in operations from the retina to the rectum.

This offers patients minimal invasive surgery instead of a much more major open operation. Using robots, the surgeons can use their skill and judgement while the robot does things they find difficult. Robots have tiny 'writs' at the end of probes, which allow them to make delicate movements through keyhole incisions that would not be possible for humans using long-handled instruments and also abolishes hand tremors.

In cancer surgery it has been used to remove tumours deep inside the brain, from the womb, prostate, kidneys etc.

Very skilled surgeons can operate the robot from a distance. In one case an operation was carried out in Strasbourg, Germany by surgeons in a New York business centre. 15 robot devices have already been bought in UK hospitals at a cost of £1,000,000 each including St. Mary's Hospital in London.

It is claimed in 10 years' time, surgeons will no longer be putting hands onto patients.

Secondary Treatment

If surgery cannot completely cure the local cancer, or if it has spread to other parts of the body, other treatments may be incorporated such as chemotherapy, radiotherapy, hormonal therapy or immunotherapy.

Geopathic Stress

It is important that you are not Geopathically Stressed before you have surgery, to ensure you heal better afterwards (see page 14).

Reconstruction

Surgery can be used to restore:

Appearance - such as reconstruction after a breast cancer operation (detailed information in chapter on breast cancer).

A part of the body - such as creating a new bladder.

After your surgery

To drain away any fluid from your wound, a tube may be inserted. Usually the tube can be removed within days when the fluid has been drained off.

Your recovery period will depend on the type of surgery. With good pain control, you should try and get up as soon as possible and do exercises to get your lymph system going again and to prevent chest infection and blood clots.

The use of a powerful high spinning magnetic apparatus used directly on the operation scar will enable it to heal much quicker and prevent any infection. **Q10** is very good to boost your heart and body cells.

Even though some may not recommend you take **AlliTech 100% stabilised allicin,** it is a derivative of garlic, therefore has some of the side-effects of garlic e.g. causing bleeding. The manufacturers claim they have not heard of anybody having had any side-effects after taking allicin after an operation over the last ten years it has been on the market. Allicin is a very strong immune booster. It is also very powerful at dealing with viruses which antibiotics cannot tackle, and bacteria including MRSA.

When you return home, make sure you take your usual supplements and also get as much exercise as possible, particularly on a rebounder especially if you cannot get out for daily walks straight away. If you have a MagneTech (see page 232), use it direct where the surgery has been carried out, to heal the scar and the whole area much quicker and prevent any scar tissues and adhesions.

Long term complications

Most people do not have long term complications after cancer surgery. However, I suggest you ask your surgeon before you have the surgery.

Nerve damage

Ask your surgeon if the operation is likely to cause nerve damage. Surgeons will always do their best to leave any nerves intact. Now and again you may have some nerve pain after surgery.

Lymphoedema

If a large number of lymph glands have been removed during surgery and particularly if you have also had radiotherapy, you may get swelling of the arms and hands to the armpit (see details under breast cancer) or feet after groin surgery. It can also happen to other parts of the body, like the face. The earlier lymphoedema is recognised, the easier it is to control.

RADIOTHERAPY

More than half of all people who have cancer treatment will receive some type of radiotherapy, either as the primary treatment or in combination with other treatments. Radiotherapy affects both normal and cancerous tissues, but almost all cancer cells are more sensitive to radiotherapy than normal cells, which can usually repair themselves. Also radiotherapy can be directed accurately at a tumour with minimum of damage to normal cells near the treatment area or elsewhere in the body.

SUMMARY

Radiotherapy

- When is Radiotherapy given?
- Planning your treatment
- Monitoring your treatment
- Types of Radiotherapy Treatment
  - External Radiation -
    - Skin marking
    - Radiotherapy mask
    - Radiotherapy Machines
    - Dosage, Treatment, Specialised Techniques
    - Cyberknife Treatment
  - Internal Radiation -
    - Brachytherapy radiation
    - Cervix, womb (uterus) or vagina treatment
    - Radioisotope
    - Caesium or Iridium Wires
    - Safety measures
    - Treatment for prostate cancer
    - Interoperational
    - Total body radiation
- Side Effects from Radiotherapy
  - Skin
  - Head and neck
  - Chest
  - Stomach and pelvis
- Sex Life and Fertility
- Lack of Appetite

Radiotherapy

Radiotherapy treatment began over one hundred years ago when X-rays and radium were discovered. Subsequently, researchers discovered the curious fact that X-rays and radium did more damage to cancerous tissues than normal healthy tissues. Radiotherapy has made great advances during the last twenty five years, due to improved equipment and use of computers.

Radiotherapy uses a high voltage X-ray machine linear accelerator, (producing tens of thousands of times, the amount used in ordinary chest X-rays) and radioactive isotopes such as cobalt-60 and iodine-131, which emit gamma rays.

The patient is carefully shielded with lead, so only the area of the tumour is irradiated.

When is Radiotherapy given?

- **Before surgery** to shrink a tumour.
- **Instead of surgery** to avoid disfiguring surgery or when surgery is not possible, due to pre-existing conditions.
- **During surgery** to prevent lengthy radiotherapy sessions after surgery, as in breast cancer cases. This is called **inter operative radiotherapy.**
- **After surgery** to stop any cancer cells that may remain from growing.
- **Together with chemotherapy** after surgery or instead of surgery.
- **To treat symptoms of cancer** such as to reduce pressure, bleeding or pain.

Planning your treatment

To make sure your radiotherapy treatment is as effective as possible, it is important a careful plan of your treatment is made.

On your first visit to the radiotherapy department, a CT (computerised tomography) scan, will take lots of images from different angles to build up a three dimensional picture of the area to be treated. This may take up to one hour.

You may also need an MRI scan, which uses powerful magnetic fields to give additional information about the area of your body to have radiotherapy. A PET scan may also be carried out.

In cases of planning for treatment of the pelvic area, a liquid which shows up on X-ray, may be passed into your rectum, into your bladder or a tampon may be used to show the exact position of the vagina. These procedures may be slightly uncomfortable, but are only used for planning.

You may have the first treatment the same day, or you may have to wait up to two weeks while the physicist and the oncologist prepare the final details of your radiotherapy treatment.

Monitoring your treatment

The effect on you is monitored in various ways, mainly by checking on the rate of blood cell production by the bone marrow, which is sensitively affected by radiation.

Radiation damages the DNA of the cancer cells, so they are unable to reproduce and form new cancer cells. However, cancer cells are sometimes able to repair their DNA damage, which is why radiotherapy must be given repeatedly on a continuous basis.

Types of Radiotherapy Treatment
External Radiotherapy
Skin marking

When the area to be treated has been identified, ink markings are usually made on your skin to pinpoint the exact place where the radiation is going to be directed. If the markings rub off later, do not redraw them yourself, tell your radiographer. Often two or more pinpoint-size tattoo marks will be made on your skin. These tattoo marks are also useful later, after your sessions of treatment, to show the area where radiotherapy treatment was given, to prevent giving future treatment in that area.

Radiotherapy mask

To prevent movement during treatment, mainly when treating head and neck areas, a mould or shell is made on which markers can be made.
A plaster cast is first taken of the body part from which a clear Perspex or other plastic mask is made. Sometimes a plastic mask is used, which becomes soft in warm water - it will be moulded to your body and hardened after a few minutes, ready for use.
Moulds covering your face will have holes cut for the eyes, nose and mouth. You will only have a mask on for a few minutes at a time.

Radiotherapy machines

Radiotherapy is mainly given by machines called linear accelerators (Lin.Acs), except in skin cancer cases. Treatment time varies depending on the type of machine, from a few seconds upwards. Usually treatment takes 10-15 minutes or less on any type of machine, including the time to position you.

Dosage

The amount of radiation given used to be measured in **rads**. The term used now is **centigray** (cGy). One cGy is equal to 100 rads.
Calculating the correct dosage is a balance between delivering the maximum effective dosage to the visible tumour and any invisible tumour cells that might be nearby, while protecting the surrounding normal tissues as much as possible. The total dosage necessary is then divided on a daily basis over a specific period.
Different organs tolerate a maximum dosage without harming normal tissues as follows: lungs 2000 cGy, kidneys 1800 cGy and liver 3000 cGy. Higher dosage can be given to smaller parts of any one of theses organs.
To give the normal cells a chance to recover, radiation is given daily, three to five days a week over a period of one to eight weeks. It is usually given as an outpatient.. External radiotherapy does not make you radioactive, so it is perfectly safe for you to be with other people, including children, during your treatment period.

Radiotherapy Treatment

During the treatment, you will lie on a fairly hard couch. If you are uncomfortable, let the radiographer know and they can usually arrange for you to have some foam pads underneath you.
Most radiotherapy machines can give treatment from different angles, by rotating around your body. Once you are in the correct position, the staff will leave the room to prevent them from being exposed to any unnecessary radiation during treatment.

Specialised Techniques

New radiotherapy machines have been developed called multi leaf collimators to target the cancer tumours more precisely, so higher doses of radiation can be given, but affecting the surrounding healthy cells less. Metal sheets fixed to the radiotherapy machine can be adjusted individually to ensure more accurate shaped beans.

Three dimensional IMRT (3D-IMRT) also multi leaf collimator, which are moved during treatment to enable the shape of the treatment beam to be even more precise and allows the dosage to be altered in different parts of the area to be treated.

Research studies has shown that the above methods have less side-effects than traditional radiotherapy, but microscopic cancer just outside the treated area may not be destroyed and causes the cancer to come back - so take care of the BIG FOUR.

Cyberknife or gamma knife is another new method of applying radiotherapy very accurately, greatly reducing side-effects. It uses a movable robotic arm which is attached to a miniaturised radiotherapy machine. This gives enormous manoeuvrability, firing hundreds of pencil-thin beams of radiation from thousands of angles around the patient which converge on the tumour. This allows tumours (also odd shaped ones) in critical places to be targeted extremely accurately with little damage to surrounding healthy tissues. This allows higher doses to be given over a longer period than conventional radiotherapy, which lasts 10-15 minutes. But only one to three sessions are needed, instead of up to 30, but each session can take up to five hours. The machine has a sophisticated software that tracks the location of the tumour with multi metre precision every few seconds, using tiny gold markers as guides. This means the robot can follow tumour movements as the patients breathes in and out. The first cyberknife has been in operation at Guy's and St. Thomas' Hospital in London, but up to five machines will be in use in the UK during the year.

Internal Radiotherapy Treatment

This is mainly used to treat cancer in the head and neck area, the prostate glands, the cervix, womb (uterus), vagina or the skin.

Treatment is given either by Brachytherapy or Radioisotope treatment.

Brachytherapy

In this treatment, a solid radioactive material, normally caesium 137, is placed close to or inside the tumour for a limited period of time. Once removed, the radioactivity disappears and it is safe to be with other people.

The advantage of Brachytherapy treatment is that it gives a higher dose of radiotherapy direct to the tumour, but does not affect the surrounding normal tissues very much.

Treatment for cervix, womb (uterus) or vagina

One or two **applicators** are filled with caesium and inserted into the vagina while you are under a general anaesthetic or sedation in the operation room. Often a urinary catheter is put into the bladder, so you will not have to get on and off bedpans, which could dislodge the applicators. An X-ray will check the applicators are in the right position. The applicator is kept in place by cotton or gauze padding inside your vagina. If this is uncomfortable, you may need regular painkillers.

Many hospitals have a machine called **Selectron**, or similar name, which passes a small radioactive ball into the applicator through tubes. If somebody needs to go into your room, the machine is switched off and the radioactive balls go back into the machine. The time you spend on the machine is usually between 12-48 hours.

A machine called a **Microselector** gives the radiotherapy in a few minutes and you can go home the same day.

To keep your vagina clean after treatment, it is suggested that you use vaginal douches for a few days after treatment.

Sometimes women are given both internal and external radiotherapy for maximum effect.

Radioisotope

A radioactive liquid is either given as a drink or injected into a vein. The radioactivity will gradually disappear and you will only stay in isolation until the radiation has broken down in your body. You will be allowed home when most of the radiation in your body has gone. Your belongings will also be checked. You should be able to carry on your life almost as normal as soon as you leave hospital, apart from staying away from children and pregnant women for a few days.

Caesium or Iridium Wires

This treatment is for treating tumours in the **mouth, legs, cervix and breast.** Very thin radioactive needles, wires or tubes are inserted under general anaesthetic in the operation room. An X-ray is sometimes taken to ensure the radioactive material is in the right place. The wires are usually removed after 3-8 days.

Safety Measures for the above Internal Radiotherapy

To prevent unnecessary radiation exposure to hospital staff and your friends and relatives, certain safety measures have to be taken:

- You will be nursed in a separate room alone or with somebody else having similar treatment. To protect other people from any radiation, lead screens may be placed either side of you.
- Doctors and staff will only stay in your room for a short time.
- If visitors are allowed in, (no children or pregnant women), they can only stay for a short time by sitting at the end of the bed. The may be allowed to talk to you from outside the room through an intercom.

A Geiger counter may be used to check the radiation in the room. A small radiation counter is sometimes worn by staff.

Treatment for prostate cancer

Small radioactive seeds are implanted into the prostate through the perineum (the area between the scrotum and the anus). It involves an overnight stay and is done under general anaesthetic. Only one treatment is required.

The seeds are not removed, but stay in the prostate tissue. The radioactivity gradually fades away over one year. The radioactive seeds only affect an area within a few millimetres, so will not affect other people.

The incidence of incontinence and impotency problems is less than for surgery or external radiotherapy, but there are other possible side-effects such as urinary retention (5-10% of cases), urinary frequency and urgency, and possible rectal problems. It is quite normal to get blood in your urine. If you get a lot, let your doctor know. Drink plenty of water to flush out the blood.

Interoperational Radiotherapy

This is external radiotherapy given during an operation for cancers of the breast, colon, rectum, stomach, brain, pancreas and gynaecological organs.

During surgery, after the tumour has been removed, radiotherapy is given direct to the area. The operation is then completed. Inter-operative radiation can deliver a single high dose directly to any remaining tumour or to the immediate surrounding area, where there might still be cancer cells. As any organs nearby will be sensitive to radiation such as skin, intestines and liver, they can be held aside or shielded. Often interoperation radiotherapy saves lengthy external radiotherapy sessions later on.

Total Body Radiation

In preparation for bone marrow transplantation, the whole body may be treated with radiation.

In **semi body radiation,** a large single dose of radiation is given in a single treatment to about half of the body, either the upper or lower half. It is usually used if there is a large amount of local disease in the gynaecological area or the abdomen. It may also be used in cancer of the lung, oesophagus, prostate or digestive system.

Side-Effects from Radiotherapy

The treatment itself is painless, but may later cause uncomfortable side-effects. Radiotherapy affects people in different ways. Some can carry on working; others feel too tired and have to stay at home.

Skin All external radiation has to go through the skin. Most skin reactions appear as a redness, gradually tanning and then peeling. In bad cases, the skin will weep.

100% stabilised allicin gel, applied direct to the area being treated several times a day, will deal with any skin damage caused by the radiotherapy, even when the skin is weeping. Apply during and after radiotherapy treatment.

Head and Neck Radiotherapy to the mouth may cause dental problems, so you may need frequent check-ups at the dentist. It is important that you tell your dentist that you have had radiotherapy before having any dental work later on. To prevent any damage to your gums, make sure that you take Q10 all the time.

Your mouth may become sore, dry and your taste buds may be affected, as your mouth is very sensitive to radiotherapy. The treatment can also cause infections such as thrush and sticky mucus.

Using the powerful high spinning magnet MagneTech (see Part Five) by the mouth daily, has shown to alleviate some of the above problems.

My wife Lena, who had throat cancer, was given the strongest radiotherapy possible-ten times over two weeks. When she came home, she felt as if her head was exploding. I held the MagneTech at the back of her head for 10 minutes, which made her head feel normal again. St. Thomas' Hospital radiotherapy department staff said they had never come across a patient who could take radiotherapy of the neck so well. They even gave her two extra days' radiotherapy. Lena was the only patient smiling in the waiting room.

During any cancer treatment, it is important that you do not lose your appetite and lose weight. But this can be especially difficult until your mouth feels better. If it becomes too painful or difficult, a thin tube may be passed into your stomach through your nose.

Another way of giving liquid food is by passing a tube, called a PEC or RIG tube, through the wall of your abdomen into your stomach. Very nutritious liquid is then passed during the night, when you are asleep.

You may also lose your hair on a permanent basis within the treatment area.

Chest A common reaction to radiotherapy is to make your chest feel tight, making it difficult to swallow solid food, so you may have to rely mainly on high calorie drinks.

Stomach and pelvis If your treatment is near your stomach, you may feel sick and vomit. Anti- sickness drugs are usually very effective.

You may also get diarrhoea and will be given anti diarrhoea drugs. Devils claw tea has also shown to be a very effective natural product. It is also important to take capsules with billions of good bacteria to replace the ones often killed by radiotherapy.

When treatment is given to the prostate, womb, colon, rectum or bladder, you may become constipated, so take capsules which give your body lots of oxygen. If you have piles, this may become more irritating. Applying direct 100% stabilised allicin gel and a powerful magnet apparatus several times a day, has been found by many people to give great relief. Your bladder might get inflamed during radiotherapy to the lower abdomen and you might feel a burning sensation when passing urine and have a need to go to the toilet more often. It is most important that you drink, preferably water and try to avoid drinks which irritate your bladder, such as alcohol, tea, coffee and acidic fruit juices, in particular orange juice. Cranberry juice and lemon barley water often helps.

Sex life and Fertility

Radiotherapy may not affect your sex life or it may temporarily or permanently change it. It is perfectly safe to have sex during radiotherapy treatment. If you find it too embarrassing to talk to hospital staff about such intimate things, (don't forget they are used to dealing with such issues), then contact **Macmillan Cancer Support** or the **British Association of Sexual and Relationship Therapy**, Tel: 020 8543 2707, Website basrt.org.uk. Very often it is much easier to talk to a specialist.

Women Unless radiotherapy is given to the ovaries, most radiotherapy treatments will not affect your ability to have healthy babies. Most specialists recommend you wait two years to try to get pregnant after radiotherapy. It is most important if you are of childbearing age, to use effective contraception during your radiotherapy treatment, as the treatment can not only cause a miscarriage but a child could be born with abnormalities.

Treatment to the ovaries will bring on the menopause, with the normal signs of dry skin, hot flushes and dry vagina.

Men Radiotherapy to the prostate, bladder and rectum may cause impotence sooner or later. You may also be too tired during treatment to wish to have sex, or you may temporarily be unable to have an erection.

Sperm production can be reduced permanently if radiotherapy is given to the bladder or prostate. In cases of the most common cancer in young men, testicular cancer, radiotherapy to the testicles can be avoided.

Sperm banking Is when sperm is stored frozen until the couple are ready to have children.

Lack of Appetite

It is most important that you do not lose weight during and after radiotherapy. You may only be able to have liquid food due to treatment to your mouth or neck, as described before. Try and have a light meal or snack before radiotherapy, unless your doctor advises you otherwise. Don't try too hard to eat if you do not feel like eating, due to side-effects. Try and eat small amounts more often. On the day that you feel good, eat regular meals. You need a balanced high protein diet to maintain your strength.

CHEMOTHERAPY (Chemo)

Chemotherapy uses drugs and hormones mostly on rapidly dividing cancer cells. It works on its own in cases of leukaemia and lymphoma. Sometimes it is used before surgery to try to reduce the tumour, and often after surgery or radiotherapy as a secondary or preventative treatment. During and after chemotherapy, it is vital to incorporate complimentary remedies to reduce the side-effects chemotherapy nearly always causes and to ensure the chemotherapy works better. It is also vital to boost your weak immune system, which caused your cancer in the first place and which will be further weakened by the chemotherapy treatment.

SUMMARY
- Chemotherapy
- Should I agree to Chemo treatment?
- How is Chemo given?
- Advantages of Chemo
- Disadvantages of Chemo
- Medicine and Supplements to take and to avoid while having Chemo
- Tests during Chemo
- Side-effects from Chemo
- How long do side-effects last?
- Lack of Appetite
- Tiredness, Infection and Bleeding during Chemo
- Will I lose my hair?
- Side-effects from Chemo you should report to your doctor
- Holidays
- Alcohol
- Sex Life and Fertility
- How to boost your immune system during and after chemo

Chemotherapy (Chemo)
There are 50 different chemo drugs and new ones are continuously being developed. Some new drugs will kill cancer tumour cells, without destroying normal cells. Some are given on their own, but often several chemo drugs are combined (combined chemotherapy).

I highly recommend **MacMillan Cancer Support** booklets on chemo and that you contact the nurses in the Support Service on 020 7739 2280 or freephone 0808 800 1234, weekdays 9 am to 8 pm.

Chemo was first derived from so called mustard gas (cyclophosphamide) when it was discovered in the late 1940s and was found to have the ability to kill rapid dividing living cells such as those in the lymph system, bone marrow and intestinal tract. So scientists worked out they could use mustard gas in modified form to poison cancer, which consists of the most rapidly dividing cells of all. This is why most chemo drugs are so toxic and nurses administering chemo must always wear protective gloves.

Should I agree to Chemotherapy treatment?

The decision to have chemo can be a very difficult one, to consider the damage the treatment does to your body and the often very harsh side-effects. Many people who have been advised to have chemo have survived after deciding not to, but it is very difficult to resist the advice of most doctors specialising in cancer. Research has often proved chemo does not do any long-term good. In fact, it does more harm in cases of the most common cancers, which kill 90% of cancer patients today. Chemo has shown to be most successful with three types of cancer - ovarian, small cell lung cancers and acute non-Hodgkin's lymphoma. The following cancers have also shown to respond well to chemo and result in people living longer:

Hodgkin's disease, intermediate - and high-grade non-Hodgkin's lymphoma, some germ cell tumours, testicular cancer, localised cancer of the small intestines and certain cancers in children, such as Wilms tumour, acute lymphocytic leukaemia and choriocarcinoma.

In many cases cancer patients, given chemo, will only survive a few extra months, but with disastrous effect on their quality of life.

When you first go and discuss chemo treatment with your doctor, take your partner or a good friend with you to make a note of what your doctor tells you, as you may well not be able to remember much when you come home.

How is chemotherapy given?

Chemo may be given in several ways to reach the cancer cells.
(A) • capsules or tablets taken orally.
   • liquid applied to the skin in cases of skin cancer (melanoma).
   • by injection into muscles, veins or under the skin.
   • through an internal or external pump into the blood stream.

Your treatment may be daily, weekly or monthly. You normally have some rest time between treatments to give your healthy cells and tissues a chance to recover. Some chemo treatment may take one or two months, but some may be on and off for several years.

(B)   Injected direct into the fluid around the spine or into particular cavities in the body, such as the pelvic cavity or bladder, where the chemo tends to stay in the area in which it is given and does not affect cells in other parts of the body.
(C)   Chemo cream may be used direct on skin cancer (Melanoma) areas.

Advantages of Chemotherapy

Can cure some cancer which has spread, reduce tumours before surgery or prevent cancer coming back. As the chemo is mainly carried in the blood, it can stop cancer cells dividing anywhere in the body. The chemo will also affect healthy cells, but they can replace themselves. Cancer cells cannot repair themselves, so they hopefully die.

Disadvantages of Chemotherapy

- As well as affecting cancer cells, certain parts of the body which also have rapidly dividing cells are especially sensitive to chemo, such as hair follicles, bone marrow, the lining of the mouth and the digestive system.
- Have side-effects.
- Less effective on large tumours.
- Some tumours develop a resistance to chemo.
- Chemo can sometimes increase the risk of cancer later in life, especially when given to children.
- When chemo has not solved the problem in the first place, and the cancer is not destroyed or the cancer comes back later, higher doses of chemo may be given with even more severe side-effects. This will usually destroy large parts of the bone marrow which manufactures your immune system.

So you see how important it is to deal with the cause of the cancer in the first place.

Medicine and Supplements not recommended to be taken during Chemo

Here is a list of medication you may not take during chemo - check with your doctor:
Antibiotics, anti-coagulants, anti-seizure pills, aspirin, barbiturates, blood pressure pills, cough mixture, diabetic pills, hormone pills, sleeping pills, some herbs, tranquillizers and diuretics.

Tests during Chemo

There are several ways of measuring how well your chemo treatment is working including physical examination, scans and X-rays. Blood count will be used to adjust the doses of chemo.

Side-Effects from Chemo

The most common side-effects of chemo are: nausea, vomiting, hair loss, fatigue and bone marrow suppression which decreases the body's ability to make red blood cells that carry oxygen to various parts of the body and white blood cells that help to fight parasites, viruses, fungal and bacterial infection and platelets which help blood to clot. If any of these three blood counts become too low, your treatment may be delayed until your count is up again. The feeling of nausea can often be reduced by taking ginger, including ginger chewing gum.

How long do Side-Effects last?

Some (such as nausea and vomiting) can occur with each treatment, and last for a relatively short time. Tiredness comes on gradually and can take some time to go away, due to lack of red blood cells. Some chemo can cause permanent changes such as damage to the lungs, kidneys and other organs.
As soon as your treatment is over, most normal cells recover quickly and the side-effects start to disappear as healthy cells have a chance to grow normally.

The time will vary from one person to another and will depend on the chemo you had and how your own physical condition is and whether you have taken account of the BIG FOUR.

Lack of Appetite

It is most important you do not lose weight during and after chemo treatment. Try and have a light meal or snack before having chemo. Don't try too hard to eat if you do not feel like eating due to side-effects. Try and eat little and often. On the days you feel good, eat regular meals. You need a balanced high-protein diet to maintain your strength.

Tiredness, infection and bleeding during chemo treatment

As explained before, your bone marrow will be weakened by the chemo lowering your blood count of red and white blood cells and platelets causing:

Tiredness - caused by fewer red blood cells - will mean you may feel tired, weak, dizzy, and sometimes short of breath. You gradually feel less fatigued after the end of your chemo treatment. The following will help:

- Try and rest when you feel tired during the day and get more sleep during the night (in a Geopathic Stress-free place).
- Cut down on your daily activities.
- Eat well, including iron-rich foods such as green leafy vegetables and red meat. Take plenty of supplements.
- Don't forget to ask family, friends and neighbours to help with housework, shopping, childcare, driving etc.
- Get up slowly from a seated or lying position.

Infection - caused by fewer white blood cells which will make it difficult for your body to fight infection, so you should take the following precautions:

- It is very important, the first two weeks after starting chemo when your white blood cells are low, to avoid contact with anybody who has a cold, flu or any other disease. If you get a cold, and/or flu, signs of infection on your lips, nose, in your eyes or in the genital or rectal area, contact your doctor and do not take any medicine not prescribed by your doctor.
- Be careful not to cut or nick yourself and do not scratch or squeeze spots.
- Ensure you wash and apply antiseptic on any cuts or wounds. Wash your hands as soon as you come home. Also before eating and before and after going to the toilet. Protect hands before doing any dirty or heavy work.
- Take warm showers and baths, not hot then use good body lotion all over afterwards. Use a soft toothbrush.

You need to contact your doctor if you have the following signs of infection: fever, sweating, chills, cough, sore throats, redness or swelling around sores, pimple or boils, unusual vaginal discharge or itching, burning feeling when passing water, loose bowels which may be due to chemo.

Will I lose my hair?

The rapid dividing cells which make up your hair roots (follicles) are sensitive to some chemo.

If your doctor says you are likely to lose your hair with the chemo, then it is not so big a problem for men, as it is quite fashionable nowadays for men to shave their heads.

However, for women it can be very distressing when the hair becomes thinner or falls out completely.

Hair loss in other body areas is much less common.

If you have long hair, the weight may hasten the loss, so consider cutting it short. Use a soft bristle brush and a mild shampoo. Do not use rollers and avoid electric styling products. Some women find changing the style of their glasses/sunglasses can help disguise the loss of eyebrows and eyelashes.

If you decide to have a wig, buy one before you start chemo and lose your hair. Bring a friend along for a second opinion. A good synthetic wig washes better, is less expensive to maintain, cooler and costs less than real hair wigs. You will often find you look really good in a wig.

Your hair will start to grow back as soon as your chemo stops and sometimes it will look better than before.

A study has shown that 69% of chemotherapy patients who took 700 mg of Vitamin E per day, for a week before and then all through their treatment, avoided losing their hair.

Side-effects while having chemo you should report to your doctor

- High temperature, shaking, chills, sweating, sore throat or cough.
- Unusual bleeding or bruising including gums and nose.
- Blood in urine or stools.
- Severe diarrhoea.
- Difficulty in breathing.
- 'Pins and needles' in your hands and feet.
- Continuous pain, including headaches.
- Swelling of hands, feet or eyelids due to allergic reaction or rash.
- Continuous pain or soreness where the chemo was injected.
- Small spots under the skin.
- Unusual vagina discharge or itching.

Case history re very sore vagina

Anne H. in Brighton "Allicin Gel has proved to be of huge benefit for my particular problem. After chemotherapy and radiotherapy, I was prescribed a course of Anastrozole (Arimidex) tablets. Unfortunately, these had the side-effect of a very sore and uncomfortable vulva and vagina. I had tried all the usual creams for this problem, with no effect at all. Fortunately, I was recommended Allicin Gel, and the difference has been unbelievable! I no longer have any discomfort! I was also suffering from frequent bouts of bacterial vaginosis, which is accompanied by an unpleasant odour. So far, after using the Gel, this has not recurred.
I cannot thank you enough for your help and do hope other women, with similar problems, will be able to benefit too".

Holidays

It is most important you do not have any 'live virus' vaccines before going abroad while you are having chemo.

Alcohol

The occasional alcoholic drink during chemo will not affect most people. Check with your doctor.

Sex Life and Fertility

Chemo may not affect your sex life or it may temporarily or permanently change. It is perfectly safe to have sex during chemo. Your cancer cannot be passed on to your partner and sex will not make your cancer worse. If you have a partner, you should both go along and discuss it with your doctor or contact a cancer support service nurse at Macmillan Cancer Support or contact the British Association of Sexual and Relationship Therapy, Tel.020 8543 2707, website basrt.org.uk. Very often it is much easier to speak to a specialist.

Women

Menopause

Chemo can bring on an early menopause causing dryness of the vagina and less interest in sex.

HRT (Hormone Replacement Therapy) can prevent or reduce the menopause. Many doctors are concerned about giving HRT, particularly in cases of breast and uterine cancer.

Contraception

Chemo can harm the foetus if you become pregnant, so you should use a reliable method of contraception, such as condoms or the cap, not the pill, during the whole course of chemo treatment. Chemo cannot pass into semen or vaginal fluids.

Monthly periods

During chemo, your monthly periods may become irregular or stop, causing hot flushes, dry skin and dryness of your vagina.

Pregnancy

If you were already pregnant before your cancer was diagnosed, it may be possible to delay chemo until after your baby is born, depending on your type of cancer, how aggressive it is and how advanced your pregnancy is.

*Caz C (Devon) was diagnosed as having **cancer in several places,** when she was four months pregnant. As no conventional treatment like chemotherapy and radiotherapy could be given, Caz's only option was to use a powerful high spinning magnetic apparatus direct on her lung and neck cancer. X-rays showed the cancer did not spread during her pregnancy and Caz gave birth to a very healthy 10lb (4.5kg) baby boy.*

Men

Some chemo may make you temporarily or permanently infertile. You may have to consider placing your sperm into a sperm bank for later use. In most cases, you will be able to get an erection and have an orgasm as before your chemo.

How to boost my immune system during and after Chemo?

It is vital you take the BIG FOUR into account when you are having chemo to ensure you strengthen your immune system the chemo is destroying and to obtain the full benefit of the chemo.

Geopathic Stress It is very important that you sleep and sit in a Geopathic Stress-free place, so your body can 'repair' itself all the time.

A mother contacted me to say her little boy could not take the full strength chemo he needed to treat his leukaemia. I found he was sleeping in a very Geopathic Stress place and advised her where to move his bed into a Geopathic Stress-free place. Very shortly after moving his bed, he could take the full doses of chemo needed. Some time afterwards, he was declared free of cancer.

Micro-parasites Most chemo kills off parasites, but I still advise people to take 100% stabilised Allicin Liquid from garlic, which is one of the strongest immune boosters. It also helps fight any infection and superbugs you may get in hospital.

Q10 As the liver is affected by the chemo, it cannot produce enough Q10 to revitalise itself to produce enough Q10 to give energy to every one of your good billions of cells, including your heart which needs the most. So, it is very important you take up to 500 mg per day during chemo treatment. Some doctors will prescribe Q10, so you can get it free on NHS. Otherwise, 100 mg per day is better than nothing if you cannot afford 500 mg per day.

I have heard of cases where doctors have said that you must not take Q10 during chemotherapy. This is like saying you must not drink water. Chemo weakens your liver so that it cannot produce enough Q10. If you do not have enough Q10, you will die. Q10 is an enzyme which your body cannot function without. Also the liver's ability to produce Q10 diminishes with age.

Acid/Alkaline Balance Chemo treatment plays havoc with your pH level. Read the chapter on Acid/Alkaline balance on how to correct your pH balance.

Magnetic Therapy Use an apparatus with high speed spinning magnets daily to revitalise your body. Use on your solar plexus (just above your navel), where 70% of your immune system is stored, on your reflexology points under your feet, on your kidneys and liver. Any one of these points you can treat up to 20 minutes. Also one minute or so on your thyroid and thymus (it matures your T cells which attack any infection). Maximum one hour each session, but you can do it several times a day. Very effective in healing mouth ulcers, which chemo can cause. As magnetic therapy kills toxins, it is best not to use magnetic therapy until three days after a chemo session.

Rebounder It is the most effective, safe and easy way to exercise. It is claimed, one minute on a rebounder will double your white blood cells, which are reduced during chemo. This increase in white blood cells does not last long, so you need to exercise on the rebounder several times a day.

Rebounding also helps if you are depressed.

Vitamins and Minerals It is vital you keep up your intake of vitamins and minerals during chemo. Even more so if you get less from your food, if you lose your appetite. The most important to take are Vitamin E, C and D, Selenium with Zinc and multivitamins or seaweed, which is the most nutritious organic plant on earth, containing over one hundred carbohydrates/fibres, vitamins, minerals, trace elements, amino acids and betaines and helps your intake of iron and regulates your pH.

Ozonated Water

Ozone (O_3) is a very good way to reduce the side-effects from chemo, by detoxing your body and removing those toxins through a simple chemical reaction, which allows your liver and kidneys to process the waste much more efficiently. (See Part Four).

Red Grapes are claimed to protect your red blood cells, brain and heart tissues during chemo. The bioflavinoids in red grapes has a very antioxidant effect. It is reported they are 200% stronger than Vitamin C, 575% stronger than Vitamin E and about 400% stronger than beta-carotene.

Homeopathy Remedies Many of these have shown to help to minimise side-effects from chemo.

Other Therapies like Acupuncture, Aromatherapy, Bach Flower, Homeopathy, Reflexology, Hypnotherapy, Healing, Kinesiology, Radionics, Reiki, Shiatsu, Therapeutic Massage, Yoga etc. will all help your body and make you feel better.

Bach Flower Remedies When you feel upset before going to hospital, or other times including when you cannot sleep, take the Rescue Remedy which is a combination of five remedies originally selected by Dr Edward Bach. It has no harmful side-effects, is non-toxic and does not influence or is influenced by drugs.

What about my doctor's opinion?

Try not to be influenced against the above advice, just because your doctor does not fully understand or has a different view. For example, the benefits of Q10 have been known for over 30 years, supported by hundreds of scientific reports and clinical trials. Allicin from garlic has proved very successful over the last 10 years.

LASER

Laser treatment uses a narrow intense beam of light to shrink or destroy tumours. Compared to surgery with a scalpel, laser treatment is very precise, with less bleeding, swelling or scarring and in addition healing time is often shorter. Used in photodynamic therapy, lasers could save the UK millions of pounds in treating head and neck cancer. All round a much quicker treatment which also reduces the use of anaesthetic.

SUMMARY
- Laser
- Laser Types
- Endoscopic Laser Therapy
- Photo Dynamic Laser Therapy

Laser (light amplification by simulated emission of radiation)
As in hyperthermia, the laser light raises the temperature of the tumour, which damages or destroys the cancer cells. At 212° (100° C), it can vaporize tissues in a few seconds.
Laser is often used to treat inaccessible areas or where, due to health reasons, surgery, chemotherapy and radiotherapy cannot be used. Laser is used in treating many kinds of cancer such as skin, lung, oesophagus, cervical, vaginal, pancreas, stomach, colon, rectum, anus, bladder, penile and vocal cord.
It is also used to help relieve symptoms caused by cancer such as keeping vital body tubes opened, like the oesophagus for swallowing, the trachea for breathing or the colon, rectum and anus for eliminating stools.

Laser types
The three most used laser types in treating cancer are:
- Carbon dioxide laser which removes thick layers from the skin's surface in skin cancer cases without penetrating the deeper layers.
- Nd: YAG laser can penetrate deeper into tissue than other kinds of lasers such as treating throat cancer.
- Argon laser which can only pass through superficial layers of tissue. Also used in photodynamic therapy.

Endoscopic Laser Therapy
The laser is activated through a flexible tube called an endoscope, which has been passed through any opening in the body like the mouth, nose, anus or vagina. The laser operator can, through the endoscope, see the tumour directly and aim the laser precisely at the target tissue.

Photo Dynamic Laser Therapy (PDT)

A light sensitive chemical agent called Amphimex is injected three to four days before a chemotherapy drug bliomycin. Because cancer tumours have high metabolic activity and are surrounded by a proliferation of new blood vessels, the drug accumulates around the cancer cells in preference to healthy tissue. When a low-powered argo laser is shone on the tumour directly or through the skin, the light triggers a chemical reaction which enables the drug to enter the tumours and kill them.

Mr Colin Hopper, who heads the National Medical Laser Centre in London, said: "PDT is a medical miracle. You can see the tumours turn black and die in a matter of days. You destroy cancer without having to use a scalpel. We started treating mouth and oesophagus cancer and it has been proved in head and neck cancer. We also know that it works in lungs, prostate, stomach, breast and in the difficult to treat cancers such as cancer of the pancreas. It is completely painless and the cancer is destroyed in a very short time".

Unfortunately, only a handful of UK hospitals use this treatment, which kills cancer in one treatment in less than one hour. PDT is often performed on an outpatients basis or may only requires a short stay in hospital. It removes the need for surgery and/or lengthy chemotherapy and radiotherapy. PDT is presently carried out at University College Hospital, London.

It is still called a 'pioneering' treatment although it has been used successfully thousands of times in different countries. It is claimed that by using the PDT treatment throughout the UK could save the NHS £1 billions a year in treating cancer, even though not all types of cancer tumours can be treated.

This may have saved my wife from dying of throat cancer over nine years ago as she refused a major operation to remove a large part of her throat and tongue.

HYPERTHERMIA-Heat therapy

The idea of using heat to help destroy cancer tumours has been around for a long time. Hyperthermia can be used on its own or in combination with radiotherapy, chemotherapy and biological therapy.

SUMMARY
- **Research**
- **Types of Hyperthermia treatment**
  - **Superficial**
  - **Interstitial (inside the tumour)**
  - **Combination**
  - **Regional**
  - **Whole body**
- **Side Effects**
- **Hyperthermia Trials**

Research

Over one hundred years ago there were medical reports of tumour shrinkage and even complete remission after a high body temperature. Only during the last forty years has the effect of hyperthermia seriously been studied. It has been found elevated temperatures in the range of 39° to 42°C (102° to 107°F) make tumours more sensitive to radiotherapy and allow a better delivery of chemotherapy and biological therapy to tumours. Temperatures as high as 50°C (122°F) are sometimes applied on its own direct to a tumour such as High Intensity Focused Ultrasound (HIFU) used to treat prostate cancer (see next page).

Types of Hyperthermia treatment

Superficial equipment that supplies different types of heat energy-ultrasound, microwave or radiofrequency is connected to a box, which is placed close to a tumour in or near the skin.

Interstitial (inside the tumour) heat is applied to a small area direct to the tumour. This may be carried out by using ultrasound beams, high frequency or infra red energy. The focused beam raises the temperature to destroy the cancer cells in the targeted area, without damaging the surrounding tissues. The process is repeated until the area of cancerous cells has been destroyed. (See prostate cancer).

Combined works with other therapies, such as radiotherapy, because heat is especially destructive to certain tumours which are sensitive to radiotherapy by preventing the tumours from repairing themselves after radiation treatment. It works best if the two treatments are given simultaneously or perhaps within one hour of each other. Hyperthermia treatments are often only given once or twice a week, because cancer cells may resist subsequent heat treatment for up to three days.

Regional is carried out by heating an organ or a limb by magnets or other devices that produce high energy. This can also be carried out by heating blood removed from the patient and pumped into the region to be heated internally.

Whole body heating uses warm water blankets, hot mat induction coils - similar to those used in electric blankets or thermal chambers. Such treatment is particularly useful with chemotherapy or biological therapy. This treatment and/or reginal hyperthermia can also be used with interstitial heat treatment to improve tumour heating.

Side Effects

Complications or side effects from radiotherapy do not usually increase by combining it with hyperthermia. However, using hyperthermia on its own can cause discomfort or even significant local pain. Also it can cause blisters which generally heal quickly. In a few cases it can cause burns, which tend to heal very slowly unless very powered high spinning magnets are used directly (see Page 232).

Hyperthermia Trials

Trials in Europe have proved the benefit of superficial hyperthermia, in combination with radiotherapy for chest wall recurrence of breast cancer, as well as metastasis melanoma in the skin, lymph nodes or tissues under the skin. In the USA using hyperthermia with radiotherapy with a variety of superficial cancers proved the complete response rate was 50% better than when radiotherapy was used on its own. Regional hyperthermia combined with radiotherapy has also shown benefits in treating certain soft tissue sarcomas, pelvic tumours, cervical and bladder cancer. Most success in the UK has been with prostate cancer.

HIFU (High Intensity Focused Ultrasound) has now treated more than 3,000 patients worldwide with a range of cancers including liver, bone, breast, kidney, pancreas and uterus. The energy generated by HIFU is ten times more powerful than conventional ultrasound. It heats the tumours up to around 85-100°C and the cancer cells just die, leaving healthy tissues near the tumour undamaged. Any remaining tumour can then be removed by surgery. Because great accuracy is required, patients usually have a general anaesthetic, so they do not move while the energy is being targeted at the cancer. Dr James Kennedy at Churchill Hospital, Oxford has carried out many successful HIFU treatments over the last two years on liver and kidney cancer.

HORMONAL and BIOLOGICAL TREATMENT and BONE MARROW TRANSPLANT

Hormonal Treatment is used for cancers that depend on hormones for their growth. The treatment either removes or adds hormones to your body. It may include the use of drugs to block your body's production of hormones or surgery to remove the hormone-producing organ.

Hormonal treatment is mainly carried out in cases of breast, prostate or thyroid cancer. See details under the individual cancers.

Biological Treatment uses your own body's defences against the cancer. It boosts directly or restores normal defences using agents occurring naturally in your body or made in a laboratory. Usually it is used in combination with other treatments. (See how your immune system works in Part Five). Discuss with your oncologist the biological agents available as new ones are being developed all the time. *Interferons (IFN's)* have been shown to be able to fight a number of different cancers including melanoma, kidney cancer and leukaemia. *Interleukins IL-2* is also used for treating kidney cancer and melanoma.

Bone Marrow Transplant is mainly used in cases of leukaemia. After the patient has been pre-treated with chemotherapy and/or radiotherapy, bone marrow is extracted from the marrow cavity of the pelvis or breastbone of the donor and injected into one of the recipient's veins, to enable new healthy blood cells to be produced. See full details under leukaemia (see Page 148).

PART THREE

CANCER

Cancer is a general term for the abnormal growth of cells.

We all experience two normal situations in which our body tissues grow much more rapidly than they usually do. We grow from a single cell to a perfectly formed human being in nine months. Then we grow into a normal size adult over the next sixteen years or so. Also when we injure ourselves and need rapid repair, restoration and replacement of damaged tissues, our body can produce many new cells in a very short time.

When growth or healing is complete, a set of genes tell the cells to 'switch off'. But mainly if our immune system is weak, some cells continue to divide and double in an uncontrollable way. After many months, sometimes years, the doubling process has occurred many times before a tumour can be detected. As an example, a 6 mm (¼ inch) lump in the breast is about the smallest lump that you can feel with your fingers. Such a tumour contains over one billion cells and has undergone thirty doublings since it first became an abnormal cell.

6 mm tumour

BENIGN TUMOURS

These may appear in any part of the body like freckles, moles, or fatty lumps in the skin. This is a growth that is not cancerous. It can usually be removed for cosmetic reasons and in most cases does not return. (Read also about benign tumours under breast cancer). Benign tumours do not spread to other parts of the body. Most do not endanger life unless they are growing in a confined area such as in the brain. In most cases benign tumours will not become cancerous. However there are lesions that are considered precancerous such as a thickness of the lining of the mouth or cervix. This should be addressed before any cancer develops.

MALIGNANT TUMOURS

These have two significant characteristics:
*   They have no wall or clear cut border. They put down roots and directly invade surrounding tissues.
*   They have the ability to spread to other parts of the body. Small parts of the malignant tumours may break away and travel to other tissues and sometimes start similar growth.

TYPES OF CANCER

Carcinoma   (*Carcin* - means 'hard' and - *oma* means 'a lump')   About 80% of cancers are carcinomas, which may occur in the skin, the stomach, the colon (large bowel), the rectum (lower end of the bowel), the bronchial tubes, the breast, prostate, kidneys, liver, the ducts of the pancreas or gallbladder etc. Any lining surface, anywhere in the body, can become the site of a carcinoma.

Myeloma   Originates in the bone marrow in the blood cells that manufacture antibodies.

Lymphoma   Originates in the lymph system.

Leukaemia   Involves the blood forming tissues and blood cells.

MAIN WARNINGS SIGNS OF CANCER

- A lump that does not go away.
- Unusual bleeding or discharge.
- Change of bowel or bladder habits.
- A sore that does not go away.
- Persistent hoarseness or cough.
- Indigestion or difficulty in swallowing.
- Change in a wart or mole.

Unfortunately some cancer symptoms seem so trivial and are similar to other less serious illnesses that they are often ignored by most people. For example, continuous coughing when everybody around you seems to be coughing could be the first sign of lung cancer. Also irregular vaginal bleeding can be due to a whole list of causes, but could be the first sign of cancer of the uterus. Read about symptoms of specific cancer under individual chapters on cancers. Any suspicious symptoms that persist for longer than two weeks should be investigated by your doctor. GPs are not cancer specialists, so if you are not satisfied with your doctor's diagnosis, get a second opinion or insist on seeing an oncologist (cancer specialist).

How To Reduce The Likelihood Of The Cancer Returning

First of all take care of the BIG FOUR (Part One) - Geopathic Stress, Micro Parasites, Q10 and Acid-Alkaline Balance (pH).

1. Of the thousands of cancer cases I have been asked to check out, all had Geopathic Stress lines through the areas during sleep where the cancer started. So first of all ensure you sit and sleep in a Geopathic Stress free place.
2. Next, it is important you boost your immune system, which orthodox treatment has weakened, often causing you to feel below par for a long time and may even cause pneumonia and heart problems. 100% stabilised Allicin from garlic will boost your immune system, so you feel better and prevent any micro parasites coming back. There was a 90% chance micro parasites were present when your cancer was first diagnosed.
3. Recommend taking 100 mg Q10 per day. Your liver converts the lower Co-enzyme Qs into Q10, which can be absorbed by your body and is vital to your entire cells energy metabolism ('your cells' starting plugs'). Your liver needs Q10 to operate 100%. Unfortunately Geopathic Stress creates a vicious circle. Your liver becomes weak, so it cannot produce enough Q10, which it needs to function normally. The liver's ability to produce Q10 diminishes with age. Read more about Q10 in Part One including case history of remission of breast cancer in 32 'high risk' patients.
4. Most people diagnosed with cancer have a very low Acid-Alkaline balance (pH). See Part One on how to obtain a healthy pH.
5. Malnutrition is present in most cancer patients and a stay in hospital can make it even worse. So a good nutritional supplement, e.g. an easily digested drink packed with calories, protein, minerals and vitamins is initially essential, followed up with various supplements especially Vitamin D. See Part Four.
6. Ensure you take as much exercise as possible. See Part Five.
7. Attitude - ensure you have the right attitude 'I will kill this cancer and make sure it does not come back'. Laugh, talk and pamper yourself.
   There may be specific additional recommendations under individual cancers.

FEMALE CANCERS

Breast cancer is by far the most common cancer in women accounting for 30% of all new cases and affecting about one in nine women.
Approximately another 10% is cancer of the female reproduction system.
40% more men die of cancer, excluding breast and prostate cancer than women, mainly due to the fact that women are more inclined to see their doctor if they feel something is wrong, so any cancer is diagnosed earlier, making treatment more successful.
Also on average women are more likely to believe in complementary remedies.

SUMMARY
- Breast cancer
- Cancer of the female reproduction system
- Ovaries and fallopian tubes
- Endometrial - uterus or womb
- Cervix - cervical
- Vagina
- Vulva

BREAST CANCER (Females) [1]

Breast cancer is not only the most common cancer in women (30%) but also the cancer which most affects women emotionally. To many women breasts are a very important part of their body and mutilating them unnecessarily by surgery can prevent them feeling comfortable with their bodies again. The earlier you detect cancer the more chance there is of preserving the breasts intact. 15% of women diagnosed with breast cancer will not develop invasive cancer [2] and therefore need no treatment.

[1] 1% of Breast Cancers occur in men [2] Invasive cancer or a tumour's ability to metastasise - to spread throughout the body - is the hallmark of genuine cancer.

The emotional side of breast cancer

I have often been told that health professionals seldom accept the extreme emotional reaction that women have after being diagnosed with breast cancer. There is a very complex emotional response, simply because the cancer affects the breast which is part of a woman's femininity. Even those who have experienced cancer in other areas of the body are unlikely to understand the emotions associated with breast cancer. One in five breast cancer sufferers are engulfed by feelings of hopelessness.

There is a very good chance that you will live the rest of your natural life without the cancer returning if you follow my advice and deal with what caused the breast cancer in the first place.

Symptoms

A lump, thickening, swelling or enlargement [3] of your breasts; dimpling; retraction of nipple; change in the skin of the breasts such as dimpling or puckering; redness, skin or nipple discharge, feeling hot; enlarged lymph nodes under arm and along top of collar bone.

Research

There are over 100 new breast cancer cases diagnosed in the UK every day – over 40,000 per year. Breast cancer is the biggest killer of women aged 35 to 50. Even though figures show that over 75% of women survive more than 5 years after orthodox cancer treatment, the survival rate is much lower after 10 or 20 years as the cancer often returns.

All right, so you say 20 years is not bad, but what if you get breast cancer in your early thirties with young children – do you not want to live to see your grandchildren?

About 13,000 women die of breast cancer every year in the UK.

Some women after surgery, chemotherapy and radiotherapy (which is the common standard treatment today) get breast cancer again within two years and find the cancer may even have spread further so may be advised to take 50% stronger chemotherapy the second time around. Isn't it about time you did something serious to improve your ineffective immune system, to enable your body to destroy pre-cancerous cells in the first place? Take account of The BIG FOUR.

Remember a 'healthy' diet, keeping slim, not smoking, regular visits to the gym and no history of cancer in your family, will **not** prevent you from getting cancer.

When the famous singer Carly Simon, was told she had breast cancer a few years ago, her doctor said there are two types of cancer patient. The first say they are scared that they'll die. The other type says "cure me". My sister-in-law, who survived cancer four times, always said "I have not got time to die" and carried on a very active life, including regular swimming for many years.

Even though the survival rate has increased over the last 20 years, many more people are diagnosed with cancer, so just as many people die each year. As I have mentioned many times before, the increase in cancer cases is often due to thousands of additional chemicals in many of our food, drinks and beauty products. Major contributory factors are also dairy products, diet, obesity, parasites, environmental pollution and Geopathic Stress. Geopathic Stress has increased many times during this period.

[3] The only exception here is if you are pregnant because the breasts tend to become enlarged and tender in preparation for the baby.

Geopathic Stress slows down the absorption of vitamins, minerals, trace elements etc. from your food, so many cancer patients are malnourished, which alone can be a major cause of death.

Breast Pain (Mastalgia)

It has been found that the worse the breast pain the less likely it is to be cancerous. There are two types of breast pain:

1 Cyclical, which is associated with menstrual periods
2 Non-cyclical, which may originate in the breast or in the nearby muscles and joints. (90% of women who suffer with breast pain are much more worried about the possibility of breast cancer than about the pain itself. Breast pain is a reassuring symptom, since its presence all but excludes breast cancer).

Breast pain is commonly associated with swelling, hardening and a feeling of tenderness in the breast. Breast lumpiness may or may not be associated with pain and again does not indicate there is cancer.

It is still common for doctors to prescribe ineffective remedies – diuretics or even antibiotics, to treat mastalgia. Some doctors suggest evening primrose oil in high doses, which takes several months to become effective. The most effective treatment for breast pain is treating the breasts direct with very powerful high speed magnets. The manufacturers give a full refund if the treatment does not work and there has been no case of any side effects over the last 17 years that the apparatus has been on the market.

Cancer and the Faulty Genes

Cancer researchers say 5-10% of cancers are caused by faulty genes inherited from one or both parents.
They claim the presence of faulty genes, known as BRC1 and BRC2 increase the risk of getting breast cancer by the age of 55 by up to 85%. Cancer researchers also claim about 61% of women who carry the faulty genes will get ovarian cancer by the age of 75.

Women who have the faulty gene and who have a strong family history of breast cancer are often tempted to have double mastectomy and/or have their ovaries removed later in life. Mothers, who conceive using IVF treatment will be able to screen and reject embryos that have the faulty genes. However, does the chance of getting cancer warrant denying someone the right to live, when there are some basic things you can do to prevent cancer? Even though breast and ovarian cancer represents about 25% of women who die of cancer, a double mastectomy does not prevent you developing other types of cancer.

In all cases where women claim they got breast or ovarian cancer because their mother, grandmother or sister had cancer, I found they all slept in a Geopathic Stressed place. So before you decide to mutilate your body, find out if those family member(s) slept in Geopathic Stressed bed(s).

A typical case was reported in 'The Times' July 3rd 2004. Kerry at 24 decided to have a double mastectomy and reconstructive surgery, as her mother, grandmother, great aunt and her great aunt's daughter has all died of cancer. On checking, all slept in GS beds, at the time their cancer was diagnosed, as follows:

Mother's bed

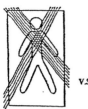

Mother's bed when she was 28 and first had breast cancer and when she died of breast cancer at 34

Grandmother's beds

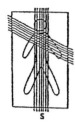

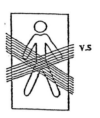

When she first developed breast Cancer in her early thirties (she had a single mastectomy).

Grandmother's bed when she died of ovarian cancer.

Great Aunt's bed

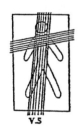

Great Aunt's Daughter's bed

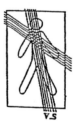

Great Aunt's (her grandmother's sister) bed, when she died of ovarian cancer.

Great Aunt's daughter's bed, when she died of cancer.

Kerry's bed

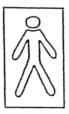

Geopathic Stress-free

(Key: **S** = Strong GS line **VS** = Very strong GS line)

Not knowing about Geopathic Stress and parasites, Kerry has psychologically taken the right decision. However, my advice is, if you have the faulty genes, check on Geopathic Stress,
parasites and the other BIG FOUR before contemplating mastectomy and removing your ovaries.

I feel so strongly about the misunderstanding with faulty genes that I herewith give two more cases.

Case two was reported in the 'Daily Telegraph' 23 November 2004. Diana believed from the age of 19, when her mother died at 51 of breast cancer, that she had an increased risk of getting breast cancer herself, particularly since breast cancer also caused the death of her grandmother.

Grandmother's bed   Mother's bed   Diana's bed

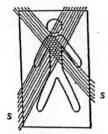 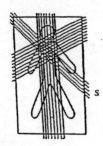 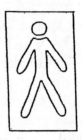

Geopathic Stress lines through their beds   Geopathic Stress-free
when they were diagnosed with cancer.

Case three was reported in 'The Daily Telegraph' 28 December 2004. Sally's grandmother died as a young mother of breast cancer. Her mother had breast cancer when she was 50 and died of a secondary cancer when she was 73. Therefore Sally believed that she had an increased cancer risk because of her family history. She is now having regular Ductal Endoscopy (see later) and helps with a research programme.

Grandmother's bed   Mother's bed   Sally's bed

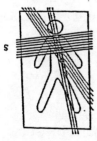 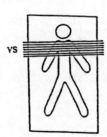 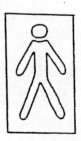

Geopathic Stress lines through their beds   Geopathic Stress-free
when they were diagnosed with cancer.

Ductal Carcinoma In Situ (DCIS)

This is an early form of breast cancer confined within the milk ducts in breasts. It is not strictly cancer, like a tumour, and the cancer cells are 'non-invasive' – they have not spread to the other parts of the body and it is not known if or when the cancer cells might develop and invade.

If you have been diagnosed with DCIS, some doctors feel you should have preventative surgery – lumpectomy or mastectomy, as frequent ordinary mammogram X-rays might encourage cell growth. Have they not heard of many other ways of testing for cancer successfully? - such as BSM, digital mammogram and ultrasound. In other words wait and see if the cancer develops – there is a strong possibility it will not if you ensure you do not sleep in a Geopathic Stress place, prevent parasites, adopt a dairy free diet, take exercise, take Q10 and other vitamins including Vitamin D and minerals as described elsewhere, also ensure acid/alkaline balance is high.

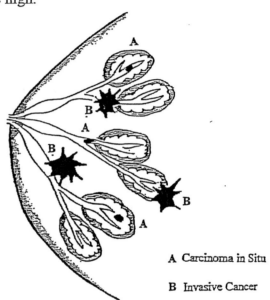

A Carcinoma in Situ

B Invasive Cancer

Of all the women screened and found to have breast cancer, 20% have DCIS. Of this, only one in four will develop invasive cancer in their lifetime and they will all be Geopathic Stressed. **In other words 15% of women diagnosed with breast cancer, will not develop invasive cancer and most of them will be subjected to traumatic surgery.**

The only advantage with surgery for DCIS, is that as it is not a true cancer, chemotherapy and radiotherapy are not part of the recommended treatment.

Checking for Breast Cancer
Breast Self Examination (B.S.E.) and Medical Examination

Research has shown that women who carry out self-examination have a positive attitude to life and employ preventative health measures. B.S.E. should commence from the time you develop breasts and continue until you die.

If you do not think doing B.S.E will inevitably lead to finding cancerous lumps, you will not feel nervous about doing it.

Britain's Chief Medical Officer reports that 90% of breast tumours are found by women themselves.

Remember

The vast majority of breast lumps are non cancerous, (9 out of 10). Unfortunately, 90% of women do not do B.S.E and there are many reasons for this:

1. Good information on B.S.E is hard to find. [4]

[4] One of the best informed books on B.S.E is 'Women's Health Handbook' by Dr Miriam Stoppard – one of the leading authorities on women's health. Published by Dorling Kindersley 2003 at £9.99.

2. Many women are embarrassed about touching their breast except in the shower or bath, or when breast feeding[5] They are therefore unaware for a long time of dramatic changes or developments of large tumours.

3. They feel that if they find something wrong, it must be cancer - yet only a few lumps turn out to be cancerous. Even if it is cancer, early detection greatly improves the success of a cure.

Basic Guidelines for B.S.E

Examine your breasts at regular intervals, both visually and by physical examination. Look in the mirror for anything unusual (see under symptoms).

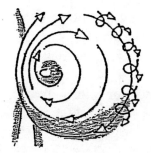

Examine your breasts by lying down in a relaxed position and put your right arm behind your head. This will flatten your breast tissues against your chest wall and shift your breasts towards the centre. If your breasts are very large, put a pillow under your left shoulder. Use your left hand to examine your right breast. Firmly press the breast tissues with your fingers in a circular pattern from the edge of the breast towards the nipple or use your own pattern as long as it is systematic. Check armpit and along top of collar bone for swollen lymph nodes which feel like lumps. Next, put your left arm behind your head and examine your left breast with your right hand.

The majority of cancerous lumps are found in the upper outer quadrant of breasts, (see details later on 'Breast Cancer and Bras'). Examine yourself; say every month, in a very relaxed way at different times of the month to get used to your breasts, as they change in consistency and texture during the menstrual cycle [6]
Post-menopausal women might choose a specific day each month (e.g the first day of the month) to ensure consistency.

Women, who have had a mastectomy or lumpectomy, should inspect the incision to feel for any lumps or skin changes. Remember B.S.E has its limitations. You will not be able to detect a tumour if it is pea-sized and is located deep inside your breast tissue or a cancer located in the milk ducts, [7] so an ultrasound and digital mammography might be a good idea at regular intervals.

It is important to get used to normal lumpiness which comes and goes during the menstrual cycle. When you are examining your breasts, you are mainly only looking for one thing: a new discrete lump that is constant in size, usually hard, irregular, non-tender, fixed in position and does not vary with your menstrual cycle. If you find such a lump, take extra care to examine your armpits and the top of the collar bone, where you main lymphatic system drains into your bloodstream. If you find a symmetrical lump on the other breast, it is nothing to worry about, as it is just the way your breasts are shaped.

Lumps which are painful, absence of hardness, easy mobility and presence of multiple nodules, usually mean there is no cancer tumour.

[5] Some women find it more comfortable to let their partner examine their breasts

[6] Most women find their breasts get small lumps in the second half of their menstrual cycle. The lumps are separate, tender if squeezed and the size of orange pips, these are swollen milk glands ready to develop if you become pregnant.

[7] In one survey of breast cancer cases, 44% (of whom 70% were aged 40-59) discovered the cancer through self-examination, 37% through mammograms or ultrasound tests and 8% through a doctor's examination.

There are three main reasons for seeing your doctor:

1 The lump is a new one.
2 It is very distinct, not just a thickening of the breast tissue.
3 It is unchanged through a couple of menstrual cycles.

If you cannot decide whether something is serious or not, see your doctor anyway.

Olivia Newton-John said "thanks to self-examination, I found my breast cancer early enough for it to be treated successfully 12 years ago, **I touched, I felt and I lived**".

A hand-held **Breastlight** [8] emits a safe LED-powered light which picks up as dark patches any tiny lumps - as small as 7 mm - which cannot normally be felt during physical examination.

The user stands in a darkened room holding the torch underneath and to the side of the breast against the skin.

Women under 50 are not eligible for the national breast screening program, yet younger women get more aggressive tumours than older women and have dense breast tissue which makes mammograms less effective. **Breastlight** is claimed to have a success rate higher than a mammogram, but should not be the only test if a tumour is suspected. **Breastlight** may also be ideal for thousands of women who are uncomfortable about performing regular breast checks.

Checking out a Breast Lump by a Doctor
Before you go to see your doctor, ask a friend to go with you for moral support.
To check out a lump, most medical tests will involve the 'triple assessment' approach, which is:

    a) A manual examination, more or less as described under B.S.E.
    b) Ultrasound and, if a mammography, ensure it is digital mammography.
    c) Fine-Needle Aspiration Cytology - FNAC (see later).

Size of Breast Tumours found by Ultrasound, Mammography and breast Self Examination

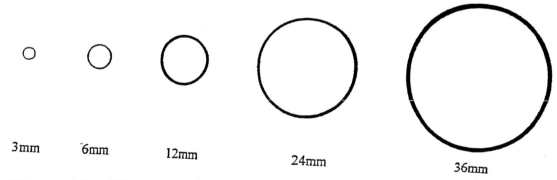

3mm   6mm   12mm   24mm   36mm

Ultrasound or Mammography
3mm (⅛ inch) and 6mm (¼ inch)
found by regular ultrasound or mammogram.

(8) Breastlight costs about £85. Stockist information at www.breastlight.com Tel: 0845 3011452

B.S.E
12mm (½ inch) found by women who do regular B.S.E
24mm (1 inch) found by women who do occasional B.S.E
36mm (1½ inches) found by women untrained in B.S.E

Diagnosed Stages 1 to 4 of Breast Cancer - see end of chapter

Standard Mammogram

This is a type of X-ray of the breast, which can pick up small tumours and other abnormalities that neither you nor your doctor can detect through manual examination. Mammograms can detect 90% of breast tumours often 6 months to 3 years before they can be felt manually. A mammogram is recommended as a routine check every three years for women over 50 as breast cancer is comparatively rare in women under 50. The NHS is now being asked to extend routine mammograms from the age of 47 to 73. The radiologist compresses each breast twice in turn between two plates, so that a good image is obtained. The procedure is painless but might feel uncomfortable. Each X-ray takes about 10 to 15 seconds.

A specialist radiologist interprets the plates and results are normally available in a few days. It can be worrying if you are asked to have a further test, but in 90% of these call-backs, the first readings are simply not clear because of dense overlapping breast tissue interfering with the results.

Remember in 70-80% of cases where mammograms are positive, no cancer is found after a biopsy has been taken.

Disadvantages with Standard Mammogram Tests

Some doctors maintain that even low dose X-rays can be potentially damaging. Others say the benefit of mammogram screening outweighs related low-risk radiation. More worrying is the report [9] that mammograms can rupture in-situ cysts in the breast(s) and spread the incidence of carcinoma in-situ (CIS), which now represents about 20% of all breast cancers, which has increased by 38%, and 200% of this increase is due to the use of mammograms [10]

When I was in the USA during Breast Cancer Awareness Month (BCAM) held throughout October (called pink ribbon campaign in the UK), I was astonished to see the main advice to prevent cancer was to have a mammography at least every three years between 20 and 39, and every year from then for the rest of your life. Are the manufacturers of X-ray films behind the promotion of mammography tests where there is a potential of selling half a billion dollars' worth in the USA alone?

The routine practice of taking four films of each breast annually results in approximately 1 rad (radiation absorbed dose) and is about 1000 times greater than that from a standard chest X-ray. Over 11kg (25lb) pressure is applied to each breast during a mammogram test, which could cause the spread of any cancer cells. Is it any wonder many specialists maintain that mammogram tests increase your chance of getting breast cancer? On balance, I feel it is much safer to use ultrasound or digital mammography.

The study in the journal 'Archives of Internal Medicine' compared 100,000 women who had received regular two-yearly standard breast mammograms over six years with

[9] **Reported in the Lancet in April 1994, JP Netten of the Royal Jubilee Hospital in London**
[10] **The Lancet July 1995**

100,000 similar women who had not. At the end of the study, the cancer tumour rate of the women who had regular screening was 22% higher.

Lately, both Swedish and Danish studies have shown that there has been no decrease in cancer deaths due to mammography screening since they were first recommended over 20 years ago. Many doctors now maintain a monthly B.S.E combined with a yearly clinical breast examination (C.B.E) by a trained health professional is at least as effective as mammograms in detecting early tumours and so much safer.

Digital Mammography
This is much less invasive than a standard X-ray mammography and better at detecting tumours in young women who have dense breasts. Images can be manipulated and magnified, which can immediately highlight tiny and subtle tumours reducing the need for recalls. Digital images can be transmitted instantaneously from centre to centre if several experts are involved. The NHS is now going to spend £100 million on installing digital mammography all over the UK. Do insist on a digital mammography in future for a more speedy, accurate and safer test.

Xero-Mammography
Similar to standard mammograms, but produces the image on paper rather than on film. Accuracy depends on the experience of the radiologist whatever method is used.

Ultrasound
Patterns are produced by the echoes of sound waves, which vary in intensity according to how solid the tissues are they bounce off. The advantages over a standard mammogram are:

1 Very useful for examining young women, who have very dense breasts.
2 It can tell the difference between large solid lumps and lumps filled with fluid.
3 It can detect a rich blood supply to a lump which usually occurs in cancerous tumours.

Unfortunately, ultrasound largely depends on the skill of the operator as the images can be hard to read and are open to misinterpretation causing many cases to be wrongly diagnosed. Don't be shy to ask when the equipment was last serviced, and if the operator is a radiologist specialist and to enquire about his/her accuracy rate. Ultrasound is less than 80% accurate.

Molecular Breast Imaging (MBI)
Standard mammography detects breast cancers by looking for areas in normal tissues that may turn out to be tumours. However, MBI can be inaccurate, particularly when detecting small, early tumours or in women who have dense breasts (as the difference in density between normal and abnormal tissue can be undetectable on X-ray photos). About one in three women has dense breast tissue. A newer type of Molecular Breast Imaging provides photographs of gamma-ray emissions given off by cells, to find molecules in breast cancer tissues that behave differently from healthy breast tissues. This technique can 'see' through dense tissue to detect any abnormalities.

Thermograph
Infra-red photographs are taken of breasts after they have been uncovered for a little while so the breasts have become cooler. Cancer cells are rapid growing and dividing, which creates a higher temperature than the surrounding cells. This can be detected by a

thermograph temperature map. This is a less common test than mammograms and ultrasound and never used as a first time investigation, but less dangerous than standard mammograms.

Fine-Needle Aspiration Cytology (FNAC)

This is a test to sample cells from a lump. Under ultrasound guidance, if the lump cannot be felt, a fine needle is inserted into the lump. If fluid is withdrawn, the lump is a cyst and the fluid can be drawn off and the cyst will disappear. If the lump is solid, a sample of cells is removed for microscopic examination.

Biopsy – Cutting Needle

As FNAC only produces tiny samples of cells, it is impossible to tell whether they originate from in-situ cancer or an invasive cancer. A cutting-needle biopsy provides a core of cells that can be analysed to make this distinction. Under local anaesthetic a special fine-notched needle is inserted to withdraw a fine core of tissue for detailed examination. In most cases there is hardly any discomfort and the skin is left virtually intact, but in about a quarter of cases a wound is left causing problems such as infection or haematomas. In such cases use a powerful high spinning magnetic apparatus to solve the problem.

Biopsy - Open

This is an alternative to a cutting-needle biopsy. The skin is cut away to reveal the lump which is removed with a margin of surrounding healthy breast tissue. If the lump is found to be cancerous, open biopsy nearly always means removing the whole lump (lumpectomy). This is carried out in hospital under general anaesthetic.

Sentinel Node Biopsy

If a cancer tumour has been detected, sentinel node biopsy involves removing the first lymph node in the armpit, which drains the tumour, to find out if it contains any cancer cells. If it is clear, you probably will not need additional surgery or radiotherapy to your armpit. This, in turn, can help to avoid lymphoedema. This then can be done on the NHS. It may take some time to arrange, but can ensure you get the least invasive treatment.

If a mastectomy is suggested after a cancerous tumour has been found, give yourself time to agree to this procedure in case you wish to follow an alternative route.

Ductal Endoscopy

This is a very new technique to detect the very earliest signs of breast cancer. A tiny fibre optic telescope the size of a pinhead – is inserted into each of the six milk ducts in both breasts. The ducts are examined for signs of minute changes in the lining and build up of the tiniest early cluster of malignant cells. One day no doubt breast tumours could be treated directly through the telescope, without the need for surgery as we understand it today.

Benign Lump

If tests show the lump is benign (non-cancerous) there is no need to remove it surgically if:
1 Mammography or ultrasound scan show that the lump is harmless.
2 On examination the lump feels smooth and is mobile.
3 FNAC finds no cancer.

4   There is no change in the size of appearance of the lump during follow-up examinations after three or six months. If your doctor does not require a follow-up examination, you should always request one if you notice any change.

You have the right to keep your lump undisturbed if benign.

Treatment

When you see your consultant for the first time, make sure you have a friend with you, who can take notes or record the conversation (if your doctor agrees). In most cases, you will remember very little of what your doctor told you, due to the shock of being told that you have breast cancer.

Surgery

Removal of the breast cancer tumour is the standard procedure in most cases of breast cancer (See Part Two). Breast cancer surgery can be carried out at a day surgery clinic. Surgery sites are often joined externally with surgery 'super glue' to minimise scars. Cryosurgery has now also been carried out. (See under Prostate Cancer).

Lumpectomy or Mastectomy

Your doctor should give you time to think over whether you should have a lumpectomy or mastectomy. If you agree to go ahead, no doubt your doctor will explain everything in detail.
The mastectomy with reconstruction could take several hours.

Lumpectomy

In this operation, where only the breast cancer tumour is removed, unfortunately both chemotherapy and radiotherapy are often recommended afterwards to ensure the cancer does not spread.

Mastectomy

This is surgical removal of the breast. Over the last 20 years, a **simpler mastectomy** has been implemented, so less reconstruction is required afterwards.

Radical mastectomy This was the former standard procedure where the whole of the breast and affected lymph nodes in the armpit were removed.

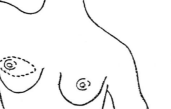
incision for
simple
mastectomy

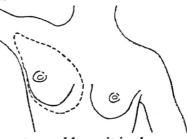
incision for
radical
mastectomy

If you are pre-menopausal and having a mastectomy operation, try and have it in the second two weeks of your cycle, rather than the first two weeks, as research has found you will have almost double the long term survival rate.

Surgeons have now started to give strong radiotherapy direct to the area, where the cancer tumour was, before closing up the operational area. This not only prevents long sessions of radiotherapy after the operation, but also prevents the damage from radiotherapy gamma rays as they travel from the skin to the previous cancer area. However if the surgeon is satisfied that all the cancer has been removed, chemotherapy and radiotherapy are often unnecessary afterwards.

Lymph nodes

When breast cancer spreads it moves first to the lymph nodes in the armpit. This occurs in around 33% of breast cancer cases. Traditionally surgeons have removed all these nodes (there are about 20 in each armpit), in an attempt to eliminate any migrating cancer cells. But this can have severe side effects including lymphoedema (described later).

About 15 years ago doctors discovered the tumour drained first into the sentinel node. But until recently this could only be identified during surgery by injecting a blue dye close to the nipple or near the tumour. After a few minutes the dye passed into the lymph system and on to the first lymph node (sentinel node) before removing it for testing.

Women then faced an agonising wait of up to two weeks to find out whether all the lymph nodes needed removing and may then face further surgery if the cancer had spread.
This involves 3,000 secondary surgeries each year in the UK. Why the sentinel node cannot be tested for cancer with a fine needle before surgery to see if it is cancerous, I do not understand.

A new **one stop nucleic acid amplication (OSNA)** test involves analysing the glands under the armpit during surgery to check if the cancer has already spread, so it can be dealt with at the same time as the surgery is carried out on the breast tumour and while the patient is under general anaesthetic.
So far over 750 patients have had the OSNA test in total at Alexandra Hospital in Portsmouth and The Royal Surrey County Hospital in Guildford.

Reconstruction

After a single or double mastectomy, most surgeons carry out reconstructive surgery at the same time. In the most common procedures, the doctors put sacs in the breast(s) and every week add more saline solution to stretch the skin and muscle until the required size has been achieved. After about a year, an operation is normally carried out to replace the saline solution with silicone which is permanent.

Some surgeons carry out a Latissimus Dorsi Flap (own tissue implant) reconstruction, where muscle, fat and skin from the back are cut away and tunnelled under the arm to form a 'breast'. The flap keeps its artery and blood vessels intact even after it has moved to the new site. Normally, one surgeon works on the back, while the other focuses on the breast(s). Some surgeons take the flap from the stomach, but this can leave patients with other complications.

The latest procedure involves taking fat, skin and muscles from the base of the woman's buttock, which leaves less scarring and is less painful. The feeder artery is severed, so that the flap can simply be placed in the position without tunnelling. Micro surgery is used to connect its blood vessels to those in the chest muscles. The nerves slowly grow in, so with blood circulating through, it feels softer and warmer, to the patient like a normal breast. Whatever type of surgery is carried out, scars normally reduce to thin white lines after a time. Lipmodelling involves taking the patient's own body fat, say from the abdomen and reinjecting it into the breast to form a completely natural breast, but this entails extremely precise surgery.

Often you have a breast care nurse to visit you regularly, so you can ask questions you do not like asking the doctor. Some women are quite happy not to have any reconstruction done.

Massaging Scar Tissue

Once the mastectomy incision (with or without reconstruction) has healed, scar massage is often recommended. This is performed directly over the scar or any lumpy area using the fingers lubricated with a good quality organic moisturiser. A powerful rotating magnetic apparatus applied direct has shown to heal operation scars very quickly.

Suitable Bra

Many recommend you do your 'homework' on buying a good quality bra before any surgery, so you have all you need beforehand. This will prevent you having to be measured and 'pulled about' immediately afterwards when you may be sore and tired. "Amoena" is a leading worldwide provider of post-surgery lingerie, 0800 0726636, Amoena - online.co.uk. Other suppliers are John Lewis, 08456 049049, John Lewis.com, Nicola Jane, nicolajane.com and Marks and Spencer.com

Chemotherapy & Radiotherapy after a Breast Cancer Surgery

After surgery, doctors often recommend chemotherapy and radiotherapy just to make sure all the cancer has been destroyed. (See Part Two).

High-dose chemotherapy has been tried mainly in the USA, to blast out the breast cancer, but has shown to be of no greater benefit than ordinary chemotherapy. High-dose chemotherapy simply increases the side-effects without offering any clear benefits. This was the controversial treatment unsuccessfully tried by the late Linda McCarthy, wife of the ex-Beatle, Paul. I tried, in vain, at the time to contact Linda to tell her she was sleeping in a very Geopathic Stress place and she would have had a far better chance of surviving if she had taken the danger of Geopathic Stress seriously.

In the majority of studies, the most important question of all: "does chemotherapy help you to live any longer than you would if you don't get the treatment?" is never asked. There is very little evidence to support the use of chemotherapy for breast cancer. In one of the few reviews of all studies comparing chemotherapy with tamoxifen, chemotherapy proved no better. The majority of the 46,000 women diagnosed with breast cancer in the UK each year are treated with chemotherapy, usually anthracycline, but it is only effective in about a quarter of the patients[1]. Hopefully, new tests under trial, will confirm if the chemotherapy is effective within 24 hours, rather than at the end of gruelling sessions of treatment.

Apart from the usual side-effects caused by chemotherapy, like nausea, vomiting and hair loss, the less reported side-effects is the increased risk of developing leukaemia, particularly among women who receive certain forms of chemotherapy or drugs combined with radiation for breast cancer. This treatment, not only kills cancerous cells, but normal ones too, including those of the bone marrow - the foundation of the immune system - of the intestinal walls and hair follicles. If you agree to chemotherapy and/or radiotherapy, it is vital you take the BIG FOUR into account to ensure your treatment does not damage you too much and prevent the cancer returning, often in a different place.

Radiotherapy has shown to cause problems in over 40% of reconstructive surgeries, such as pain and feeling unwell compared with just 10% with women who had no radiotherapy.

In another study, over 60% of women who received radiotherapy for breast cancer, developed lung cancer on average 17 years later and in most cases in the lung on the same side as the breast which had radiotherapy. Breast cancer patients also risk soft tissue cancer of the breast after radiation.

[1] Source Macmillan Cancer Research UK

The British Radiotherapy Action Group Exposure (RAGE), has been formed by women who have experienced catastrophic arm injuries, like lymphoedema, caused by radiotherapy. They probably did not need the radiotherapy in the first place.

Hormone Therapy

This is a type of systemic therapy to treat breast cancer. Systemic therapy means it treats the whole body. Also called endocrine therapy.

What are hormones and how are they linked to breast cancer?

Hormones are chemical messengers that are produced in organs called endocrine glands, for example, the pituitary gland in the brain and glands in the ovaries. Hormones are carried around the body in the blood to other organs or tissues where they influence growth and nutrition.

When, why and who will be offered hormone therapy

- If your tumour is oestrogen sensitive. About 75% of breast cancer in post-menopausal women is oestrogen sensitive and about 50-60% in pre-menopausal women.
- An oestrogen receptor test (an examination for sensitivity to oestrogen) is now routinely carried out on the tumour following surgery. Those who have a high oestrogen receptor are most likely to benefit from hormone therapy. If you have a low oestrogen receptor, your doctor will weigh up the benefits against the potential risk of side effects.
- New 'wonder drugs' like Herceptin, which might stop cancer cells dividing, are only for 25% of women who show positive for the HER-2 gene.
- Hormone therapy can cause a variety of side effects, from mild to severe. Some diminish after some time; others last for ever, even after discontinuing taking the drug. Typical side effects are nausea, hot flushes and night sweats,
- Vaginal dryness, mood change, loss of libido (sex drive) and weight gain are further side effects depending on the individual response and which drugs you are taking.
- Hormone therapy may be prescribed as:
  - *Neo-adjuvant therapy.* Used before surgery to try and reduce the tumour. *Adjuvant therapy.* After surgery with or without radiotherapy or chemotherapy (usually after chemotherapy).
  - *Recurrence or secondary breast cancer.* This is often the first choice of treatment for secondary breast cancer to control the spread of the cancer if you are oestrogen receptive.
    You will probably be offered a different type of hormone therapy, if you are already on one.
  - *Primary hormone therapy.* This can be given as the only treatment, for example, for women who have other illnesses, such as lung or heart conditions which mean they are unable to have surgery or radiotherapy. It may also be an option for those who do not want surgery.

Various Drugs

MacMillan Cancer Support has fact sheets that give more detailed information about the individual drugs.

Tamoxifen (including Nolvador, Tamoxifen and Noltam) has been the most popular hormone therapy drug for over 20 years. This drug is not normally given for more than 5 years after cancer treatment.

If you take Tamoxifen, ensure you have regular tests on your eyes, liver and womb (endometrium) and take other drugs or radiotherapy for the shortest time possible. Not all women benefit from Tamoxifen. BRCAZ positive women may be less likely to develop breast cancer if they take Tamoxifen, but BRCAI positive women derive no protection from taking the drug. No studies have proved that Tamoxifen will work on pre-menopausal women.

Unfortunately research has now discovered that the drug can cause an aggressive and difficult to treat cancer in the other healthy breast. Research from the Fred Hutchinson Cancer Research Centre reviewed the progress of 1,103 women with breast cancer who had taken tamoxifen most of the time. Of these, 369 women developed a second breast cancer.

Femara This drug can be taken by post-menopausal women for a further three years after having taken Tamoxifen for five years. Also used as a first line of treatment for women with secondary breast cancer. It is claimed Femara reduces cancer by 42% and reduces the risk of cancer spreading to other parts of the body. Femara may increase the chance of getting osteoporosis, which may be prevented by taking Shark Cartilage at the same time.

Armasin (Exemestane). This may be used as the second or third line of treatment, when other drugs are no longer effective for post-menopausal women with secondary cancer. This drug costs about £4,000 per month.

Zoladex (also known as Goserelin). Experts believe Zoladex could benefit up to 5,000 women who develop breast cancer each year before the menopause. The drug is given once a month as an implant under the skin of the stomach, instead of chemotherapy, without having to endure unpleasant side effects and the risk of losing their fertility. This hormone therapy drug called LHRH, works by stopping the pituitary gland from producing a hormone which stimulates the ovaries, to manufacture oestrogen. About two-thirds of pre-menopausal patients have hormone-sensitive breast cancer. Once treatment has ended, the ovaries usually begin functioning normally again after about two years.

A new British study, which combined results from trials involving 12,000 women, found LHRH used on its own to treat early breast cancer, was as effective as chemotherapy.

Anastrozole known as an aromatase inhibitor, acts by cutting the level of oestrogen circulating in the bloodstream in post-menopausal women with hormone sensitive early breast cancer.

Compared to Tamoxifen, those taking Anastrozole had a 15% better chance of surviving more than 5 years. In addition, the amount of time that passed before the breast cancer recurred, rose by 25% and there was less cancer spread. Anastrozole was approved for use on the NHS in August 2007.

Herceptin This is a new type of 'targeted' medicine which might stop cancer cells from dividing. The treatment costs about £20,000 per year. Herceptin can only be used for 25% of breast cancer patients who show positive to HER-2 gene.

None of the hormone therapies works 100% of the time, nor are they suitable for all breast cancer patients. Most only give some protection for 5 years, while others give a few more years protection afterwards. So, ensure you take care of the BIG FOUR.

Lymphoedema

This can develop in as many as one in five women who have had surgical or radiotherapy for breast cancer, where lymph nodes in the armpit have been removed or damaged. Lymph nodes are part of the lymphatic system which carries the fluid (lymph) from the soft tissues back into the bloodstream.

Lymphoedema can affect the whole arm or only a limited portion such as the hand, the wrist area, the area below the elbow or, much less often, the area above the elbow.

Lymphoedema can also affect the breast area, if the lymph nodes have been damaged or removed because the fluid from this area also needs to drain via the breast back to your bloodstream. The condition is debilitating, is often painful and can show signs of swelling. It can start immediately and last for life or may occur for a while then disappear, but may recur or reappear years later.

What does lymphoedema feel like?
- A feeling of tightness and hardness in the arm which may result in difficulty of movement.
- A gradual thickness of the skin on the arm. Lymph may also leak through the skin as the condition worsens.
- Deep aching pains or shooting pains up the arm.
- Pins and needles in the arm.
- A feeling of tightness, tenderness or pain in the elbow.
- An intolerance to heat in the affected arm (climatic, saunas, baths).

Even though your first port of call will be your GP, I also suggest you contact the Lymphoedema Support Network (LSN), visit website or contact St. Luke's Crypt, Sidney Street, London, SW3 6NH. Breast Cancer Haven (www.breastcancerhaven.org.uk) can also be of great help. Tel: London - 020 7384 0099, Hereford - 01432 361061, Leeds - 0113 237 3017.

Main points to note with your arm which has Lymphoedema:
- Moisturise your skin frequently.
- Regularly rest your arm in an elevated position. Must be supported.
- Don't carry heavy objects with your affected arm. Do not wear handbags from the shoulder, watches or other jewellery.
- Don't permit the skin to be pierced for any reason i.e. injections, drawing blood or vaccinations. (Don't trust anyone, not even your personal doctor or nurse to remember which your at-risk arm is).
- Use a powerful rotating magnetic apparatus on a daily basis on your arm to help your lymph flow freely (see Page 232).
- Also contact the above lymphoedema breast cancer website.

Breast Cancer and Bras
The lymph system fights infection and drains the toxins into the blood stream to be cleansed by the kidneys. The main entry from the lymph system in the upper chest area is into the subclavian vein running from your arm up near both sides of your neck - so when modern women wear bras for long periods, their shoulder strap is restricting the flow from the lymph channel into the subclavian vein. The horizontal strap is also restricting the flow of the lymph channels and nodes under the armpit. This observation was confirmed by Sidney Singer and Sonia Grismeijer who presented compelling evidence for the connection between bras and breast cancer in 'Dressed to Kill' (Avery 1995). They conducted a three year study of 4700 women living in cities throughout the USA.

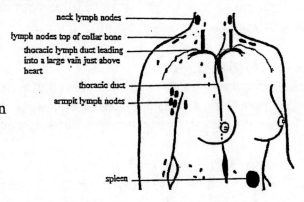

Women who wore their bras over 12 hours daily but not in bed – the majority, were 21 times more likely to develop breast cancer compared with women who wore their bras just a few hours a day. On extreme ends of the bra-wearing spectrum, women who also wore bras to bed have a 125 fold greater chance of getting breast cancer than did women who refrained from wearing them altogether.

Most breast cancer tumours start at the top of the breast roughly outside where the bra shoulder strap is fastened onto the bra again restricting the lymph glands.

As for under-wired bras, the metal crosses acupuncture meridians and so can block the normal flow of the body's energy or *chi*. According to the Chinese, this blockage can cause stagnation and disease.

Bras which squeeze the cleavage to make women appear bustier are the worst bras to wear.

I am not suggesting women should not wear bras, but I do suggest the following:

1) Exercise your arm without a bra each day.
2) The best exercise is on a Rebounder, which is smaller and stiffer than a trampoline. By rebounding you increase gravity by 25% both on the down and the up movement revitalising your lymph system (which has no pump) and your whole body. If you can build up your exercise on the Rebounder to 10 to 15 minutes a day, use 3 to 5 minutes exercising your arms (see more details under exercise). However, some women may not be able to rebound in comfort without a bra.
3) Massage yourself or get somebody to do it for you around the lymph area where it enters the subclavian veins.
4) When convenient, wear wide shoulder bra straps, or padded pieces under the bra straps, at the shoulder. This is particularly advisable if you have already had breast cancer.
5) Use a powerful rotating magnetic apparatus both at your lymph/subclavian veins and under your armpits for a few minutes a day. This is the best way to break up stagnation and create a rapid improvement to your lymph system.
   A woman had suffered for 30 years with breasts full of lumps, bumps and gravel. Each breast was treated 10 minutes per day for four days with powerful rotation magnets, which unblocked the lymph glands in her breast and brought them back to normal.

The chance of a woman getting breast cancer a hundred years ago was 1 in 500, now, it is 1 in 8. A hundred years ago few women wore a bra – coincidence? (I know food contained more minerals and was not filled with chemicals, women died younger, people were often not told it was cancer etc).

Breast Implants
Implants for breast enlargement may not in themselves contribute a higher risk of cancer, but to support larger breasts the bras will cause a larger strain on the lymph system, so daily exercise is more important without the bra on.

Underarm Deodorant
Your body emits a lot of toxins through the apocrine sweat glands in your groin and arm pits. The material is broken down by bacteria to form odorous substances. You need to kill the bacteria without blocking the glands; otherwise the toxins go back into your

lymph nodes, many of which are near the upper outer part of your breasts, where the larger numbers of breast cancer tumours develop.

Using a traditional antiseptic deodorant stick or spray may still block your sweat glands and may contain propyl alcohol which can encourage micro parasites (see Part One). An even quicker way for propyl alcohol to enter the blood stream under your armpit is when shaving because you can accidentally cut the skin and expose blood vessels.

Use instead a total natural and traditional antiseptic deodorant, which uses the property of pure alum minerals salts, a natural occurring mineral with astringent and antiseptic qualities, which neutralises bacteria and therefore helps to control body odour normally for 24 hours. Put your perfume somewhere else!

Dairy Products

The main change in your diet is to cut out all dairy products immediately (see Part Four). Professor Jane Plant CBE, one of Britain's most eminent scientists, had cancer recur five times (initially breast cancer), before she discovered the relationship between dairy products and breast cancer. Her last tumour, a lymph node in her neck, disappeared within five weeks, after she stopped consuming dairy products. Before, she was given only months to live. It is now over ten year since Professor Plant had cancer.

Plant explains in her international best selling book, 'Your Life in Your Hands', [11] the problems caused by hormones and growth factors in cows and goats milk and how the calcium you need is much better supplied from vegetable matter, which is the same source cows and goats obtain their calcium from.
In Plant's book, written with Gill Tidey, 'The Plant Programme' [11], she gives practical and comprehensive advice on how to avoid dairy products and include a full range of menus for many delicious meals.
Breast cancer cells are still breast cancer cells, when they occur in secondary cancer tumours, in other parts of your body such as lungs or liver.

How to ensure a high success rate and reduce the likelihood of the cancer returning

It is most important that you take care of the BIG FOUR - no Geopathic Stress, destroy any microbes, mainly micro parasites, take adequate Q10 and ensure a high acid alkaline balance in your blood.
Take the necessary vitamins, minerals etc. modern food no longer provides to prevent you suffering from malnutrition. Also take at least 20 mcg daily of the vital Vitamin D. Also get enough exercise. Ideally exercise daily on a rebounder to vitalise your lymph system and help dispose of toxins from your body. Two minutes on a rebounder will double your white blood cells for one hour.
About 90% of people who get cancer have a thyroid which is out of balance. Using a MagneTech for one to two minutes direct daily will revitalise it. Do the same on the thymus, which matures your T-cells and say 20 minutes on your solar plexus where 70% of your immune system is located. Most importantly, use the MagneTech daily for 20 minutes directly on the breast to heal it and any scar tissues. Also underarm if you have

[11] **Published by Virgin Publications Ltd**

had any lymph nodes removed, if you are to prevent lympheodema.

A Russian Medical study by N.G. Bakhmutskii examined the effects of a rotational magnetic field on a group of 51 breast cancer patients. The magnetic field was applied mainly direct to the breast tumours. The results showed a significant, positive response in 27 of them (SOV Med(7) 1991 p.25-27).

Ensure you go on a non dairy diet.

You have got to take charge of your own health.

Breast Cancer and Geopathic Stress Cases

The following diagrams show where the Geopathic Stress lines were in the beds of breast cancer cases, when the cancer was first detected.

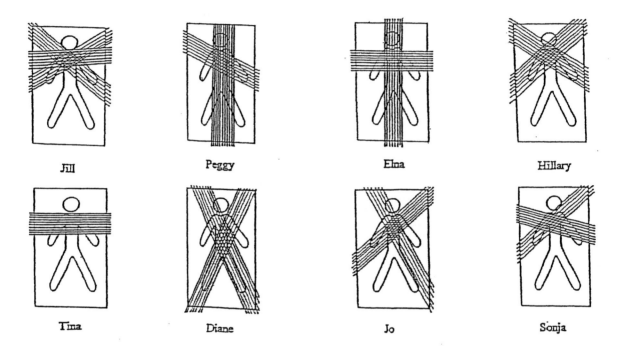

| Jill | Peggy | Elna | Hillary |

| Tina | Diane | Jo | Sonja |

Case Histories

Case reported by Practitioner JMA 4.20.94

Edith A. had several 15-20 mm hard breast cancer tumours. Her bed was moved out of the Geopathic Stress and she treated herself with strong rotating magnetic therapy on vertebrae (7 cervical down to 5 thoracic to increase flow of blood etc.) and direct on tumours for up to 20 minutes per day. Also took 150/180 mg Q10 per day. Tumours softened up and disappeared within one and a half months. No orthodox treatment was given.

Jessica R was diagnosed with breast cancer, but did not want conventional treatment. Apart from Vitamin C and B17, she took 400 mg of Q10 per day. Within a few months, the tumour had shrunk from 3½ cm to 1½ cm and her surgeon did not suggest surgery as this might spread the cancer. Jessica now takes a maintenance program of 200 mg of Q10 per day.

It must be strongly emphasised that the above described treatments etc. may only help a few people.

Stages of Breast Cancer

Stage 1   Cancer tumour is less than 24 mm (1 inch) across and has not spread outside the breast.

Stage 2A Cancer tumour up to 48 mm (2 inches) across and has spread to lymph nodes under arm (or) cancer tumour is bigger than 48 mm (2 inches) across and has not spread to lymph nodes under arm.

Stage 2B Cancer tumour is bigger than 48 mm (2 inches) across and has spread to lymph nodes

Stage 3A Cancer tumour can be over 48 mm (2 inches) across and has spread to lymph nodes under arm and the lymph nodes are attached to each other or to other structures.

Stage 3B Cancer has spread to tissues near breast - skin or chest wall including ribs and muscles in chest (or)
Cancer has spread to lymph nodes inside chest wall along breast bone.

Stage 4   Cancer has spread to other organs of the body, most often the bones, lungs or brain (or)
Cancer has spread to lymph nodes in neck near collarbone.

Photo Dynamic Laser Therapy (PDT)

This is the latest treatment for breast cancer which is a painless, non invasive way of destroying breast cancer tumours in less than one hour and can often be carried out on an outpatient basis (see page 45).

Menopause

Eight out of 10 women aged 50 plus, suffer from menopausal symptoms linked to fluctuation in hormone levels as fertility comes to an end. These symptoms include hot flushes, memory loss, mood swings and vaginal dryness. If these symptoms become intolerable, particularly if you are in a full-time job, it may be worth considering hormone replacement therapy (HRT) as in my opinion the 0.6% chance that this may cause breast cancer is even less likely if you take care of the BIG FOUR.

Breast Cancer Haven

This charity was started in 1997 by Sara Davenport who was concerned by the lack of emotional support and information available to people with breast cancer. Sara believed "no-one should have to face breast cancer alone".
At the Breast Cancer Havens in London, Hereford and Leeds, integrated healthcare is specifically designed to support people through their treatment. The centres provide up-to-date support, counselling, information, complementary therapies and a place for meeting others going through a similar experience. Visitors can benefit from the expertise of specialist nurses, hair and make-up classes and bra fitting sessions. Each Haven has a cafe area, a library and a relaxation area. All services are **free of charge**.
Breast Cancer Haven Centres
Effie Road, London, SW6 1TB   Tel: 020 7384 0099
37 St Owen Street, Hereford, HR1 2JB   Tel: 01432 361061
4-5 The Gateway, West East Street, Leeds   Tel: 0113 284 7829

Please note details on other charities who also deal with breast cancer patients are on pages 261 to 265.

CANCER OF THE FEMALE REPRODUCTION SYSTEM

> Since so many of the cancer problems that occur in this part of a woman's body are silent, regular checkups are advisable even though a pelvic examination can be a nuisance and also embarrassing. I am convinced that if you take full account of the BIG FOUR, your chance of getting cancer in the first place will be much reduced.

Cancer of the Female Reproduction System (Gynaecological)

What you need to know?
- Many operations for this kind of cancer may affect your ability to have children. They may also affect your ability to have sexual relations.
- Since each part of the female reproduction system is unique, treatment varies depending upon the location of the tumour.
- Make sure you understand exactly what is going to be done to you, what organ will be affected and what side effects you can expect before you have any treatment.
- A Pap test can accurately detect cancer of the cervix. It is not a test for detecting cancer of the uterus (womb), fallopian tubes or ovaries.
- Keyhole surgery is now widely used to cause minimal invasive surgery and less time in hospital.
- Human papilloma virus (HPV) infections are found in the majority of cancers of the cervix, vulva and vagina.

What areas are involved?
- Ovaries and fallopian tube
- Endometrial - uterus or womb
- Cervix - cervical
- Vagina
- Vulva

Female Reproduction System

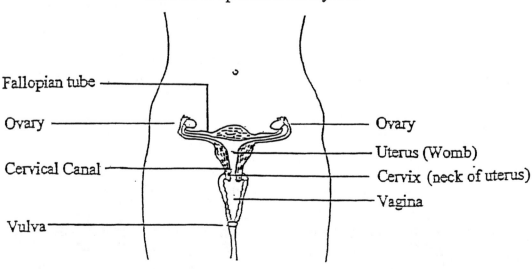

Emotional and sexual relations

Most women feel shocked and upset by the idea of having treatment to the most intimate and private parts of their body. Anger, fear and resentment are normal emotions when these strong feelings are also combined with the trauma of cancer diagnosis, surgery and other treatments. You may find the normal closeness of your relationship is also affected. It is therefore important to give yourself and your partner time to deal with your emotions and feelings, which may bring you closer together.

Everyone has their own way of coping with difficult situations. There is no right way to cope. Some prefer to keep their feelings to themselves or talk to family and friends or outsiders. See useful organisations below.

When you first have sexual intercourse after having treatment you will probably worry about pain and think that your sex life will never be the same again. You may have to make adjustments. Tell your partner if you feel pain.

If you have had your cervix and uterus removed and had a vagina reconstruction, it may not be possible for you to have vaginal orgasm. However, surgery to the vagina does not affect the clitoris, so it will be possible to have an orgasm through oral sex and masturbation.

Remember that no matter what kind of cancer treatment you have, the ability to feel pleasure from being touched will almost always remain. Even if some aspects of sexuality have changed, pleasure is still possible.

Useful organisations

British Association for Sexual and Relationship Therapy
PO Box 13686,
London SW20 9ZH
Tel: 020 8543 2707
Email: info@basrt.org.uk
Website: www.basrt.org.uk
Offers counselling and psychotherapy and can give details of local counsellors.

DES Action UK
PO Box 128, Blaydon LDO
Tyne & Wear NE40 3YQ
Tel: 0191 489 2257
Email: mail@des-action.org.uk
Website: www.des-action.org.uk
Gives support and information to women exposed to DES.

Gynae C
1 Bolingbroke Road,
Swindon,
Wiltshire SN2 2LB
Tel: 01793 322005
Email: Gynae_C@yahoo.com
Website: www.communigate.co.uk/wilts/gynae
A national helpline offering support to women with gynaecological cancer.

OVARIAN CANCER

Ovarian cancer is often referred to as the 'silent killer' because it usually only becomes apparent at an advanced stage, when it may well have spread to other parts of the body, resulting in a low survival rate. However early stage diagnosis results in a high survival rate, but survival after treatment for severe ovarian cancers can be vastly improved with simple lifestyle changes. However, prevention in the first place is obviously best.

SUMMARY

- **Symptoms**
- **Research**
- **Who is most likely to get ovarian cancer?**
- **The Ovaries**
- **Diagnosis**
- **Types of Ovarian Cancer**
- **Treatment**
- **How to ensure a higher success rate and reduce the likelihood of the cancer returning?**
- **Case History**

Symptoms
Often few symptoms. Abdominal swelling. In rare cases vaginal bleeding. Women over 40 may experience generalised digestion discomfort, unexpected weight loss.

Research
Most people will say they knew somebody who has had breast cancer, but when it comes to ovarian cancer, most people will say they know of somebody who's died of it. Out of the 7000 UK women who are diagnosed every year, about 5000 will die of it.

Who is most likely to get Ovarian Cancer?
Ovarian cancer can occur at any age but most likely in women over 50, with over 60 year olds at highest risk. In addition:

- women who have never had children
- women who have had breast and colon cancer
- women who have taken postmenopausal oestrogen
- women who are affected by the BIG FOUR, eat dairy products and are low in Vitamin D.

The Ovaries

Ovaries are the size of an almond and are located in the pelvis, one on each side of the uterus. During the menstrual cycle one ovary releases an egg that travels through the fallopian tubes to the uterus.

The ovaries are the body's main source of female hormones - oestrogen and progesterone, which regulate the menstrual cycle and pregnancy. These hormones are central to the development of the female's bodily characteristics such as the breasts, body shape and body hair.

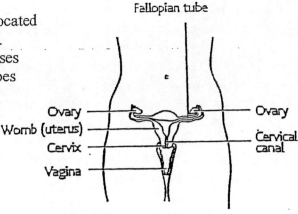

The ovaries and their surrounding structures

Diagnosis

Ultrasound of the ovaries is normally used to help differentiate between healthy tissues, fluid-filled cysts and tumours. Ultrasound is carried out by inserting an instrument which produces sound waves into the vagina. The pattern of the sound waves, produce a sonogram (a picture of the ovaries on a computer screen). A CT scan may also be carried out as well as an intravenous pyelogram (IVP). This is a series of X-rays of the kidneys, urethra and bladder to help determine if the cancer has spread. A blood test to measure a substance that is produced by the ovarian cancer cells called CA-125 may be carried out.

The cancer antigen test has proved useful for monitoring the success of ovarian cancer treatment, indicating whether a tumour has shrunk or if it has re-occurred. This test works less well at detection, missing about half of all early tumours. If cancer is suspected the only sure way of testing is to have a biopsy to examine a sample of the ovarian tissue under a microscope.

Types of Ovarian Cancer

Epithelial ovarian cancer accounts for 90% of cases and occurs in the lining of the ovary. About 15% are called tumours of low malignant potential and are treated differently than the more common and more invasive ovarian cancers of the epithelium. Germ cell tumours affect the egg-making cells, in the ovaries; are quite rare, and mostly affects young women. Also rare are stromal tumours.

Treatment

Surgery is the most common treatment. The type of surgery depends upon the extent of the cancer. A total abdominal hysterectomy and oophorectomy means that the ovaries, fallopian tubes and uterus are removed. Removal of both ovaries causes sterility and the loss of sex hormones especially oestrogen. This will not occur if only one ovary is removed along with the fallopian tube connected to the ovary being removed.

Chemotherapy is often recommended either by pill, put into blood stream intravenously or given directly to the affected area. Radiotherapy may also be used either externally from a machine or put directly into the sac that lines the abdomen in a liquid that is radioactive.

Case History

Jette had surgery to remove cancer tumours on both ovaries followed by intensive chemotherapy treatment. Her doctor told her, without hesitation, that her type of cancer most often came back and was then terminal. Jette's bed was found to be very Geopathic Stressed. She had slept there for 18 years and always had cold feet and sweated profusely each night. As soon as Jette's bed was moved into a Geopathic Stress-free place, Jette's feet immediately became warm during the night and she was no longer sweating.

She also felt so much more comfortable on her settee once it was moved out of Geopathic Stress.

Jette was also full of micro parasites when she was diagnosed, which together with Geopathic Stress, contributed significantly to her weak immune system which could not prevent her getting cancer in the first place. (The chemotherapy killed her parasites).

It is almost seven years since Jette had cancer. She is now back in a full time job, a healthy person, full of life with sparkling eyes much to the delight of her husband and children.

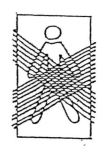

Geopathic Stress lines through Jette's bed where she use to sleep.

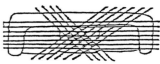

Geopathic Stress lines through Jette's settee before it was moved.

How to ensure a high success rate and reduce the likelihood of the cancer returning

It is most important that you take care of the BIG FOUR - avoid Geopathic Stress, destroy any microbes, mainly micro parasites, take adequate Q10 and ensure a high acid alkaline balance in your blood.

Take the necessary vitamins, minerals etc. as modern food no longer provides enough to prevent you suffering from malnutrition. Take at least 20 mcg daily of Vitamin D which is vital.

Also get enough exercise. Ideally exercise daily on a rebounder to vitalise your lymph system and help dispose of toxins from your body. Two minutes on a rebounder will double the number of white blood cells for one hour.

About 90% of people who get cancer have a thyroid gland which is out of balance. Using a MagneTech for one to two minutes daily direct will revitalise it. Do the same on the thymus, which matures your T-cells and say 20 minutes on your solar plexus where 70% of your immune system is located. Most importantly, use the MagneTech daily for 20 minutes directly on the problem area to heal it and any scar tissue.

You have got to take charge of your own health.

ENDOMETRIAL - lining of the UTERUS (WOMB) - CANCER

> Endometrial cancer is relatively common and also highly curable, particularly combined with complementary remedies.

SUMMARY
- **Symptoms**
- **Research**
- **Who is most likely to get Endometrial Cancer?**
- **The Uterus**
- **Types of cancer of the endometrium**
- **Diagnosis**
- **Treatment**
- **How to ensure a higher success rate and reduce the likelihood of the cancer returning**

SYMPTOMS
Abnormal bleeding after menopause, pain during sexual intercourse, difficult or painful urination, pain in the pelvis. May begin as watery blood streaked discharge.

RESEARCH
Almost 6000 new cases of endometrial cancer is diagnosed in the UK each year, with chance of survival after 5 years at over 70% before taking account of the BIG FOUR.

WHO IS MOST LIKELY TO GET ENDOMETRIAL CANCER?
- Those who are obese or have diabetes.
- Over 50.
- Those who use hormone replacement therapy.
- Those who take the drug tamoxifen.
- Those who began menstruation at a very young age or began the menopause late in life (over 52 years old).

THE UTERUS (WOMB)
The uterus is a hollow, pear shaped organ about 8 cm (3 inches) long before childbirth and larger after. It has thick muscular walls and is suspended by ligaments between the bladder and the rectum. The cervix, the lower part, protrudes into the vagina. The endometrial (the inner lining where a baby grows) is soft and velvety to the touch and contains many blood vessels and mucous glands. This lining undergoes considerable changes in the course of the menstrual cycle and much of it is cast off during menstruation. The two fallopian tubes emerge at the upper end of the uterus.

TYPES OF CANCER OF THE ENDOMETRIUM

Three quarters are several varieties of endometrial adenocarcinomas - ciliated adenocarcinomas, secretory adenocarcinoma, papillae or villoglandular, adenocarcinoma with squamous differentiation, adenocanthoma or adenosquamous. Other types include mixed (account for 10%), urine papillary serous (less than 10%). Clear cell carcinoma (about 4%) and mucous, squamous and undifferentiated (each account for 1% or less).

DIAGNOSIS

Your doctor will examine your pelvis, checking the uterus, vagina, ovaries, fallopian tubes, bladder and rectum. Routine laboratory tests, including blood test and urinalysis. A Pap test may also be done. A uterine biopsy (endometrial biopsy) can either be performed by your doctor by inserting a tube through the cervix into the uterus. Tissue samples are then taken from the uterine lining. The other way of doing a biopsy is where the uterus is scraped by a gynaecologist on an outpatient basis. Biopsy samples are then examined under a microscope.

Further tests may be carried out by transvaginal ultrasound.

If tests show you have cancer, further tests are needed to determine the extent of the cancer, such as X-rays, CT (computerised tomography) and MRI (magnetic resonance imaging).

TREATMENT

Surgical hysterectomy in cancer cases involves the removal of the uterus, fallopian tubes, ovaries, the upper third of the vagina and the lymph nodes in that region.

Sometimes hormone tablets are given in addition to surgery or if surgery is not feasible.

No ill effects arise as a result of the slight shortening of the vagina during surgery, as the structure of the vagina is very elastic and stretches easily. Sexual intercourse is best avoided for about six weeks after a hysterectomy operation.

How to ensure a high success rate and reduce the likelihood of the cancer returning

It is most important that you take care of the BIG FOUR - avoid Geopathic Stress, destroy any microbes, mainly micro parasites, take adequate Q10 and ensure a high acid alkaline balance in your blood.

Take the necessary vitamins, minerals etc. as modern food no longer provides enough to prevent you suffering from malnutrition. Take at least 20 mcg daily of Vitamin D which is vital.

Also get enough exercise. Ideally exercise daily on a rebounder to vitalise your lymph system and help dispose of toxins from your body. Two minutes on a rebounder will double the number of white blood cells for one hour.

About 90% of people who get cancer have a thyroid gland which is out of balance. Using a MagneTech for one to two minutes daily direct will revitalise it. Do the same on the thymus, which matures your T-cells and say 20 minutes on your solar plexus where 70% of your immune system is located. Most importantly, use the MagneTech daily for 20 minutes directly on the problem area to heal it and any scar tissue.

You have got to take charge of your own health.

CANCER OF THE CERVIX (CERVICAL)

Since the NHS set up the screening program 20 years ago, the cases of cervical cancer has halved. The smear (Pap) test enables the cancer to be detected early and is therefore highly curable. Vaccination in young women will hopefully also reduce future cervical cancer cases.

SUMMARY
- **Symptoms**
- **Research**
- **Type of cervix - cervical cancer**
- **Who is most likely to get cervix cancer?**
- **The cervix - cervical**
- **Vaccination to prevent cervix cancer**
- **Diagnosis**
- **What is human papilloma virus?**
- **Treatment**
- **How to ensure a higher success rate and reduce the likelihood of the cancer returning**

SYMPTOMS
There are usually no visible symptoms or signs in the early stages of cervical cancer. As the cancer grows, there may be unusual bleeding or discharge. You may have longer menstrual periods, a heavier flow, bleeding between periods or after intercourse or after menopause. The bleeding is usually bright red and unpredictable as to when it appears, its amount or its duration. Although these symptoms may not be cancer, they should be checked out by your GP.

RESEARCH
About 3,000 women get cancer of the cervix in the UK each year, with a five year survival rate of over 60%. The age varies when women usually get cervical cancer, with the peak for cancer *in situ* between 25 and 35 and invasive cancer between 45 and 50. However cervical cancer may occur at any age. About 25% occurs in women under the age of 35. Women as young as 20 have been known to have cervical cancer.
UASA trials are being carried out to see if folic acid can lower the risk of women infected with HPV (see later) which is implicated in 99% of cervical cancers.

TYPES OF CERVIX - CERVICAL CASES
There are two main types of cervical cancer. The most common kind resembles the squamous (scales) part of the cervix and is therefore called **squamous carcinoma.** Some tumours show a different appearance, the most common of these resemble a glandular lining and is called **adenocarcinoma.** These cells produced mucus. In most cases the type of cancer is not important, as the extent of the cancer and other features of its appearance

under the microscope, such as invasion into the blood or lymph vessels.

WHO IS MOST LIKELY TO GET CANCER OF THE CERVIX?
Women who:

have papilloma virus (HPV) infection in the genitals and began having sexual intercourse before 16 years of age.

have had many sexual partners.

have had sex with partner who has had many sexual partners.

smoke cigarettes.

have been infected with HIV.

THE CERVIX
The cervix connects the uterus (womb) with the vagina.

VACCINATION TO PREVENT CANCER OF THE CERVIX
Both Gardasil and cervarix vaccination works by mimicking the structure of the live HVP strain 16 and 18 and stimulates an immune reaction in the body which will enable it to fight the real infection at a later date. The vaccine does not contain live strains of HPV and tests so far show it cannot cause the disease. There is no significant date on how long the vaccination will be effective.

Girls 12 to 13 will now be offered the injection at school and 17 to 18 years old will receive the injection as a 'catch-up' before they leave school. For the vaccination to work, it has to be administered before the girl has been infected by HPV. As around 1 in 10 girls under the age of 16 already has the virus, it was thought best to vaccinate girls before they were likely to have had sexual activity. If your daughter wishes to have the jab and you don't, the final decision is legally yours for your daughter until she is 16 years old.

DIAGNOSIS
The main diagnosis is the liquid based cytology (Pap) smear test, which is simple, nearly painless and can be carried out by your GP, in a clinic or a hospital. Living cells are collected in and around the cervix, usually with a small cervical brush or a wooden spatula and stored in liquid and sent off to a laboratory for examination.

The percentage of misinterpretation has shown to be quite high. If no change is found, the test is called 'negative'. If the lab finds changes in the cells, the test results are called 'positive'. Half the time the changes are caused by minor infected tissues that are swollen, changes in your menstrual cycle or changes that are part of growing old. The other 50% are a sign of the human papilloma virus. So if you first test 'positive', you will be asked to have a second Pap smear test. It is obviously a very anxious wait before you have the second test results which can take up to five weeks, but bear in mind if it is bad news, modern treatment is very successful. Fortunately most second tests prove to be 'negative'. On the other hand, some Pap smear tests called 'normal' are not, but this seldom happens .
NHS offers screening for over 25 women, but the starting age for women in Scotland, Wales and Northern Ireland is 20.

Doctors advise that every woman should have a Pap smear test within a few years of starting sexual activity. If the results are 'normal', every three to five years until the age of seventy. After that probably every five years. Your own doctor may advise you otherwise.

A hand held device could slash the time it takes to diagnose cervix cancer to just a couple of minutes and reduce false alarms, this will hopefully be on the market within four years.

It has been developed by Sheffield University and manufactured by Zilico Limited. An APX pen-like probe is placed on the surface of the cervix and an electric current is generated, which is completely painless. The probe is linked to a computer programme that can recognise abnormal patterns of electrical flow caused by pre-cancerous cells. Cancerous cells tend to have much lower levels of impendence, which means they conduct electricity at a faster rate than healthy cervix cells. The device has already been tested on more than 500 women as part of a major European clinical trial. Let's hope the Zilico test equipment proves successful for the benefit of the millions of UK women who have the Pap smear test every year and for women all over the world.

WHAT IS HUMAN PAPILLOMA VIRUS

Human Papilloma virus often referred to by its' initials HPV including some 100 similar viruses that tend to cause warts, including the fairly common warts that grow on hands and feet. About 30 of the wart strains affect the cervix with about 12 of them known to cause cancer of the cervix. Almost all of the HPV of the cervix is passed through sexual interaction and can be spread through skin contact with any part of an infected person's genital area. So it is men who should be vaccinated!! A girl who began having sex before 18 is more likely to get HPV because her cervix is much less mature. Luckily most of the time women with HPV do not end up with cervical cancer, as 90% of infections are cleared by the immune system within two years.

TREATMENT

The size of the tumour and whether the cancer has spread will be the main factor in deciding what treatment is appropriate for you. It may also depend if you are of child bearing age.

Treatment may involve the following:

Radiotherapy - either external beam radiation and/or brachytherapy, where a pencil size tube is inserted into the vagina and uterus, whereby the radiation is concentrated on the area of the cancer.

Conization Also called **cone biopsy** where a cone shape piece of tissue is removed from the cervix by laser or **harmonic scalpel** using ultrasound vibrations to cut tissues and seal. The edges of the cervix may be sutured (stitched) together or sealed with electric current. Conization may lead to increased risk of miscarriage and possible infertility because the cervix may be weakened. The scar tissue may also interfere with labour resulting in childbirth by caesarean. Conization may be used to preserve the uterus and **avoid radiation.**

Loop diathermy or LLETZ (large loop extension of the transformation zone) Your cervix will be numbed; the loop is inserted into the vagina and the precancerous cells are removed and sent for further analysis. Your wound is treated with a medical paste that hastens healing. Your cervix is completely healed within two to three months.

This technique is less costly, can be done in a GP surgery, and has a shorter recovery time with fewer complications when done by a well trained physician.

Cryosurgery uses liquid nitrogen or carbon dioxide to destroy tissues by freezing.

Hysterectomy to remove by surgery just the cervix and uterus or also ovaries, part of the vagina along with lymph nodes in pelvic area. This may be followed by Radiotherapy and or Chemotherapy which will bring on the menopause. **Radical trachelectomy** just removing the cervix without removing the uterus.

How to ensure a high success rate and reduce the likelihood of the cancer returning

It is most important that you take care of the BIG FOUR - avoid Geopathic Stress, destroy any microbes, mainly micro parasites, take adequate Q10 and ensure a high acid alkaline balance in your blood.

Take the necessary vitamins, minerals etc. as modern food no longer provides enough to prevent you suffering from malnutrition. Take at least 20 mcg daily of Vitamin D which is vital.

Also get enough exercise. Ideally exercise daily on a rebounder to vitalise your lymph system and help dispose of toxins from your body. Two minutes on a rebounder will double the number of white blood cells for one hour.

About 90% of people who get cancer have a thyroid gland which is out of balance. Using a MagneTech for one to two minutes daily direct will revitalise it. Do the same on the thymus, which matures your T-cells and say 20 minutes on your solar plexus where 70% of your immune system is located. Most importantly, use the MagneTech daily for 20 minutes directly on the problem area to heal it and any scar tissue.

You have got to take charge of your own health.

VAGINAL CANCER

> This type of cancer is uncommon, highly treatable and curable,
> particularly if combined with complementary therapy.

SUMMARY

- **Symptoms**
- **Research**
- **Types of vaginal cancer**
- **Who is most likely to get vaginal cancer?**
- **The vagina**
- **Diagnosis**
- **Treatment**
- **How to ensure a higher success rate and reduce the likelihood of the cancer returning**

SYMPTOMS

Blood stained vaginal discharge, bleeding after sexual intercourse, blood in the urine and pain. Sometimes frequent passing of urine including during the night. Pain in the rectum.

RESEARCH

Fewer than 300 women are diagnosed in the UK per year.

WHO IS MOST LIKELY TO GET VAGINAL CANCER?

- squamous cell vaginal cancer is most often found in women between 60 and 80.
- adenocarcinoma vaginal cancer is most often found in women between 12 and 30. The female children of women who took a hormone drug **diethylstilboestrol (DES)** between 1940 and 1970 to prevent miscarriages, have an increased risk of developing clear cell adenocarcinoma **(CCA).**
- women who have had genital warts caused by the **human papilloma virus (HPV)** have a slight risk.
- a woman who has had radiotherapy to the pelvic area is at slight risk.

THE VAGINA

It is a muscular tube that extends from the opening of the womb (cervix) to the folds of skin (vulva) between a woman's legs. It is the birth canal through which babies are born. It also allows blood from periods (menstruation) to pass out of the body.

DIAGNOSIS

The specialist will carry out a full pelvic examination including the inside of your vagina to check for any lumps or swelling. Your groin and pelvic area will also be checked for any swollen glands. Your back passage (rectum) may also be checked.

A cervical smear test may also be taken to check for any abnormalities in the cells of the cervix.

A colposcopy, which is a pencil thin lighting instrument with a low powered microscope, may be used for a closer examination of the whole vagina. The vagina may be painted with a liquid that makes any abnormal areas show more clearly.

A biopsy will be carried out by taking a small tissue sample from any abnormal areas for examining under a microscope.

The above test may show cell changes in the vagina known as **vaginal intraepithelial neoplasia (VAIN),** sometimes called **carcinoma-in-situ. VAIN** is not cancer and the treatment is not the same as for cancer.

If the above test show that you have cancer, further tests may be necessary to find out whether any cancer cells have spread in the body either through the bloodstream or the lymphatic system. Such tests would involve a chest X-ray and blood test to see if the cancer has spread to your lungs.

CT (computerised tomography) scan and MRI (magnetic resonance imaging) scan may be used to see if the cancer has spread to other parts of the body.

TYPES OF VAGINAL CANCER

Primary vaginal cancer There are two main types of cancer that start in the vagina itself and are named after the cells from which they develop.

- **Squamous cell** which is the most common type of vaginal cancer and is usually found in the upper part of the vagina.
- **Adencarcinoma**

Other very rare types of vaginal cancer include melanoma, small cell carcinoma, sarcoma and lymphoma.

Secondary vaginal cancer is more common than primary vaginal cancer and usually comes from the neck of the womb (cervix), the lining of the womb (the endometrium) or from nearby organs such as the bladder.

TREATMENT

Treatment will depend on your age, general health, how advanced the cancer is and the type of cancer.

You may have one or a combination of radiotherapy, surgery and chemotherapy.

Radiotherapy may involve external radiation or internal radiation (see PART TWO for more details of these treatments and the affect they have on you).

Radiotherapy causes shortening and narrowing of the vagina. To prevent this, your doctor or nurse will advise you to have a **dilator** (a plastic or glass tube) inserted into the vagina to keep it open. The **dilator** should be used daily during and some time after treatment.

How to ensure a high success rate and reduce the likelihood of the cancer returning

It is most important that you take care of the BIG FOUR - avoid Geopathic Stress, destroy any microbes, mainly micro parasites, take adequate Q10 and ensure a high acid alkaline balance in your blood.

Take the necessary vitamins, minerals etc. as modern food no longer provides enough to prevent you suffering from malnutrition. Take at least 20 mcg daily of Vitamin D which is vital.

Also get enough exercise. Ideally exercise daily on a rebounder to vitalise your lymph system and help dispose of toxins from your body. Two minutes on a rebounder will double the number of white blood cells for one hour.

About 90% of people who get cancer have a thyroid gland which is out of balance. Using a MagneTech for one to two minutes daily direct will revitalise it. Do the same on the thymus, which matures your T-cells and say 20 minutes on your solar plexus where 70% of your immune system is located. Most importantly, use the MagneTech daily for 20 minutes directly on the problem area to heal it and any scar tissue.

You have got to take charge of your own health.

CANCER OF THE VULVA

> This cancer is rare and when detected early is very curable.

- **Summary**
- **Symptoms**
- **Who is most likely to get cancer of the vulva?**
- **The Vulva**
- **Diagnosis**
- **Ovarian Cancer**
- **Treatment**
- **Is sexual intercourse possible after Vulvectomy?**
- **How to ensure a higher success rate and reduce the likelihood of the cancer returning**

SYMPTOMS
Itching, burning, bleeding, pain and a lump or growth on the vulva.

WHO IS MOST LIKELY TO GET CANCER OF THE VULVA?
- 75% of women who get vulva cancer are over 50.
- Almost all cancer of the vulva develops slowly over the years from carcinoma **in situ** found in women from 30-35 years old.
- It is thought that the **human papilloma virus (HPV)** is responsible for 50% of vulva cancer.
- Cigarette smoking and HIV infection.

THE VULVA
The Vulva is the outer part of the vagina and looks much like a pair of lips. It is made up of several structures including the clitoris, labia, hymen, vaginal opening and bladder opening (urethra).

DIAGNOSIS
Punch biopsy is normally carried out to determine cancer. Other tests may be carried out such as a cystoscopy, a pencil thin lighting instrument with a low powered microscope, which is inserted into the urethra.

CANCER OF THE VULVA
Stage O or **in situ**: found only in the vulva or surface of the skin.

Stage I: found only in the vulva and/or in the perineum (space between the opening of the rectum and vagina). Two centimetres (one inch) or less in size.

Stage II: as stage I, but more than two centimetres (one inch).

Stage III: as stage II and spread to lower part of urethra, vagina, anus and/or has spread to nearby lymph nodes.

Stage IV: spread beyond the urethra, vagina and anus into the lining of the bladder and bowel or pelvic bones, or spread to the lymph nodes in the pelvis or other parts of the body.

TREATMENT

Surgery and/or laser are the most common treatment. Also radiation, if surgery cannot be tolerated. Surgery procedure can involve:

Skinning vulvectomy, which removes only the skin of the vulva that contains the cancer.
Partial vulvectomy, which takes out less than the entire vulva.
Simple vulvectomy, which takes out the entire vulva, but no lymph nodes.
Radical vulvectomy, which removes the entire vulva and the lymph nodes around it.
Pelvic exenteration, which removes the lower colon, rectum or bladder as well as the cervix and vagina.

Following surgery reconstruction with plastic surgery and a skin graft may be done to create an artificial vulva or vagina.

After a radical vulvectomy, because the large number of lymph nodes have been removed, fluid collects under the skin and may cause a problem until other lymph channels have been established. It is therefore important to start deep breathing, coughing and leg exercises immediately after surgery. Frequent irrigation with a sterile saline solution, heat lamp treatment and sitz baths (only buttocks and hips immersed in water) will promote healing.

IS SEXUAL INTERCOURSE POSSIBLE AFTER VULVECTOMY?

Intercourse is still possible though you may have to change position or technique. Removal of the vulva may cause the remaining vagina tissues to tighten, making intercourse and physical examination more difficult. Intercourse and/or stretching of the vagina right after the operation are important to make sure that the tissues will remain supple and elastic.

How to ensure a high success rate and reduce the likelihood of the cancer returning

It is most important that you take care of the BIG FOUR - avoid Geopathic Stress, destroy any microbes, mainly micro parasites, take adequate Q10 and ensure a high acid alkaline balance in your blood.
Take the necessary vitamins, minerals etc. as modern food no longer provides enough to prevent you suffering from malnutrition. Take at least 20 mcg daily of Vitamin D which is vital. Also get enough exercise. Ideally exercise daily on a rebounder to vitalise your lymph system and help dispose of toxins from your body. Two minutes on a rebounder will double the number of white blood cells for one hour.
About 90% of people who get cancer have a thyroid gland which is out of balance. Using a MagneTech for one to two minutes daily direct will revitalise it. Do the same on the thymus, which matures your T-cells and say 20 minutes on your solar plexus where 70% of your immune system is located. Most importantly, use the MagneTech daily for 20 minutes directly on the problem area to heal it and any scar tissue.

You have got to take charge of your own health.

MALE CANCERS

As mentioned before more men die of cancer than women, generally they are more reluctant to visit a GP, so any cancer is diagnosed at a later stage, making successful treatment less likely. Men on average are also less likely to believe in complementary remedies, which may have prevented the cancer in the first place.

MALE CANCERS

- **Prostate cancer - the most common in men**
- **Penile cancer - very rare**
- **Testicular cancer - young men's cancer**

PROSTATE CANCER

Prostate Cancer is the most common cancer in men (20%). Most cases are 'pussy cat' which means the cancer is slow growing. In these cases mild or no orthodox treatment is best and you will die <u>with</u> prostate cancer not <u>of</u> it, especially if you make some simple changes to your life style.

In 'tiger' cases, even if the cancer is growing quickly, you must take time to discuss the most suitable treatment for you. Unlike most other types of cancer you may have the choice of up to 20 different types of orthodox treatment. Some treatments can make you incontinent and/or impotent. As in all cases of cancer you must take charge of your own health and do vital things before, during and after any orthodox treatment (which your doctor may not tell you about), to ensure success.

Symptoms

Urinal difficulties such as in starting and stopping, narrow stream, burning, painful and frequent. Urgent feeling especially at night. Sometimes blood in urine. Tenderness over the bladder. Dull ache in the pelvis and back. Nearly all these symptoms are similar to simple prostate enlargement, which most men in the West over 50 have, mainly due to our diet.

Research

Prostate cancer is the second most common cancer in men in the Western world. Over 30,000 cases are diagnosed each year in the UK and it now kills about 10,000 men a year, - about one man each hour - but 82% survive for more than 5 years.

One in six men will develop prostate cancer by the age of 60, but more young men are being diagnosed in their 50s, 40s and even late 30s. Men of Afro-Caribbean origin are especially at risk.

Localised disease, where the cancer is confined within the prostate, is generally curable and a much wider choice of treatment is available.

Poor diet, including lack of essential vitamins, minerals and trace elements, particularly Q10 and Selenium have been blamed for the increase in prostate cancer. But Geopathic Stress - which has been associated with over 95% of cancer cases - has, as mentioned before, increased many times over the last few years. So do something NOW to prevent prostate cancer.

Dairy Products Prostate cancer can affect one in three men during their lifetime, but in China it is as low as one in 200,000. Why is there such a difference? The Chinese do not eat dairy products.

As soon as men from China move to western countries and adapt western diets with a very high dairy product content, they soon get prostate cancer in the same proportion as local people. The average USA diet contains over 40% of dairy products.

One of the problems is the growth factor and hormones in dairy animals, which have been added to the animal feed to increase milk production and which have increased by over 300% during the last few years. Research has shown these additions promote growth in breast and prostate tumours. See chapter on Dairy Products.

The Prostate

The prostate is a sex gland found only in males. It is walnut sized and lies at the base of the bladder surrounding the tube called the urethra, which carries urine and semen to the end of the penis. During sexual intercourse, at orgasm, the prostate responds to muscular contractions to bring together the component elements of semen (sperm, lubrication and nutrients) and cause them to pass down the urethra. A healthy prostate is essential to full sexual functions. As men age, the gland becomes enlarged and can thus squeeze the urethra, giving a reduced urine flow. This can lead to problems and diseases including cancer.

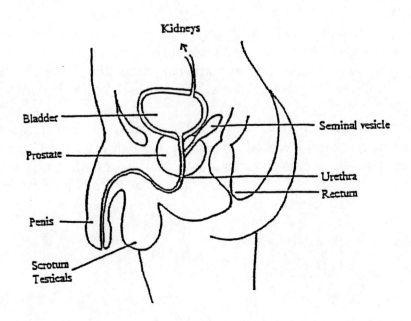

Checking for Prostate Cancer
Rectal Examination

This is often the simplest and first examination for prostate cancer. Your doctor inserts a gloved finger into your rectum to feel your prostate. The difference can readily be felt between a simple enlargement and a diseased prostate gland, which will feel hard and knobbly. This examination is painless.

PSA (Prostate Specific Antigen) test

PSA is produced by the normal prostate and secreted into the seminal fluid in large quantities. Prostate cancer changes the cellular barriers that normally keep PSA within the ducting system of the prostate and causes it to be released into the bloodstream. A blood test will measure the amount of PSA in the blood. The results are calculated in mg/ml (milligrams per millilitres) - a very tiny amount.

'Normal' PSA depends on your age as follows:

40-49 yrs	= 2.5 mg/ml
50-59 yrs	= 3.5 mg/ml
60-69 yrs	= 4.5 mg/ml
70-79 yrs	= 6.6.mg/ml

A high reading would be up to and over 10 but can be as high as 100 and above.

The problem with the PSA test is that it not only misses up to a third of all prostate cancer cases, but also produces a large number of 'false positives' with up to three out of four tests turning out to be negative.

The PSA reading can also be high due to an inflamed prostate (prostatitis), enlarged prostate, benign prostate disease or a high intake of dairy products. Taking exercise or sexual intercourse before a PSA test can also give a high reading.

When I had a routine PSA test some years ago, it registered 20. As I had recently had an AMAS test which had not detected any cancer, I decided not to have further tests immediately. When I had a further PSA test six months later, it registered 5. I asked the consultant why it had been so high initially and he said that I probably had an infection at the time. The USA AMAS test is not available in the UK at the moment.

Ideally after cancer treatment the elevated PSA number drops (eg from say 25 to 0.4) indicating that the cancer has been eliminated. If a retest is carried out some time later and the numbers are again elevated, this may indicate the cancer has reoccurred in the prostate and may have spread to the lymph nodes or bones, which are the most common areas of mestastasis in prostate cancer.

Ultrasound (TRUS)

A trans-rectal ultrasound is sometimes carried out to inspect the prostate.

Biopsy

Following any abnormality indicated by the above tests, a biopsy of the prostate is usually recommended. This is done at your hospital as an outpatient. The test itself normally takes no longer than about ten minutes. As this test can be a little uncomfortable, a local anaesthetic is given. An ultrasound probe is inserted through the back passage in order to provide a 'map' of the prostate. The doctor will then pass a fine needle through the prostate from the rectum to extract from 6 to 12 samples of tissue. These are sent for examination to a pathologist, who will then determine whether any cancerous tissue is present, and if so, a Gleason Score will be awarded. There may be some blood in the urine and/or the back passage for a few days or more rarely up to three weeks after a biopsy and blood in the semen for 4-6 weeks.

Personally, I did not find the biopsy I had prior to my operation on my enlarged prostate too unpleasant and I had none of the after effects described above.

Recent research suggests that it is possible that prostate biopsies may underestimate the extent of the disease, due to sampling error.

Cystoscopy

This is a short test lasting no more than five minutes in which the doctor passes a thin flexible tube through the urethra to examine it and the bladder. Local anaesthetic is sometimes applied. There can be a little bleeding for a short while afterwards.

In order to ascertain whether the cancer has spread beyond the prostate, imaging tests are often recommended. These are:

Nuclear Bone Scan

This test is to show whether the disease has spread to the bones. A small amount of low dose radio-active material is injected into the arm about three hours before the scan. The scan takes about 45 minutes. Images of any bones showing the disease will show up on the scan. A bone scan will not usually be carried out unless the PSA score is greater than 10 and the Gleason score is high. It is painless and quite harmless.

CT Scan (Computerised Tomography)

This test uses a rotating x-ray beam to scan the body from several angles. The test is primarily used to check whether the lymph nodes are enlarged, which is often an indication that the disease has spread to them. Again, this test is usually done where there is a possibility that the disease has spread to other organs.

MRI Scan (Magnetic Resonance Imaging)

This scan creates a cross-section of a selected part of the body by using magnetic fields. The test is a further check to see whether there is any spread outside the prostate. The scanning machine locates your body in a tunnel. Some may find this a little claustrophobic, but the head usually remains clear of the tunnel. The machine can seem rather noisy and you are asked to keep as still as possible during the process. It is possible to speak to the radiographer through a microphone/headphone system. The procedure is quite harmless.

Bone Density Test

A bone mineral density test (BMD) is an X-ray scan that measures bone mass and helps to determine calcium levels, bone strength and brittle bone disease which could increase the risk of fractures.

The Gleason Score

This is the system used for grading the aggressiveness of prostate cancer cells. A 'Gleason' score rating is given as a result of examining cancerous tissue under a microscope by a pathologist. It is most often obtained from a needle biopsy. The grades of the two most common patterns are added together to give a score from 2 to 10.

> Scores of 2-4 are considered the least aggressive
> Scores of 5-7 are considered as moderately aggressive
> Scores of 8-10 are considered as the most aggressive

TNM (tumour/nodes/metastasis[1] - staging of Prostate Cancer.
Presently the most favoured system of clinically staging prostate cancer is the TNM system.
T stage of the disease refers to the form of the primary tumour within the prostate. This rating is perhaps the most relevant.

T1 = Small cancerous tumour found inside the prostate.
T2 = When your physician can feel the tumour in one or both the lobes of the prostate during physical examination with a finger (DRE - digital rectal examination).
T3 = When the disease has extended through the prostalic capsule to the surrounding tissue on one or both sides of the prostate. It may also have extended into one or both seminal vesicles.
T4 = When the tumour has escaped from the prostate and has invaded one or more of the following: the bladder neck, the external sphincter (which helps to control urination) and the rectum. The tumour may also have invaded the levator muscle and/or may be fixed to the pelvic wall.
N stage disease is rated from 0 to 3 depending on the size of the cancer found in the pelvic lymph nodes. N1 being up to 2cm, to N3 being greater than 5cm.
M stage disease is rated 0, M2a, M2b, M2c, depending on whether the disease has spread beyond the lymph nodes to the bones or other sites.

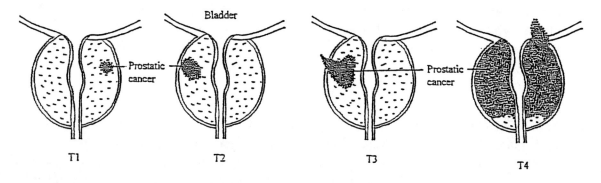

[1] Metastasis is the spread of the cancer to other organs

Pre-treatment Discussion

You are no doubt in shock when you have been diagnosed with prostate cancer, so read 'Questions to ask your consultant about your treatment' Part Two to get the full benefit from your consultation. I recommend you take a good friend with you who can take notes.

You may only recall 10% if you are under severe stress. Your friend may also get a different view of what was said.

In addition to the questions listed in the above mentioned chapter, the following questions relate to prostate cancer:

1. What are my readings on the PSA test and Gleason Score?
2. As far as you know, is the cancer confined to my prostate?
3. Will the treatment recommended make me incontinent and/or impotent? Will I be able to have intercourse?

Making the right choice of treatment
Watchful waiting

This is if your cancer is the 'pussy cat' type, either for older men where the disease may grow so slowly that it may not affect the person's quality of life, or for those whose health may not allow them to undergo radiotherapy or surgery. It will involve continuously monitoring once or twice a year with PSA and DRE tests. More active treatment such as hormone therapy can be considered if the levels of the tests go up. Strong magnetic therapy on a continuous basis at home, has shown good results. Again it is vital to change your lifestyle as described later so you can live out your natural span.

Watchful waiting is sometimes used to describe 'active surveillance' and this can cause confusion. Please ask your doctor or consultant whether it involves regular DRE examination or other tests or whether it involves a more pro-active approach with more frequent checks and repeat biopsies. 60-80% of men on 'active surveillance' will never need treatment for their prostate cancer.

Treatment options
Surgery

The operation, suitable for organ-confined prostate cancer, is called a **radical prostatectomy**. It removes the whole prostate and the seminal vesicles that help to produce semen. It is a major operation and only carried out on men able and fit enough to cope with the recovery. The operation is carried out through a large incision in the abdomen or through the perineum (the area between the anus and the scrotum). The operation takes 2-3 hours performed under general anaesthetic and entails significant blood loss. It requires 5-7 days in hospital and at least 6 weeks off work. An option is **laparoscopic** or keyhole surgery with less trauma, less blood loss, less post-operational pain and quicker recovery. This complex operation, however, is only undertaken by very few surgeons, who should have proven experience in the technique. Further information from Mr Christopher G. Eden MS. FRCS (Urol), The Hampshire Clinic, Basing Road, Old Basing, Basingstoke, RG24 7AL Telephone 01256 329877. Even newer is **robotic surgery**. The robot allows the surgeon to see all the tissues magnified ten times in '3D' and the robot arms have such remarkable dexterity and precision that the chances of damaging surrounding structures is minimised. This technique is at present only available in a few hospitals. Further information from St. Mary's Hospital, Paddington or Robotic Urological Surgery Ltd. Tel: 08700 796796.

Some incontinence and impotence are the main likely side-effects of surgery.

The advantage of surgery is the cancer may well be completely eradicated and you will know exactly how far the cancer has developed. It will also eradicate any BPH (Benign Prostate Hyperplasia) the age related benign swelling of the prostate.

External Beam Radiotherapy

This common option uses radiation to destroy the cancer cells. It usually involves sessions of 10 or 15 minutes a day for five days a week for several weeks. As with surgery, there are side-effects such as bladder or rectal irritation, tiredness and nausea.

The newer Radiation Therapy (IMRT) is far more precise in which the beam is shaped and directed at the body typically from five different angles. Very good results have been reported on this new technique.

Brachytherapy

This is a newer form of radiotherapy in which radio-active seeds are implanted into the prostate through the perineum (the area between the scrotum and the anus). It involves an overnight stay, and is carried out under general anaesthetic. Only one or two treatments, at short intervals, are required. The incidence of incontinence and impotence problems is less than for surgery or radiotherapy, but there are other possible side-effects such as urinary retention (5-10%), urinary frequency and urgency and possible rectal problems.

Cryosurgery

Cryosurgery, or Targeted Cryo-ablation of the Prostate (TCAP) involves inserting, under ultrasound guidance, a number of probes into the prostate gland. A gas (e.g. Argo) is passed down these probes under pressure and, at the tips, it is allowed to expand and flow back out other channels of the probes.

This rapid expansion of the gas at the tips causes a significant cooling, known as the Joule-Thompson effect. An ice ball is formed which destroys the tissues and tumour in close proximity at the tips and suitable positioning of these probes, the whole tumour. The process often also involves the use of a second gas (e.g. helium) to actively thaw the area. Several freeze/thaw cycles may be used. Additional probes are used to measure the temperature to ensure adequate control.

Cryosurgery is often suitable for those with localised tumours where the cancer is contained within the prostate and when radiotherapy has failed, but the cancer is still in the prostate. This operation is not suitable for cases of an over-enlarged prostate.

Trans-rectal ultrasound is used for insertion and guidance of the five to eight needles. This is done under general or spinal anaesthetic and lasts about 1-2 hours. You will normally be in hospital for 2-3 days after treatment and have a catheter in place for a couple of weeks.

It is a relatively non-invasive technique with minimal blood loss. There is a short recovery time and the operation can be repeated if not totally successful. It is only available at a few centres in the UK. For further information contact Mr John Davis (Consultant Urological Surgeon), Royal Surrey County Hospital, Egerton Road, Guildford, GU1 3TB, Tel: 01483 51122 x 4878, private patients 01484 567517.

Photo Dynamic Laser Therapy (PDT) (see page 45)

High Intensity Focused Ultrasound (HIFU)

This treatment involves a probe, which emits an ultrasound beam and is placed in the back passage. The focused beam raises the temperature to destroy the cells in the targeted area without damaging the surrounding tissues. The process is repeated until the area of cancerous cells has been destroyed.

HIFU is non-invasive and aims to retain a good quality of life. It is suitable for locally confined prostate cancer T1 or T2. The technique is relatively new, but has been performed on over 6,000 patients in France, Germany and the USA.

It may have less post-treatment side effects of incontinence and impotence than conventional methods. Repeated treatments are possible if the cancer recurs. As the prostate swells immediately after treatment and there may be temporary post-treatment urinary retention or urgency, a catheter is needed for a couple of weeks.

Normal activity can be resumed within a few days.

For further information contact Mr Mark Emberton, University College Hospital, Institute of Urology, 48 Riding House, London, W1N 7EY or Mr Simon Brewster, Churchill Hospital, Old Road, Headington, Oxford, OX3 7LI.

A Photo Dynamic Laser Therapy (PDT) involves injecting a light sensitive drug and later a laser which destroys the cancer tumours in less than one hour. It requires only a short stay in hospital and will save surgery, radiotherapy and chemotherapy (see page 45).

Hormone Treatment

It seems that, in order to grow, most prostate cancers need the male hormones (androgens), the most common of which is testosterone. By inhibiting the generation of testosterone, the cancer will be starved and shrink. This treatment is often used when the cancer has spread beyond the prostate or has recurred after treatment. It is also used in combination with radiotherapy to shrink the tumour so that the radiotherapy is more effective. Hormone treatment alone does not cure the cancer, but it can shrink and control it for several years before the cancer becomes 'androgen independent'.

Orchidectomy This is the surgical removal of the testicles, which thereby substantially stops the generation of testosterone. This is effective, the least toxic and least expensive procedure, but understandably is not favoured by most men and especially young ones.

LH-RH (Luteinising hormone-releasing hormone) analogues. These drugs can decrease the amount of testosterone produced by the testicles as effectively as surgical removal. These drugs are administered by the injection of a slowly dissolving pellet either monthly, quarterly or once a year. When first administered, these drugs cause an initial surge of testosterone, which is counteracted by a short course of anti-androgen tablets shortly before and after the first injection. Unfortunately you will be impotent and lose your sex drive; the effects are reversible if you stop taking the drugs. Side-effects can include hot flushes, which can be reduced by taking a short course of an anti-androgen drug.

Anti-androgens These drugs do not stop the production of testosterone, but block the effects of both testicular and adrenal androgens. They are usually taken in tablet form, which makes it far less drastic than the removal of the testicles and LH-RH with less side-effects. They can however cause stomach upsets, swelling and increased sensitivity of the breasts.

Anti-androgens can be used as a stand-alone therapy referred to as 'anti-androgen monotherapy' or can be used in combination with LH-RH analogues referred to as 'maximum (or total) androgen blockage'.

Other hormone drugs If the 'first line' hormone drugs lose their effectiveness, there are others which have been shown to be effective although only for a limited period of time. These include oestrogen, a female hormone which suppresses the effect of testosterone. These 'second line' hormone drugs are often used in conjunction with the 'first line' hormone drugs.

Intermittent hormonal therapy In this process hormone treatment is given for a limited period. This is followed by a period when no treatment is given, but the PSA is monitored and if there are signs that the disease is recurring, the treatment is repeated. Side-effects are reduced and hopefully it will extend the time period for which this treatment is effective.

Chemotherapy Unfortunately a high percentage of men with adrenal prostate cancer will eventually develop hormone-refractory prostate cancer that does not respond to hormone drug therapy.

However doctors are now advocating new types of chemotherapy. Taxotiven combined with Prednisolone has shown for men with hormone-refractory, metastatic prostate cancer, a 24% reduced risk of death. It also shows an improved patient response to PSA results by 43% and improved pain response by 59% related to the earlier drug 'Mitoxa-trone'.

Unfortunately, chemotherapy can also destroy up to 30% of your immune system, so you must ensure you have a good nutritious diet. If you do not feel hungry, take food in a liquid form. Your supplements should include vitamins C, D and E, selenium and zinc, garlic capsules with high allicin content and multivitamins or seaweed, which contains most vitamins, mineral trace elements etc. in a natural form.

All Under One Roof

Guy's Hospital in London is the first to offer several different types of treatment for prostate cancer under one roof. Currently the unit has two Consultant Urologists, two Radiation Oncologists, two Prostate Specialist Nurses and two Junior Doctors. The treatment includes:
three types of surgery - open, keyhole and robotic keyhole. HIFU (high intensity focused ultrasound) and Brachytherapy.

How to ensure a high success rate and reduce the likelihood of the cancer returning

It is most important that you take care of the BIG FOUR - no Geopathic Stress, destroy any microbes, mainly micro parasites, take adequate Q10 and ensure a high acid alkaline balance in your blood.
Take the necessary Vitamins, minerals etc. modern food no longer provides to prevent you suffering from malnutrition. Also take at least 20 mcg daily of the vital Vitamin D.
Also take regular exercise. Ideally exercise daily on a rebounder to vitalise your lymph

system and help dispose of toxins from your body. Two minutes on a rebounder will double your white blood cells for one hour.

About 90% of people who get cancer have a thyroid which is out of balance. Using a MagneTech for one to two minutes direct daily will revitalise it. Do the same on the thymus, which matures your T-cells and say 20 minutes on your solar plexus where 70% of your immune system is located. Most importantly, use the MagneTech daily for 20 minutes direct on the prostate to heal it and any scar tissues.

You have got to take charge of your own health.

PENILE CANCER

This is a very rare cancer and highly curable when diagnosed early.

SUMMARY

- **Symptoms**
- **Who is most likely to get cancer of the penis?**
- **Treatment**
- **How to ensure a higher success rate and reduce the likelihood of the cancer returning**

Symptoms
A pimple or sore on the penis, a small nodule, white thickened patches, a raised velvety patch, wart or ulcer, especially one that is painless. Bleeding associated with erection or intercourse, persistent, abnormal erection without sexual desire, foul smelling discharge or a lump in the groin.

Who is most likely to get cancer of the penis?
It is almost exclusively found in uncircumcised males between the ages of 50 and 70.
Some cancers from the prostate, lung, pancreas, bladder, kidneys, testicles or urethra can spread to the penis.
Males who have the human papilloma virus (HPV).
Cigarette smokers.

Treatment
Almost 90% of cancers of the penis are found in the early stage and the tumour removed by microsurgery or laser surgery and sometimes also the removal of the foreskin. In more widespread cancer of the penis, part or the entire penis is removed. If the cancer has spread to the groin, some lymph nodes may be removed and radiotherapy and chemotherapy are sometimes used.

How to ensure a high success rate and reduce the likelihood of the cancer returning

It is most important that you take care of the BIG FOUR - no Geopathic Stress, destroy any microbes, mainly micro parasites, take adequate Q10 and ensure a high acid alkaline balance in your blood.

Take the necessary Vitamins, minerals etc. modern food no longer provides to prevent you suffering from malnutrition. Take at least 20 mcg daily of the vital Vitamin D.

Also take enough exercise. Ideally exercise daily on a rebounder to vitalise your lymph system and help dispose of toxins from your body. Two minutes on a rebounder will double your white blood cells for one hour.

About 90% of people who get cancer have a thyroid which is out of balance. Using a MagneTech for one to two minutes direct daily will revitalise it. Do the same on the thymus, which matures your T-cells and say 20 minutes on your solar plexus where 70% of your immune system is located. Most importantly, use the MagneTech daily for 20 minutes directly on the penis to heal it and any scar tissues.

You have got to take charge of your own health.

TESTICULAR CANCER

> **Any lump, swelling or other changes round the testicles can be checked on a regular basis by you. If testicular cancer is detected early, the success rate if over 95%.**

SUMMARY

1. **Symptoms**
2. **Research**
3. **Who is most likely to get Testicular Cancer?**
4. **Your Testicles**
5. **TSE – Testicle Self Examination**
6. **Diagnosis**
7. **Treatment**
8. **What are the implications of having a testicle removed?**
9. **How to ensure higher success rate**
10. **Preventing Testicular Cancer in the first place**
11. **Case Histories**

Symptoms

A lump found in testicles. Swelling or other changes round the testicles, or sudden collection of dull aches in the lower abdomen, groin and lower back. Tenderness or enlargement of breasts. Pain in testicles is seldom present in cancer cases.

Research

Approximately 2,000 cases of testicular cancer are diagnosed in the UK each year. This is a 100% increase over the last 20 years and is continuously on the increase. Scandinavians and Irish men have the highest incidence. In Denmark it accounts for over 6% of all cancers. It is not so common among black and Asian men. The cure rate is 95% if the cancer has not left the testes and better than 70% even if it has.

Who is most likely to get Testicular Cancer?

The peak age is 20 to 40 then it declines until age 60 when there is a slight increase. Boys as young as 15 can get it. Men with undescended or partially descended testicles are at greater risk. You are unlikely to get testicular cancer unless you are sleeping in a Geopathically Stressed place. This is why there are claims that testicular cancer is inherited, as the father slept in the same Geopathically Stressed home.

Your Testicles

The two testicles are egg-shaped glands situated in the scrotum behind and below your penis. Sperm develops in the walls of the seminiferous tubules. When the sperms are more mature they pass to the epididymis for further maturing, before passing up the vas deferens tube under pressure from more sperms below, until they reach the seminal vesicle in the prostate gland for storage. During each ejaculation millions of sperms pass out through the penis.

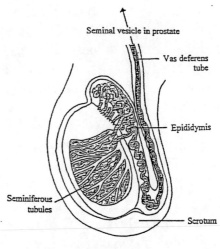

TESTICLE

TSE – Testicle Self Examination

It is easy to carry out testing on yourself once a month, after a warm bath or shower, as the testicles need to warm up. While standing, you should gently roll one testicle between your thumb and fingers checking for lumps (often painless, the size of a pea), swelling or other changes. Test the other testicle the same way. Both testicles should feel smooth except for the epididymis, the bumpy sperm tube along the top and back. Unfortunately testicles can sometimes be quite lumpy, so a good indication can be a hard lump combined with surrounding areas feeling unusual.

Very often it can be benign cysts, which must still be checked. Men are inclined to say they are too embarrassed or too busy to visit their doctor. If something bothers you go and see your doctor. The sooner cancer is detected the less treatment is necessary.

Diagnosis

Unfortunately your doctor may not find any lumps only by physical examination as your testicles may be cold, so insist on an ultrasound to evaluate any tumour. After ruling out infection and other diseases which can mimic testicular cancer, urine tests can be used to show irregular testosterone levels which can be symptomatic. An X-ray can also be carried out. If a simple biopsy is suggested ask for a second opinion. A biopsy involves cutting through the outer layers of the scrotum, which may cause the disease to spread locally.

If testicular cancer is detected a CT scan of the chest, abdomen and pelvis is usually done to determine if the cancer has spread.

Types of Testicular Cancer

There are two main types: Seminoma Cancer which is slow growing and Terationas Cancer which is fast growing.

Treatment

Most surgeons will suggest removing the testicle completely but it is possible to have only the lump removed, which can be performed under local anaesthetic. If after testing the lump turns out to be cancerous, the whole testicle will then be removed. During surgery to remove the one testicle, a biopsy will be taken of the other testicle to make sure it is free of cancer (it is very seldom that cancer is found in both testicles).

After surgery you have three options. Two oncological treatments – radiotherapy or chemotherapy, which most likely will make you sterile or be ineffective. Most surgeons believe there is a 25% risk that the cancer could return if you do not have oncological treatment but a few basic changes to your lifestyle will make the chance of cancer returning minimal – however, most doctors will not tell you that. Instead you get the sometimes horrible side-effects from oncological treatment plus the problem of building up your immune system again.

Tests will be carried out at regular intervals to ensure the cancer has not returned which may include a blood test.

What are the implications of having a testicle removed?

A man with only one testicle can still have a normal erection and produce sperm. A gel-filled implant, which has the weight, shape and texture of a normal testicle can be inserted surgically to restore normal appearance. If part of the scrotum skin must be removed during surgery, it may be difficult to restore the scrotum. Most men don't bother to have an implant.

How to ensure a high success rate and reduce the likelihood of the cancer returning

It is most important that you take care of the BIG FOUR - no Geopathic Stress, destroy any microbes, mainly micro parasites, take adequate Q10 and ensure a high acid alkaline balance in your blood.

Take the necessary Vitamins, minerals etc. modern food no longer provides to prevent you suffering from malnutrition. Take at least 20 mcg daily of the vital Vitamin D.

Also take enough exercise. Ideally exercise daily on a rebounder to vitalise your lymph system and help dispose of toxins from your body. Two minutes on a rebounder will double your white blood cells for one hour.

About 90% of people who get cancer have a thyroid which is out of balance. Using a MagneTech for one to two minutes direct daily will revitalise it. Do the same on the thymus, which matures your T-cells and say 20 minutes on your solar plexus where 70% of your immune system is located. Most importantly, use the MagneTech daily for 20 minutes direct on the testes to heal it and any scar tissues.

You have got to take charge of your own health.

Case Histories

Tom N (Bournemouth) had testicular cancer over 15 years ago. He had the cancerous testicle removed, but he had to fight a very hard battle with the consultant who insisted on him having chemotherapy.

Tom's bed was found to be very Geopathic Stressed, so he moved it into a safe place. Tom took Shark Cartilage, Pau D'Arco and plenty of mineral and vitamin supplements. Two months afterwards, Tom's blood showed he had no more cancer and he is still free of cancer today and would not dream of sleeping in a Geopathic Stress place again.

As described in my book 'Are You Sleeping In A Safe Place?' our son Mads was diagnosed with Teratomas Cancer while sleeping in Geopathic Stress accommodation while at Leeds University in January 1984. During his chemotherapy treatment, he unwittingly moved into a Geopathic Stress free place and the cancer drastically reduced. Unfortunately he moved again into a very Geopathically Stress cottage and the chemotherapy no longer worked. His cancer spread and Mads died in February 1985. At the time I knew nothing about Geopathic Stress.

CHILDREN'S' CANCER

Being told your child has cancer is devastating. It is one of the greatest challenges any parent has to face, coupled with intense emotions and fear. The survival rate in children diagnosed with cancer has gone up from 30% to 80% over the last thirty years due to better treatment and drugs. The side effects are far less, resulting in a better quality of life through childhood as well as into adulthood with fewer long term ill effects. The chance of children getting cancer in the first place is far less if parents ensure their children sleep in a place free from Geopathic Stress, which has been found present in every case of children diagnosed with cancer.

SUMMARY

TYPES OF CHILDHOOD CANCERS

Approximate % of total cancer cases diagnosed

		Page
Brain Tumours	25%	4
Germ Cell Tumours	3%	5
Langerhans Cell Histiocytosis (LCH)	6%	6
Leukaemia		
Acute Lymphoblastic Leukaemia (ALL)	22%	7
Acute Myeloid Leukaemia (AML)	7%	7
Liver Tumours	1%	10
Neuroblastoma	7%	11
Lymphoma		13
Hodgkin's Disease	4%	
Non-Hodgkin's Lymphoma (NHL)	6%	
Rare Tumours	3%	14
Retinoblastoma	3%	15
Sarcoma	8%	17
Osteosarcoma		
Ewing's sarcoma		
Soft Tissue sarcoma		
Wilms Tumour	5%	18
	100%	

General Information on Childhood Cancer

Over 1,500 children are diagnosed with cancer each year in the UK [1].

Childhood cancer is mainly diagnosed and treated in specialist departments in hospitals or specialist hospitals like Great Ormond Street Hospital in London, as some childhood cancers are difficult to diagnose and treat due to rarity of some childhood cancers.

Childhood cancer is often difficult to detect early as it develops so quickly, compared with adult cancer.

If the initial treatment for childhood cancer does not succeed and further treatment such as total body eradication - as used in bone marrow/stem cell transplantation - has to be given, studies have found the rate of new solid cancer is 8.3 times [1] higher than expected among those who survived ten or more years. It is therefore vital that the child never sleeps in a Geopathic Stress place the rest of its life. Also that micro parasites are kept at bay and the immune system is rebuilt and continuously boosted.

It is very important you read at the end of this chapter remedies, which have no side-effects, and are essential for your child's speedy recovery and give the best chance for the cancer not to return.

Cancer is not infectious and cannot be passed on to other people.

Even children diagnosed with unusually high white blood cell count are often found to have something other than cancer.

Some girls, especially around eight years old, may develop a mildly tender swelling in one or both breasts with an underlying mass. This may not be serious. The mass usually reduces and disappears within six to twelve months. Breast cancer is very rare in children. The enlargement should be inspected by a doctor. Any biopsies or surgical intervention should be delayed and the mass should only be removed if it becomes very large or the symptoms come back.

However the depth of pain you feel when told your child has cancer, you must face reality. You will most likely find your child can cope and accept the illness as well as an adult can, sometimes better.

It is highly recommended to get the free booklet *'A Parent's Guide to Children's Cancer'* from MacMillan Cancer Support which contains information about cancer in children, their diagnose and treatment and support services available. It also talks about the emotional impact of cancer for a child with cancer.

What Child is most likely to get Cancer

In all the cases of cancer in children I have come across, the mother of the child was sleeping in a bed during pregnancy which had one or more Geopathic Stress lines running across the middle part of her body. This can cause pre cancerous cells to develop during pregnancy (the first hit), which generally remain in the child's body for 10-16 years.

(1) **Cancer Research UK figures**

These cells can then turn into cancer cells (the second hit) if the child sleeps in a bed which is affected by Geopathic Stress.
(Some doctors claim a genetic 'mistake' occurs in the womb, during development of the DNA in the growing foetus).

If affected by Geopathic Stress the child has a lower absorption rate of vitamins, minerals and trace elements from its food resulting in malnutrition which causes a lowering of the child's immune system.

In most cases of childhood cancer if it is present in one child, it does not mean that a brother or sister is more likely to develop cancer, unless they are also Geopathic Stressed.

Micro-parasites are also present in most cases of childhood cancer.

Telling your Child it has Cancer

Openness and honesty are usually the best approach, depending naturally upon the age and understanding of the child. Toddlers can be told that they are sick and need to take medicine to get better. Avoid calling them "bad cells" as your child may feel the cancer is a punishment for bad behaviour. Older children need to know that cancer is a serious, but a treatable illness. Do not avoid the subject for fear of saying something wrong. It is best to deal with the question in a matter-of-fact and honest manner, so that you keep communication open.

Symptoms

Symptoms vary depending on which type of cancer they have. If your child feels unwell for one or two weeks, including high fever, being sick, losing appetite and weight, unusually angry, you should take your child to see your GP. Additional symptoms for various childhood cancers are described under individual types of cancer.

Side effects of treatments

Treatment often causes side effects and will depend on the treatment given and which part of the body is being treated.
Side effects can include:
* nausea (feeling sick) and vomiting
* loss of hair
* increase risk of infection
* bruising and bleeding
* tiredness
* diarrhoea

Clinical Trials

Often children have this treatment as part of clinical research trials, which are completely voluntary and you will be given plenty of time to decide if it is right for your child. The aim of the trial is to improve and understand the best way to treat the cancer, usually by comparing the standard treatment with new or modified versions. Research has found that people receiving treatment within clinical trials; tend to do as well or better. This does not always mean the clinical trial is better, but is probably because hospitals that carry out trials have access to more uptodate equipment and follow precise guidelines when giving treatment.

BRAIN TUMOURS

Brain Tumours are the most common solid tumours that occur in children. Children of any age may be affected. About 350 children are diagnosed with brain tumours each year in the UK. Boys are affected more often than girls.

Brain tumours can be either primary or secondary. Primary brain tumours are tumours which develop in the brain. Secondary brain tumours (more commonly called *cerebral metastasis)* occur when cancer cells from other parts of the body spread to the brain. See under Brain Tumours in adults for more details.

Primary brain tumours can develop from any of the different types of cells found in the brain. They can be either non-cancerous (benign) or cancerous (malignant).

Most primary brain tumours are benign They remain where they started and do not spread or destroy other parts of the brain, but may cause pressure on part of the brain. **Malignant primary brain tumours** are most likely to cause problems by spreading to the normal brain tissue which surrounds them. This can cause pressure and damage to the surrounding area.

The two main types of malignant primary brain tumours that affect children are:
Gliomas develop from the supporting cells of the brain (which hold the nerve cells in place). They can be subdivided into two main types in children: *astrocytomas* and *ependymomas.*
Medulloblastomas usually develop in the cerebellum at the back of the brain. They may spread to other parts of the brain or into the spinal cord.

Signs and symptoms

Brain tumours may cause a wide variety of symptoms including morning headaches, vomiting, seizures, irritability, behaviour problems, and changes in eating or sleeping habits, vision changes and changes in muscle coordination or moments of unconsciousness.

Diagnosis

A variety of tests and investigations may be needed to diagnose a specific brain tumour including CT or MRI scan, which gives a detailed image of the inside of the brain. A brain angiogram, which shows up the structure of the blood vessels in the brain, is sometimes used to help plan surgery. Careful examination of the eyes is important, as this can show if there is any raised intracranial pressure. A hearing test may also be done. A biopsy of the tumour is often taken. A chest X-ray and blood tests may be needed to check the child's general health.

Tumour Biopsy

To find out exactly which type of tumour it is, a biopsy may be carried out to remove a small sample of the tumour. A small *burn* hole is made in the skull through which a fine needle is passed to remove a piece of the tumour. This is examined in the laboratory by a pathologist. Sometimes it is not possible to identify the exact type of tumour until the whole tumour, or part of it, is removed during surgery (this is called an excision biopsy).

Having a biopsy is likely to mean a few days in hospital, as it involves an operation under a general anaesthetic.

Treatment
Surgery, radiotherapy or chemotherapy may be used alone or in combination. Steroids may be given before or after surgery or radiotherapy to help reduce the swelling that often surrounds the brain tumour. Doctors try to avoid giving radiation to children under three, because it is during the first few years that a child's brain cells develop most rapidly.

Complementary Remedies - See end of chapter

MagneTech Therapy
Powerful high speed spinning magnetic apparatus have been used on adults to prevent brain tumours growing and sometimes tumours reducing in size. As this apparatus has been successfully used on children for other health problems, without any side effects, there is no reason why they should not be used near the tumour before or after orthodox treatment.

GERM CELL TUMOURS
Germ cell tumours are a very rare type of cancer which develops from cells that produce eggs or sperm and mainly affect the ovaries or testes. Over 80% of children get cured of this cancer.

Germ Cell can also develop in other parts of the body where they can develop into tumours, such as the bottom of the spine, the brain, chest and abdomen. Benign tumours (non cancerous) do not spread, but can cause problems by pressing on nearby tissues and body structures. Malignant (cancerous) tumours can grow and spread to other parts of the body.

Signs and Symptoms
The symptoms depend on where the tumour develops, but usually a lump appears that can either be felt or lead to other problems.

Diagnosis
A variety of tests and investigations may be needed to diagnose a germ cell tumour. A biopsy will help to identify if the tumour is benign or malignant. A CT or MRI scan can detect the exact position of any tumour. Chest X-rays may be taken to see if there is a tumour in the lungs. Germ cell tumours often produce proteins (tumour markers) which can be measured in the blood before, during and after treatment.

Treatment
Treatment will depend on a number of factors including size, position and how advanced the cancer is. Usually treatment involves surgery or chemotherapy or a combination of the two. It may be necessary to remove the ovaries or testes, if this is where the tumour first developed. If only one ovary or testis is removed, your child may still be able to have children. Germ cells are very sensitive to chemotherapy, which can be given as injections or infusions into a vein.

Side effects of treatment will depend on treatment and may develop many years later, such as problems with hearing, kidneys and lungs.

Complementary remedies - see end of chapter

LANGERHANS CELLS HISTIOCYTOSIS (LCH)

LCH is not strictly a cancer, rather a cancer like condition. Histiocytosis is cells which are part of the immune system and are found in many parts of the body.

LCH

In LCH, the Langerhan's cells are abnormal and spread into many parts of the body via the bloodstream, including the bone marrow, skin, lungs, liver, lymph glands, spleen and pituitary glands, where they may cause damage. 50-100 children develop LCH each year in the UK. It can affect children of any age and is more common in boys than girls. There are two groups of LCH:

Single-system LCH when the disease affects only one part of the body, for example, the skin or the bones.

Multi-system LCH when it affects more than one part of the body.

Signs and Symptoms

The symptoms will depend upon which part of the body is affected and whether the disease is affecting more than one part of the body.

If the LCH is affecting the following areas, it can cause:

bone - pain in the bones and or swelling or lumps on the skull.

skin - skin rash, including cradle cap and nappy rash.

ear - discharge or hearing problems.

lungs or chest - breathing difficulties.

abdomen - tummy problems and possible jaundice.

lymph glands - enlargement.

pituitary glands - hormone problems, which can cause passing large amounts of urine and being very thirsty. It may also cause poor growth or delayed puberty.

Children may be unusually irritable and have poor appetite.

Diagnose

X-ray, blood tests, biopsy and MRI are the normal tests carried out.

Treatment

Single-system LCH may disappear on its own. Sometimes surgery and corticosteroids may be used.

Multi-system LCH is usually treated with chemotherapy and corticosteroids.

(Corticosteroids are hormonal substances, naturally produced in the body).

Useful organisations

Histiocytosis Research Trust, website: hrtrust.org.

The Histiocytosis Association, website: histio.org.

Both websites will give details of research, advice and put you in touch with other families who have experienced LCH.

Complementary Remedies - see end of chapter

LEUKAEMIA

More children get leukaemia than any other form of cancer, with about 400 new cases diagnosed each year in the UK. Approximately 75% get acute lymphoblastic leukaemia (ALL) and 25% get acute myeloid leukaemia (AML). ALL is most common between the ages of 1 to 6 and more common in boys than girls. AML can affect children of any age and girls and boys are affected equally.

Leukaemia is a cancer of the white blood cells. All blood cells are produced in the bone marrow. Bone marrow is the spongy substance at the core of some of the bones in the body.

Bone marrow contains and produces:
- Red blood cells which carry oxygen around the body.
- White blood cells which help fight infection.
- Platelets which help the blood clot and control bleeding.

There are two different types of white cells - lymphocytes and myeloid cells. These white blood cells work together to fight infection. Normally, white blood cells repair and reproduce themself in an orderly and controlled way. In leukaemia, the process gets out of control and the cells continue to divide, but do not mature.

These immature dividing cells fill up the bone marrow and stop it from making healthy bone marrow and blood cells. As the leukaemia cells are not mature, they cannot work properly. This leads to an increased risk of infection because the bone marrow cannot make enough healthy white blood cells.

There are four main types of leukaemia:
Acute lymphoblastic (ALL)
Acute myeloid (AML)
Chronic lymphoblastic (CLL)
Chronic myeloid (CML)

Chronic leukaemia usually only affects adults and is extremely rare in children and young people. Each type of leukaemia has its own characteristics and need a specific treatment.

ALL is a cancer of the immature lymphocytes called lymphoblasts or blast cells. There are two different types of lymphocytes - T-cells and B-cells (see further details in chapter on immune system). Often the leukaemia occurs at a very early stage in the immature lymphocytes, before they have developed as far as becoming either T-cells or B-cells. However if the cells have developed this far before becoming leukaemia, the type of leukaemia may be known as T-cell or B-cell leukaemia.

AML is an overproduction of immature myeloid white blood cells (blast cells). Cells which have started to show some of the features of myeloid cells and are said to show some *differentiation*. Cells which do not show signs of becoming a particular type of white blood cell are known as *undifferentiated*.

There are different sub-type of AML depending upon exactly which type of cell has become leukaemic, at what stage of development *(maturation)* the cells are and whether the cells are *differentiated*. Knowing the sub-type of AML is important as it helps the doctor to decide on the best treatment.

Signs and Symptoms

As the leukaemia cells multiply in the bone marrow, the production of normal blood cells is reduced. Children may therefore become tired and lethargic due to anaemia, which is caused by lack of red blood cells. Tendency to bleed or bruise easily, shortness of breath, bone or joint pains, frequent infections, abdominal pain or swelling. Sometimes tiny red dots of purple spots on the skin. Also swollen lymph glands.

Diagnosis

Blood test usually shows low numbers of normal white blood cells and the abnormal leukaemia cells. A sample of bone marrow is needed to confirm the diagnosis. A lumbar puncture is done to see if the spinal fluid has any leukaemia cells. A Chest X-ray is also done, which will show if there are any enlarged glands in the chest. Other tests may be necessary depending on the child's symptoms. These tests will help to identify the precise type of leakaemia.

Treatment

The main treatment for leukaemia is usually a combination of chemotherapy drugs. The aim is to destroy the leukaemia cell, so the bone marrow can work normally again.

The initial treatment nearly always involves two courses (or cycles) of chemotherapy drugs. A bone marrow test is taken at the end of the treatment to check if the child is in remission - no evidence of leukaemia.

If there are no signs of leukaemia cells in the blood or bone marrow, further chemotherapy treatment is given to be on the safe side and to prevent the cancer coming back.

If the initial chemotherapy treatment did not succeed in destroying the leukaemia cells or if there is a relapse (1 in 5 children have a relapse), even stronger chemotherapy and often bone marrow is needed. This may involve up to three months in isolation in hospital. 1 in 4 members of a family will be a suitable donor for bone marrow. The bone marrow is usually extracted from the donor's hip bone and injected into the patient's spine, so the patient's blood can start producing cancer free blood.

Normally treatment takes 3 years for boys and 2 years for girls.

Complementary Remedies - see end of chapter

Case histories

Bill had leukaemia from when he was born. He was still being treated when he was four years old. I told his mother to move Bill's bed into a Geopathic Stress-free place. A few months later Bill's mother rang to say the doctor had just told her "It is a miracle. Bill has no longer got leukaemia".

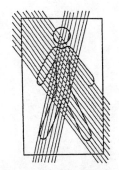

Geopathic Stress lines through Bill's bed before moving his bed into a safe place.

3 years old Olivia had a raging fever, was continuously sick, felt lethargic, angry and lost weight before being diagnosed with leukaemia. After her first chemotherapy treatment, the cancer was still found to be present. Olivia therefore had to have even more intense chemotherapy treatment to destroy the cancer. Thereafter, she had 18 months maintenance treatment of a low dose of chemotherapy in tablet form at home.

Isabella, Olivia's twin sister, is now a head taller than Olivia and is being tested for cancer at regular intervals, as doctors are worried she may also get cancer and cannot understand why she·has not got cancer, BUT then she is not sleeping in a Geopathic Stress place.

Below shows the Geopathic Stress lines through the twins' mother's bed when she was pregnant with them. Also Olivia and Isabella's beds.

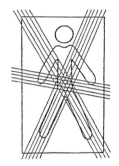
Sarah's bed during pregnancy with her twins showing Geopathic Stress lines.

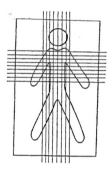
Geopathic Stress lines through Olivia's bed.

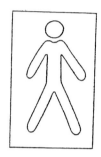
Isabella's bed has no Geopathic Stress.

LIVER TUMOURS

Cancer that starts in the liver (which is different from those that have spread to the liver from some other location) is very rare in children. If is totally confined to the liver, it is highly curable. (See full details under liver cancer in adults).

The Liver

The liver is the largest organ in the body. It is an extremely important organ and has many functions.

The Liver

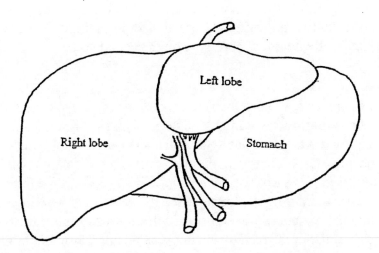

Liver cancer

Hepatoblastomas is the liver cancer most frequently found in children between the ages of new born to four, or at a later age of 12 to 15. Hepatocellular, the other type of liver cancer, is mainly found in adults.

Signs, Symptoms and Diagnosis

Some of these may be similar to liver cancer in adults.

Treatment

This will depend upon which stage the cancer is at. From stage 1, when the tumour is contained in the liver, to stage 4, when the tumour has spread to other parts of the body. Normally, it involves a combination of surgery, chemotherapy and radiotherapy.

Complementary Treatment

As the liver is weak, it needs Q10, not only to improve its vitality, but also to ensure that the liver can produce enough Q10 which is needed to boost every cell in the body. (See about Q10 under 'supplements').

NEUROBLASTOMA

Fewer than 100 children are diagnosed with neuroblastoma each year in the UK. Most children are affected under the age of 5. Neuroblastoma is a cancer of specialised nerve cells called *neural crest cells*. These cells are involved in the development of the nervous system and other tissues.

Neuroblastoma can occur anywhere in the body, but most often in the adrenal glands, which are above the kidneys. The adrenal glands release hormones to maintain blood pressure and enable us to respond to stress so are particularly affected by Geopathic Stress.

Signs and symptoms

The first symptoms are often vague such as loss of appetite and tiredness. If the tumour is in the abdomen, the child's tummy may be swollen, could cause constipation and have difficulty passing urine. If the tumour affects the chest area, the child may be breathless and have difficulty in swallowing. Less often, children may have weakness in the legs and walk unsteadily if the tumour is pressing on the spinal cord.

Diagnosis

Many tests and investigations may be needed to diagnose the cancer including X-ray, CT or MRI scans, bone marrow tests and blood tests. This will find the exact position of the neuroblastoma and whether it has spread. This is known as staging (see below). Further tests include urine tests. Nearly all children with neuroblastoma will have substances called *vanyllylmandelic acid* (VMA) or *homovanillic acid* (HVA). Your child will have VMA and HVA levels checked during treatment to see if treatment is working. A MIBG (meta-iodo-benzul guanidine) scan may also be done. MIBG is a substance that is taken up by neuroblastoma cells. It is given by injection. Attaching a small amount of radioactive iodine to the MIBG enables the tumours to be seen by a radioactive scanner. MIBG may also be used as a treatment. A biopsy of the tumour is usually taken so a small sample of the cells can be examined under a microscope.

Treatment

The treatment will depend on the age of the child, the stage the cancer is at and various other factors.

Stage 1 The cancer is contained within one area. Removal of the tumour is the normal treatment.

Stage 2A The cancer has not spread but cannot be completely removed by surgery and therefore chemotherapy may be involved.

Stage 2B The cancer has begun to spread into nearby lymph nodes. Surgery will normally remove the tumour and affected lymph nodes.

Stage 3 The cancer has spread into surrounding organs and structures, but has not spread to distant areas of the body. A combination of surgery and chemotherapy is usually carried out.

Stage 4 The cancer has spread to distant lymph nodes, bones, bone marrow, liver, skin or other organs. Treatment as under Stage 3.

Stage 5 Like Stage 4, this is found in children under the age of twelve months and will often get better on its own and no treatment may be required. The child will be monitored for the next few years. The tumour will often either disappear or may develop into a harmless benign tumour.

Case history

Ray M in Liverpool was only 9 months when he was diagnosed with neuroblastoma. He had numerous tests, including urine test and ultrasound and found that he had Stage 4. A tumour was found on one of the adrenal glands, which was removed by surgery. The cancer had spread to bones, blood, liver, skull and legs, so Ray's parents were persuaded that he have chemotherapy, which doctors told them would increase his survival rate by 10% from 40% without chemotherapy.

Timetable

June 2006 Ray was diagnosed with neuroblastoma.

July 2006 The adrenal gland, with the cancer tumour on, was removed by surgery.

July 2006 to February 2007 had chemotherapy for 5 days in hospital, then 4 to 6 weeks off before next 5 day chemotherapy session.

January 2007 Ray's mother, Jane, contacted me to check Ray's bed for Geopathic Stress. I found Ray could not have slept in a worst place. See plan. So I advised Jane to move Ray's bed IMMEDIATELY from A to B. Also advised parents' bed and Ray's two brothers' bed to be moved.

January 2008 Jane tells me that Ray has had scans every 2 months, all is clear and that his MIBG count has come down from 130 to 10. Jane also tells me she, her husband and all three boys are sleeping much better. The new baby is also sleeping well in his cot at C.

Ray was very high in parasites when he was diagnosed with cancer. The chemotherapy killed them off, but to prevent the parasites coming back, I have advised Jane to give Ray a 180 mg capsules of 100% stabilising allicin from garlic per day and make sure that Ray never gets Geopathic Stress, which could react very badly on his remaining adrenal gland. Later scans show Ray is still free of cancer.

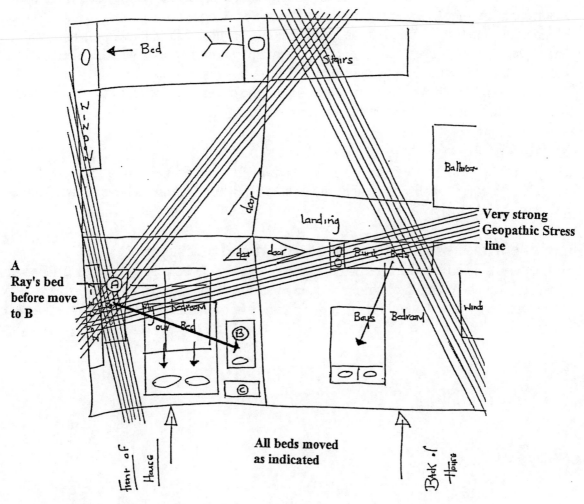

LYMPHOMA
HODGKIN'S AND NON-HODGKIN'S LYMPHOMA
Lymphoma is a general term for a group of cancers that develop in the lymph system as part of the body's immune system - in a single lymph node or in a group of lymph nodes and can spread to any part of the body. About 140 children get lymphoma each year in the UK. There is a very high cure rate for early stage lymphoma.

Although these two cancers are both lymph system diseases, with some similarities, they differ widely in cell origin, how they spread and how they are treated.

Signs and Symptoms
The first sign of lymphoma is usually a painless swelling in the neck, head, throat and abdomen. In cases of Non-Hodgkin's, it may affect the lymph nodes in the chest.

Lymph system
See details under adult Hodgkin's and Non-Hodgkin's lymphoma.

Diagnosis
In order to diagnose either Hodgkin's or Non-Hodgkin's lymphoma, a biopsy has to be carried out to remove part of a swollen lymph gland, so the cells can be examined in the laboratory. Further tests may be carried out, such as X-rays, ultrasound, CT and MRI scans, blood and urine tests to find out the exact size and position of the lymphoma and whether it has spread. Doctors may also carry out a lumbar puncture to check whether there are any lymphoma cells in the fluid that surrounds the brain and spinal cord.
'Staging' from 1 to 4 is the term used to describe the size and position of the cancer and whether it has spread. (See adult lymphoma).

Treatment
Lymphoma is normally treated with chemotherapy, but sometimes radiotherapy is also needed. For much localised disease, when the cancer has not spread beyond its original site, radiotherapy alone may be used.

Complementary remedies - see details at end of chapter
100% stabilising allicin from garlic has shown to be a great help in reducing Non-Hodgkin's lymphoma and boosting the immune system in adults. It has shown no side-effects. Why not incorporate it into your child's diet during and after treatment? See further details at end of chapter.

RARE TUMOURS

All childhood cancers are rare, but there are a number of extremely rare types. Together they account for fewer than 50 in total in the UK per year.

Types of rare childhood cancer

Tumours that normally only occur in adults These include cancers of the digestive system, the thyroid and the adrenal gland.

Rare tumours which only occur in children These include pancreatablastoma, malignant rhabdoid tumours and melanotic neuroectodermal tumours of infants.

Rare tumours in the head and neck area For example, nasopharyngeal cancer.

Rare hormonal or endocrine tumours For example, phaeochromocytoma

Rare brain tumours For example, meningioma.

Rare skin tumours These include melanomas.

In general, these rare cancers behave like the more common ones. They have the ability to keep on growing and spread to other parts of the body.

Treatment

For rare cancers, treatment may involve surgery, chemotherapy or radiotherapy, or a combination of these.

Complementary Remedies - see details at end of chapter

RETINOBLASTOMA

This is a tumour that occurs in the retina. In many cases retinoblastoma is caused by a genetic abnormality. This means that an abnormal gene has passed from the mother during pregnancy mainly, if she was sleeping in a Geopathic Stress place. The cancer can then break out if the child also sleeps in a Geopathic Stress place. This is the main contributory cause of most children's cancers. Cure rate is very high, particularly if complementary remedies are taken into account during and after treatment.

Retinoblastoma is diagnosed in about 40 children in the UK each year. Most are younger than 5 years old, although it can affect children of any age.
Retinoblastoma is a tumour that occurs in the retina. This is the light sensitive lining of the eye.

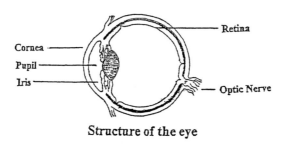

Structure of the eye

Signs and Symptoms

First signs of retinoblastoma are often a white pupil that does not reflect the light. This may be detected when a photo is taken of the child when a flash is used. The affected eye may look white in the photo. Some children may have a squint or if the tumour is large, it may cause a painful red eye.

Some children will have no symptoms and it will be picked up by screening (in children of families with a history of this condition).

DIAGNOSIS

Initial tests can be carried out by a specialist examing the eye while a light is shone into the eye from an ophthalmoscope.

Further tests may involve an examination of the eyes under anaesthetic (EUA). A biopsy to take a tissue sample is not recommended.

If retinoblastoma is diagnosed, other tests may be done to check the exact position and size of the tumour and whether it has begun to spread into surrounding structures. Such tests include ultrasound, CT or MRI scans. A lumbar puncture is sometimes carried out to collect some fluid from around the brain and spinal cord, to check if the cancer has spread into the cerebrospinal fluid. Some children may also need to have samples taken from a bone and/or bone marrow, to see if the cancer has spread to those parts.

Treatment

This will depend on the number, position and size of the tumours in the eye. The aim of the treatment is first to get rid of the cancer and secondly to try to save the sight of the eye. Depending on the treatment, some children may lose some of their sight.

Smaller tumours

For small tumours, treatment is given to the eye itself by one of the following methods:
Cryotherapy This is used to freeze the tumour. More than one session may be necessary at monthly intervals.
Laser Therapy A laser is used to vaporise the tumour. Two or three sessions may be needed at monthly intervals.
Plaque For slightly larger tumours and tumours that have not been successfully treated using other methods, a small disc containing a radioactive substance can be stitched over the tumour. The disc needs to stay in place for two to four days. The radiation destroys the cancer cells.
Thermotherapy This process uses heat to destroy the cancer cells and may be combined with chemotherapy or radiotherapy, as heat can improve the effect of these treatments. The heat is produced by a laser that is directed at the tumour.

Large tumours

These can be treated in a number of ways:
Chemotherapy may be given before the local treatment mentioned above, to help shrink the tumour. It can also be used if the cancer has spread to other parts of the body, or there is a risk it will do so.
Radiotherapy can be given to destroy the cancer cells without doing too much harm to normal cells.
Surgery if the tumour is very large and the vision in the eye is lost, the eye is removed and an artificial eye is then fitted.

Side-effects of treatment

Treatment for retinoblastoma often causes side-effects some many years later. It is, therefore, most important your child is not Geopathic Stressed and prevent your child's immune system ever becoming low again.

Complementary Remedies - see end of chapter

Useful organisations

The Childhood Eye Cancer Trust (CHECT), The Royal London Hospital, Whitechapel Road, London, E1 1BB, Tel: 020 7377 5578, Website: chect.org.uk.

SARCOMAS

There are two main types of sarcomas: bone sarcomas, such as Osteosarcoma and Ewing's Sarcoma and Soft Tissue Sarcoma, such as Rhabdomyosarcoma.

Osteosarcoma

This is the most common type of bone cancer in children and most frequently involves the large bones of the upper arms (humerus) and the leg (femur and tibia). It is more common in boys than girls and usually occurs over the age of ten.

Usually chemotherapy is given before surgery to shrink large tumours and afterwards in order to destroy any remaining cancer cells and to prevent is spreading outside the bone. Surgery usually involves taking the cancer tumour out without removing the arm or leg (limb-sparing) or removing all or part of an arm or leg (amputation). In general, more than 80% of patients have limb-sparing surgery. Studies have shown that there is no difference in survival between patients having limb-sparing and those having amputation. If part of the limb has to be removed, the bone can sometimes be replaced with a prosthetic (specially designed artificial part). This may have to be lengthened as the child grows older. Part of a bone taken from another part of the body can sometimes also be used (a bone graft).

Ewing's Sarcoma

This cancer is named after Dr James Ewing, who discovered the tumour in the 1920's. Ewing's sarcoma tends to be found in flat bones, such as ribs. It usually occurs between the age of 5 and 30. Chemotherapy is used as with osteosarcoma. Ewing's sarcoma responds well to radiotherapy and is often used after chemotherapy used before or after surgery. Radiotherapy may be used instead of surgery, if the tumour is in the spine.

Signs and Symptoms of Bone Cancer

Pain is the most common symptom of bone cancer. However, symptoms may vary depending on the position in the body and the size of the tumour. There may be some swelling in the affected area and it may become tender to touch. Bone cancer is sometimes discovered when a bone that has been weakened by cancer and breaks after the child has had a minor fall or accident.

Often very powerful rotating magnetic therapy has helped shrink tumours, so less conventional treatment has to be given.

Soft Tissue Sarcoma

Rhabdomyosarcoma is the most common soft tissue sarcoma in children. Soft tissue sarcoma is more curable than in adults. It can occur anywhere in the body, but is most often found in the head, neck, bladder, vagina, prostate, testes, arm, legs and chest. It occurs most frequently between the ages of two and six and in the teens. It is considered curable in the majority of children and treatment is usually one or a combination of chemotherapy, surgery and radiotherapy.

Symptoms

Unexplained swelling or lumps, enlarged lymph nodes, swelling in the eye, ear pain or discharge from the ear, bloody nasal discharge, vaginal bleeding, difficulty urinating or defecating, bone pain and tiredness.

Complementary Remedies

Apart from using powerful rotating magnetic therapy, (see case history under adult bone cancer). read more details at end of chapter.

WILM'S TUMOUR

This tumour is a type of kidney cancer. Specialised cells known as *metanephric blastomas* are involved in the development of the kidneys, when the child is in the womb. These cells usually disappear at birth, but if the mother was sleeping in a Geopathic Stress place during pregnancy, residual cells called *nephragenic rest* can still be found if the child is sleeping in a Geopathic Stress place.

Wilms Tumour

The kidneys are a pair of organs found at the back of the abdomen. They clean the blood to remove excess fluid and waste products which is converted into urine. Wilms tumour is named after Dr Max Wilms, who first described it. About 70 children are diagnosed with Wilms tumour each year in the UK and most are affected below the age of five.

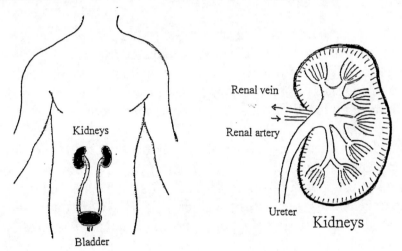

Signs and Symptoms

The most common symptoms are swelling in the abdomen - usually painless. Occasionally the tumour may bleed slightly, which can cause irritation and pain. There may be blood in the child's urine or the blood pressure may be raised. The child may also have a high temperature, upset stomach, weight loss or lack of appetite.

Diagnosis and Treatment

Various tests and investigations may be needed, such as urine and blood samples, abdominal ultrasound and CT scan. Also chest and liver scans.

Staging is a term used to describe the size of the tumour and whether it has spread.

Stage 1 The tumour is only affecting the kidney and has not begun to spread. The tumour can be completely removed with surgery.

Stage 2 The tumour has begun to spread beyond the kidney to nearby structures, but it is still possible to remove it completely with surgery.

Stage 3 The tumour has spread beyond the kidneys, either because it has burst (before or during the operation), or because it has spread to the lymph glands (nodes) or it cannot be completely removed by surgery. Chemotherapy is usually given after surgery. Radiotherapy may also be given.

Stage 4 The tumour has spread to other parts o the body such as the lungs, liver, bone or brain. Surgery, chemotherapy and radiotherapy are normally involved.

Stage 5 There are tumours in both kidneys (*bilateral Wilms tumour*). Any of the above treatments may be involved.

Follow up

Most children with Wilms tumours are cured. If the cancer comes back (*recurrent cancer or relapse*), it is usually within the first two years. To prevent this, it is most important that the child does not sleep in a Geopathic Stress place, which was partly the cause of the original cancer. Using daily a strong rotating magnetic apparatus direct, may help to shrink the tumour initially and used elsewhere on the body will improve your child's overall health. It is very important the child's immune system does not become weak again.

HOW TO ENSURE A HIGHER SUCCESS RATE

It is most important you ensure your child, who has cancer, or has had cancer, is not sleeping in a Geopathic Stress place, nor staying for long periods during the day in stressful places.
There are excellent units on the market for neutralising Geopathic Stress, but never rely only on them 100% to ensure your child is not sleeping in a Geopathic Stress place.

Even in hospital, check your child's bed is in a safe place. If found in a Geopathic Stressed place, ask for it to be moved into a safe place, particularly if your child is in hospital for a long time. If this proves impossible or you do not feel like discussing it with the nursing staff, then install a strong Geopathic Stress neutraliser. Being Geopathic Stress-free really will make all the difference to your child's recovery.

Most doctors and many nurses dismiss Geopathic Stress and say its harmful effect has not been proven scientifically. In hundreds of cases, parents have contacted me due to their baby's continuous crying most nights. After I have advised them to move the cot/bed to a Geopathic Stress-free place, the parents nearly always report that their baby sleeps peacefully the very first night after moving the cot/bed - what more scientific proof do you need!! [1]

Ensure you boost your child's immune system which any cancer treatment has weakened. The most powerful way is to take 100% stabilised allicin liquid, the very powerful part of garlic. Try mixing half a spoonful into some honey. Even 4 week old babies have taken this. In older children, mix one to two x 5ml (teaspoon) into fruit juices.

I would also recommend your child takes say 30 mg of Q10. The contents can be squashed out into some fruit juice if your child cannot swallow the capsules. Half a teaspoon of Bicarbonate of Soda in a small cup of water will help make the acid alkaline balance in the blood alkaline.

Give your child lots of cuddles, but don't forget to cuddle any other children you may have.

[1] My book 'Are You Sleeping In A Safe Place?' quotes many famous doctors on the dangers of Geopathic Stress.

BLADDER CANCER

Bladder problems are fairly easy to detect, so if the cause is cancer it can be detected early and treatments results in a fairly high survival rate over a long period. Even better results can be achieved by incorporating complementary remedies.

SUMMARY

- Symptoms
- Research
- Who is most likely to get bladder cancer?
- Your bladder
- Diagnosis
- Types of bladder cancer
- Treatment
- How to ensure a higher success rate and reduce the likelihood of the cancer returning
- Preventing bladder cancer in the first place

Symptoms

Passing of blood in the urine (haematuria), pus in the urine and a burning pain on urinating. These signs are also indicative of other less serious conditions, such as infections or bladder stones, but they should always be taken seriously, especially by older people and are a warning to see your doctor immediately. Another indication is increase in the frequency of urination.

Research

About 5000 people are diagnosed with bladder cancer including urethra and ureter cancer in the UK each year. Men are two to three times more likely to get bladder cancer than women - believed to be due to men being more likely to work in industrial environments, where toxins are present.

Who is most likely to get Bladder Cancer?

- People between the ages of 50 and 80.
- Tobacco smokers.
- White people are twice as likely to get bladder cancer as black and Hispanic people. Asian people have the lowest rate.
- Women, who have had radiotherapy for cancer of the cervix, have a higher chance of getting bladder cancer.
- Workers in industries dealing with toxins including pesticides and lorry drivers.

Your Bladder

Your two kidneys filter waste from your blood and adjust the level of various chemical substances. The surplus is urine, which is a sterile liquid that passes down the two ureters tubes to your bladder, where it is stored until discharged through your urethra tube. In women, the urethra is a short tube which opens just forward of the vagina. In men, it is longer, passing through the prostate gland and out through the penis.

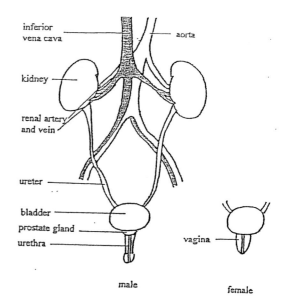

Diagnosis

First of all, a complete physical examination is carried out. Bladder tumours can sometimes be felt during a rectal or vaginal examination. Urine samples are often inspected under microscopes - *urinary cytology*, inserting a saline solution and collected through a catheter. The inside of the bladder is inspected and, if necessary, samples are taken for biopsy by inserting a *cystoscope* through the urethra. Occasionally you will need a local anaesthetic to have a cystoscopy.

Sometimes an opaque dye is injected into a vein before an X-ray is taken. The X-ray will show an outline of the kidneys, ureters and bladder. Tumours larger than one centimetre (3/8 inch) can sometimes be seen. CT scans and ultrasounds may also help to determine the extent of the cancer. Other tests may be carried out if bladder cancer is diagnosed, such as a liver function test and chest X-ray.

Bladder Cancer Tester

A NMP 22 protein is often elevated in the urine of patients with bladder cancer, even at early stages of the disease. The NMP 22 BladderChek Tester has been developed to test for high levels of NMP 22 protein in the patient's urine during a visit to the doctor. The results can be delivered during the patient's visit. The test has been approved by the FDA.

Types of Bladder Cancer

90% of bladder cancers are either papillary or non-papillary cancer. Papillary cancer is the most common bladder cancer. It is not usually invasive and is the most easily curable. The cancer tumour starts on the bladder wall, but grows into the bladder cavity and remains attached to the bladder wall, by a mushroom-like stem. The tumour may be single or multiple, the size of a pea or may fill the whole bladder. The cancer cells often look normal. Non-papillary cancer are flat legions, which develop and become invasive. Superficial bladder cancer is only in the lining of the bladder. After treatment, it may come back as another superficial bladder cancer. Invasive bladder cancer grows through the lining of the bladder and goes into the muscle wall.

Treatment

Treatment depends on the stage and the grade of the tumour, also the age and health of the patient. It may involve surgery, chemotherapy, radiotherapy or a combination of these and also laser treatment for superficial tumours and photodynamic therapy for early stages of bladder cancer. Transurethral resection (TUR) may also be used where an electric current is used to remove small growths of superficial bladder cancer. If radical surgery is used on the male, it may be necessary to remove the bladder, the prostate, the seminal vesicle, the vas deferens and pelvis lymph nodes. In women, the entire bladder, the uterus, the ovaries, fallopian tubes and part of the vagina are usually removed.

In theses cases, it may be worth considering strong magnetic therapy first, with no side effects and which may reduce the tumours, so less surgery is necessary. If the whole bladder is removed, new techniques called an orthotopic neobladder are used to remove the urine, through urine pouches made from parts of the small intestine and connected to the remaining urethra. If this is not possible, a part of the small intestine is used to make a tube through which the urine can pass out of the body through an opening (stoma). In women, the removal of the uterus and ovaries will result in instant menopause and you will not be able to become pregnant. See Chapter 'Prostate Cancer' regarding the effects on men.

How to ensure a high success rate and reduce the likelihood of the cancer returning

It is most important that you take care of the BIG FOUR - avoid Geopathic Stress, destroy any microbes, mainly micro parasites, take adequate Q10 and ensure a high acid alkaline balance in your blood.

Take the necessary vitamins, minerals etc. as modern food no longer provides enough to prevent you suffering from malnutrition. Take at least 20 mcg daily of Vitamin D which is vital.

Also take enough exercise. Ideally exercise daily on a rebounder to vitalise your lymph system and help dispose of toxins from your body. Two minutes on a rebounder will double the number of white blood cells for one hour.

About 90% of people who get cancer have a thyroid gland which is out of balance. Using a MagneTech for one to two minutes daily direct will revitalise it. Do the same on the thymus, which matures your T-cells and say 20 minutes on your solar plexus where 70% of your immune system is located. Most importantly, use the MagneTech daily for 20 minutes directly on the problem area to heal it and any scar tissue.

You have got to take charge of your own health.

Preventing bladder cancer in the first place

- Follow the points above
- Stop smoking
- If you work in a toxic environment, protect yourself with face masks and carry out a detoxifying programme at regular intervals

BONE CANCER (osteosarcoma and other types)

Cancer that begins in the bone (primary cancer) is quite uncommon. By contrast many cancers that begin in other areas of the body - such as the breast, prostate or lungs - may spread to the bones and may cause secondary tumours there. With modern orthodox treatments, the chances of a cure have increased many times over the last 20 years. The BIG FOUR are also present in most cases, so they must be dealt with to ensure an even higher success rate.

SUMMARY

- **Symptoms**
- **Research**
- **Types of Bone Cancer**
- **Diagnosis**
- **Treatment**
- **How to ensure a higher success rate and reduce the likelihood of cancer returning**
- **Case History**

Symptoms
Pain, swelling, stiffness or tenderness in the affected area which may feel warm to the touch.

These are all features that can also accompany an ordinary bruise or injury. With a bruise or injury however, the symptoms should settle down and almost disappear in two or three days. If there is a tumour in the bone, the problem will get worse over several days or weeks and be especially painful at night. Therefore a medical assessment is important if the problem does not improve within a few days.

Loss of bladder functions if the cancer is in the pelvic bones or base of spine. Tiredness, fever and weight loss.

Research
There are about 400 new primary bone cancer cases in the UK each year. There are about 40 different types of bone cancer.

Types of Bone Cancer
Primary bone cancer - This starts in the bone and generally occurs in adolescents and young adults and is usually found in the area around the knee joints, although it can occur in almost any bone.

Chondrosarcoma is a cancer of the cartilage which is the tough covering found on the ends of the bone. This cancer usually grows within a bone or on its surface. Chondrosarcoma can occur at any age and is slightly more common in men. This type of cancer is usually a slow growing tumour and the most common sites are the pelvic bone, shoulder bones and the upper part of the arm and legs.

Ewing's Sarcoma is a rare bone cancer which occurs in childhood and adolescence.

Osteosarcoma is cancers that occur almost exclusively in older children, adolescents and young adults. They are slightly more common in men than women. They are rare in the forties or beyond, except those cancers that develop in an area of bone that has been affected by **Paget's disease** for many years. In **Paget's disease** part of the skeleton becomes overactive and rebuilds itself at an abnormally fast rate in the elderly. It mainly affects the legs and the back. In many cases osteosarcoma is first diagnosed shortly after an injury.

Osteosarcoma has a tendency to spread, which it does by means of the bloodstream. Secondary cancer is most likely to appear first in the lungs (which is where the small blood vessels - the capillaries - filter the cancer cells from the bloodstream).

Diagnosis

With any suspected problems in the bone, your doctor will take a detailed history of your health, after which the following tests are likely to be done. (See Part Two for details of tests).

X-ray can give important clues about the presence of a bone tumour or confirm that there is nothing wrong. If there is evidence of cancer or anything suspicious, then almost always the next investigation is a CT scan.

CT will show the exact extent of the tumour and how much bone is involved. A CT scan may also be taken of the chest to see if the tumour has spread.

Isotope (TBC) bone scan will usually show the tumour and check that other bones are normal.

MRI scan of the tumour will show the exact size and location.

Needle Biopsy is a very important procedure in bone tumours to determine the type of cancer and what treatment is necessary.

It is important to find out if the cancer has spread to other areas of the body, particularly the lungs. Unlike most cancers, some cases of osteosarcoma can be cured even when the cancer has spread to the lungs. Tumours that begin in the legs or the arms respond better to treatment than those that begin in the spine or in the more central area of the skeleton.

Treatment

Chemotherapy may be given before or after surgery. Some osteosarcomas like periosteal are usually slow growing and treatment often does not require chemotherapy.

Chemotherapy is both given to prevent the cancer spreading and to see if the chemotherapy is effective in shrinking the tumour, as detected on a CT scan. If so, more chemotherapy is given to shrink the tumour before and after surgery.

However chemotherapy or radiotherapy is not very effective for most chondrosarcoma cancers and, therefore, surgery is the main form of treatment.

Treatment for primary bone cancer is mainly dealt with by surgery and/or radiotherapy.

The surgeon will not only try to remove the primary cancer as completely and safely as possible, but also to prevent it recurring and spreading. The surgeon will also try and reduce the affect of the operation on the function and appearance of the affected part of the body. This could involve amputating the limb up to the joint above the tumour. Sometimes radiotherapy may be involved.

Limb-sparing surgery In the past if chondrosarcoma was found in an arm or leg it was often necessary to amputate the affected limb. Today it is often possible just to remove the affected part of the bone and some of the healthy tissue around it. The bone is then replaced (prosthesis) or a bone graft (bone taken from another part of the body). If the cancer affects a bone in or near a joint, the whole joint can often be replaced with an artificial one.

Whatever type of surgery, rehabilitation after the operation is very important. Most adolescents have a remarkable ability to adapt to their new situation and are often able to continue previous active sport and to learn new ones as well.

How to ensure a high success rate and reduce the likelihood of the cancer returning

It is most important that you take care of the BIG FOUR - no Geopathic Stress, destroy any microbes, mainly micro parasites, take adequate Q10 and ensure a high acid alkaline balance in your blood.

Take the necessary Vitamins, minerals etc. modern food no longer provides to prevent you suffering from malnutrition. Also take at least 20 mcg daily of the vital Vitamin D.

Also get enough exercise. Ideally exercise daily on a rebounder to vitalise your lymph system and help dispose of toxins from your body. Two minutes on a rebounder will double your white blood cells for one hour.

About 90% of people who get cancer have a thyroid gland which is out of balance. Using a MagneTech for one to two minutes direct daily will revitalise it. Do the same on the thymus, which matures your T-cells and say 20 minutes on your solar plexus where 70% of your immune system is located. Most importantly, use the MagneTech daily for 20 minutes direct on the problem area to heal it and any scar tissues.

You have got to take charge of your own health.

Case History

On the next page is a copy of a letter from Malcolm J Ramsey of East Farleigh, Kent - as mentioned in my first chapter - who had a rare bone cancer in his lower right leg. He was only given a 20% chance of a cure without amputation above his knee. In January 2010, Malcolm is still free of cancer.

This is part of the floor plan I checked for Geopathic Stress lines in January 2007. Malcolm moved his bed from A, which was very Geopathic Stressed, to B and took my advice on the other BIG FOUR.

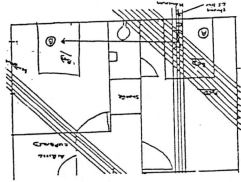

THURSDAY COTTAGE
KILNBRIDGE CLOSE
EAST FARLEIGH
KENT

31st July 2007

Dear Rolf

Further to our conversation last week I just had to write to you to say how delighted I was to discover that due to the use of the magnet that the very rare bone cancer in my lower right leg had reduced by some 80%.

I remember our conversation very well in late January when you said that after the chemo they will remark how much the cancer had reduced and it cannot just be the chemo. They were almost their exact words, they are simply amazed.

Up to two weeks ago I was due to have my leg amputated above the knee, but now after the latest scan they operated to remove the dead cancer cells and as a result my leg has been saved.

I also had secondary cancer on my lungs which again had reduced by a massive amount and as a result they are about to operate to remove the cancer spots (some 30 in number).

As a result of these operations and your wonderful Magne Tech healers I am told to expect a normal life span, very rare in most cases of this type of cancer which has spread to the lungs.

What can I say except a very big 'thank you' to you and your team, such small words but so big in their gratitude for helping save my life.

If you need any publicity, or for me to attend any meetings to speak, please let me know. I will be more than willing to help in any way, it was what I was great at!

Kindest regards

Malcolm J Ramsey

January 2013
Malcolm spoke to me about a month ago and said that he felt fine and a recent cancer check-up had shown he was all clear.

LARGE BOWEL CANCER (colon and rectal)

> After lung cancer, more people die of colon cancer than any other cancer however the survival rate is very high if diagnosed and treated early. So if your doctor does not feel you need bowel cancer diagnosed, or there is a long waiting time for a diagnosis and you are worried about bowel cancer symptoms, you can have a private scan immediately at a reasonable price.[1]
>
> Some bowel cancer patients may have several months waiting time for life saving treatment, so it is vital complementary therapy is taken seriously as it may slow the spread of the cancer or even reduce it.

SUMMARY
- Symptoms
- Research
- Who is most likely to get colon and rectal cancer?
- Your small intestines (small bowel)
- Your large bowel (colon and rectal)
- Polyps
- Ulcerative colitis
- Types of tumours in the colon and rectum
- Diagnosis
- Treatment - colon or rectal cancer
- After surgery
- How to ensure a higher success rate and reduce the likelihood of the cancer returning
- Case histories

Symptoms
Rectal bleeding (very dark red or bright blood in or on stools). Constipation alternating with diarrhoea for no obvious reason, lasting more than 6 weeks, or back passage pain or abdominal cramp, a lump in the abdomen, unexpected weight loss, loss of appetite, anaemia, weakness and fatigue, pallid complexion. Unfortunately, many cancer symptoms are overlooked in the more treatable early stages, because their symptoms are dismissed as Irritable Bowel Syndrome.

Research
About 35,000 new large bowel cancers are diagnosed in the UK every year, with about 16,000 deaths. The five year survival rate of patients whose bowel cancer tumours are caught early and surgically removed is as high as 90%. Two thirds of large bowel cancer develops in the colon and one third in the rectum.

[1] See CT scan Part Two

Who is most likely to get large bowel cancer?

- Men and women between the age of 50 and 75, but 10% are under that age and the numbers are increasing.
- Those with a personal history of ulcerative colitis, pancreatitis or Crohn's colitis.
- Women who have had ovarian, endometrial or breast cancer.
- Those who have previously had colon or rectal cancer.
- Those who have had non-cancerous growths (adenomas or polyps) in the colon.
- Those whose near families have had large bowel cancer.
- People who have slept with Geopathic Stress lines across the middle part of their body. High in micro parasites. Low in Q10 and very acid blood (low pH).

Your small intestine

The small intestine (small bowel) is a small tube about 35 mm (1 inch) in diameter and about 5 m (16 ft) long. It runs between the duodenum and the colon (large intestines) and is the main site for the absorption of nutrients into the bloodstream.

Cancer of the small intestine is very rare, mainly because the bowel contents are liquid and are not in long contact with the bowel wall.

Your large bowel

When you chew and swallow your food, it passes down your gullet (oesophagus) to your stomach where enzymes and acids help to break down your food, so it leaves in a semi solid form into your small intestine. Here essential nutrients are absorbed. The digested food then moves into your colon, where water is absorbed. The remaining waste matter (stools or faeces) are held in your colon until it is ready to be passed during bowel motions from your body through your anus.

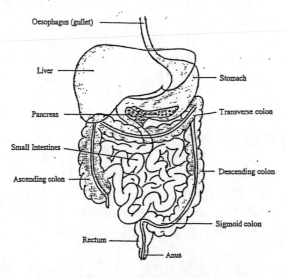

Your digestion system

The colon, (large bowel) or large intestine is 1.50 to 2.15 metres (5 to 7 feet) long in adults. It starts at the lower right part of the abdomen and is connected to your small intestine through a one-way valve called the **ileum** and defying the law of gravity, continues upward close to the liver under your ribs **(ascending colon)**. It crosses to the left side of the abdomen **(transverse colon)**. The next portion heads down the left side of your pelvis **(descending colon)**. The final section is S-shaped **(sigmoid colon)**, which along with the last section known as the **rectum**, is 20.5 to 25.5 cm (8-10 inches) long and is located in the pelvis, behind the urinary bladder.

Polyps (or adenomas)

They are benign growths that develop in the lining of the colon and can increase the risk of developing cancer. The polyps should therefore preferably be removed as soon as they develop. Not all bowel cancer starts out as polyps. Some cancers probably develop in the wall of the colon.

Ulcerative Colitis

Is a condition in which the colon becomes inflamed, in most cases due to microbes. If the condition involves most of the colon, the evidence suggests that after many years (ten or more), the chance of cancer is increased. A regular colonoscopy (once a year or so) is recommended. See Part One on how to kill microbes, including micro parasites.

Types of tumours in the colon and rectum

Most are **adenocarcinomas**, which are usually found in the lining of the colon. Other less common types of bowel cancer include **sarcomas** that begin in the connective tissues, **lymphomas**, which arise in the lymphatic tissues and rarer cancers such as **carcinoid** tumours.

Diagnosis

The sooner bowel cancer is diagnosed and treated the more likely any treatment will be 100% effective.

Unfortunately, many cases are not investigated before people have severe abdominal pain, as early signs of bowel cancer are not always easy to recognise. Therefore a new UK national screening programme for bowel cancer has been developed for people between 60 and 69 (50 and 74 in Scotland). Older people can also request the test which involves **faecal occult blood** (FOB) test every two years.

The FOB test detects tiny amounts of blood in your faeces (stool), which you cannot normally see and which can sometimes be the cause of bowel cancer or polyps.

People who have positive FOB are advised to see their GP. The doctor will feel your abdomen and examine your back passage for any lumps or swelling with a gloved finger. Any stools on the gloved finger will also be checked for blood. (Unfortunately many doctors do not perform a rectal examination when the patient complains of bleeding etc. - mainly due to embarrassment - both patients' and their own). If your GP suspects cancer, you will be referred to your hospital for further tests. Even if your doctor does not suspect any cancer, but you feel worried, you must insist on a hospital examination.

At the hospital Before examining you, the hospital specialist will ask you about your general health and repeat the rectal examination. To diagnose bowel cancer, the following test may be carried out:

Proclascopy This is a short tube which is inserted to inspect your rectum.

Sigmoidoscope is a longer tube, which can examine the first third of your colon. A tiny light and camera on the end of the tube will enable any abnormal areas to be scanned. A biopsy can also be carried out by collecting a small sample of cells for examination under a microscope.

The above tests are not usually painful, but can be slightly uncomfortable. You can usually go home straight away after the tests.

Colonoscopy uses a long flexible tube, which can easily pass around bends so most of the colon can be examined. Again a tiny light and camera at the end of the tube will enable any abnormal area of swelling to be photographed and a biopsy can be taken. Often air is blown into your colon beforehand to expand it.

Before the test, you have to follow a careful diet for a few days to enable your colon to be completely empty. As a colonoscopy test can be uncomfortable and last for about an hour, you are normally given a sedative to make you relaxed and feel sleepy during the procedure.

Barium enema A mixture of barium and air is passed into your back passage to enable doctors to watch the passage of the barium, a liquid which appears white as it passes through the colon as seen on a special X-ray screen.

On the morning of the test, you should not have anything to eat or drink to ensure your colon is empty. You will also have a bowel wash before the test at the hospital.

After a colonoscopy and barium enema test, you can normally go home after a couple of hours, but particularly after given any sedative before a colonoscopy, you should not drive yourself, so it is a good idea for somebody to accompany you.

CT colongraphy can be taken instead of a colonoscopy and barium enema using CT (computerised tomography), computer images to examine your colon, also called virtual colonoscopy. The test is only available in specialist centres so you may have to travel some way. If you need a biopsy, you still need a colonoscopy. A private clinic called Lifescan, Telephone: 01892 547341, can carry out a CT scan for about £500.

MRI (magnetic resonance imaging) scan creates sectional images of your body similar to CT scans, but instead of using radiation it uses strong magnets to take sectional images of your colon. This can help a surgeon to decide, before an operation, whether to use radiotherapy and/or chemotherapy to shrink the tumour. Sometimes a dye is injected into a vein in the arm to improve the image.

During the MRI scan, you will have to lie very still on a couch, which then travels through a fairly narrow chamber.

If you dislike enclosed spaces, mention this to the radiographer. You will be given earplugs or headphones as the scanning process is very noisy. As the MRI scan uses very strong magnets, you must remove any metal objects on you. Anybody having pacemakers, heart monitors or certain types of surgical clips must not have an MRI scan, but all this will be fully explained beforehand.

Some of the further tests may be needed if the biopsy shows there is cancer to find the size and position of the cancer and to see if it has spread.

Blood tests may be used to check your general health and to check for **carcinoembryonic antigen (CEA)** protein, which is sometimes produced by colon cancer cells.

Chest X-rays will probably be taken to check your heart and lungs.

Ultrasound scan using sound waves can be used to check inside your abdomen and, to see if the cancer has spread to other organs, such as the liver. **Endoscopic ultrasound (EVS)** test may be used by inserting a probe through your back passage to check your rectum.

CAT (computerised axial tomography) scans use a small amount of radiation (unlikely to harm you) to take X-rays which then examine the inside of your body through computerised three-dimensional pictures. This can help to show the size of the tumours in your colon and if the cancer has spread to other parts of your body. Like an MRI scan, you must lie still on a couch, which travels through a narrow chamber. The CT scan is painless and takes up to half an hour. To allow a particular area to be seen more clearly, you may be given a dye to drink or it is injected into you. A similar liquid will also be inserted by a small tube into your back passage. You must not eat or drink at least 4 hours before the CT scan.

PET (positron emission tomography) a mildly radioactive substance is injected into your vein and a couple of hours later you lie on a couch. The PET produces three-dimensional images of the body's metabolic and chemical activity.

PET/CT scan as in a PET scan, a mildly radioactive substance is injected into you and a CT scan takes a series of X-rays.

It can take up to a couple of weeks for the results of your tests to come through. These will then be discussed with you by a multi-disciplinary team of doctors and nurses to decide which is the best treatment in your case. Again take a friend along with you to record the main points discussed as you will no doubt forget over 80% of what you have been told. Telephone **Macmillan CancerLine**, Freephone 0808 808 2020, whose specialised cancer nurses will give you information on all aspects of cancer and recommend support groups during this difficult waiting period for test results.

Treatment

Cancer of the colon and rectum differ in their pattern of growth and their response to various treatments. Staging is used by doctors to describe the cancer size and whether it has spread beyond its original area. Sometimes the exact stage can only be known after the cancer has been removed by surgery.

Colon Cancer

The latest staging system for colon cancer is known as TNM

T indicates the size of the tumour and whether it has spread into the colon wall.

N indicates whether the cancer has spread into the surrounding lymph nodes.

M indicates whether the cancer has spread to other parts of the body, such as the liver or the lungs (secondary or metastasis).

Recurrent cancer is cancer which comes back after initial treatment.

Cancer cells seen under the microscope after a biopsy are normally graded as:

Low-grade The cancer cells are slow growing, look like normal colon cells and are less likely to spread.

Moderate, intermediate or high grade The colon cancer tumours are like to grow quickly, look abnormal and are more likely to spread.

SURGERY In most cases of colon cancer it is recommended to remove the part containing the cancer tumours and to join the two ends together. This is called anastomosis.

Hemi colostomy is when either the sigmoid colon - **sigmoid colectomy** or transverse colon - **transverse colectomy** - is removed. If the whole colon is removed, it is called **total colectomy**.

Surgery will usually leave you with a wound that goes in a straight line from just below your breast bone (sternum) to just above your pelvis.

Keyhole surgery More and more people are now having these operations by keyhole surgery, with four or five small cuts through which a laparoscope (a thin flexible tube containing a light and camera) is passed. Recovery from this operation is usually quick. Very early stages of colon cancer can sometimes be removed using an endoscope described earlier. The operation will just remove the cancer from the lining of the colon. If after examining the cancer cells they are found to be high grade, your surgeon may recommend a second operation.

Colostomy An operation often necessary when part of the colon has been removed and for some reason the two ends of the colon cannot be rejoined immediately. The upper end of the colon is brought through a surgical opening in the skin of the abdominal wall. The bowel contents pass out through the colostomy and are collected in a disposable waterproof (stoma) bag. An alternative is to wash out the bowel once or twice a day and cover the opening. In 85-90% of cases, a colostomy is only temporary, as the two ends of the colon can be rejoined later by a second operation.

Double-barrel colostomy In this operation the surgeon creates two separate stomas on the abdominal wall; one for draining the stools, the other for draining small amounts of mucous material.

Ileostomy Is an operation where the end of the intestines (ileum) is brought out onto the skin of the abdominal wall so the bowel contents can be flushed out or collected in a disposable stoma bag. As with a colostomy this is most often a temporary operation as the colon will be joined at a later date and the stoma removed. For advice, contact the Ileostomy Association helpline 0800 0184 724.

Magnetic Therapy Whatever operation you have, it has been found that scars heal much faster by using a high speed magnetic apparatus daily after the operation. This will also most likely prevent any scar tissues forming inside your body around the operation site. Very early stages of colon cancer can sometimes be removed using an endoscope as described earlier. The operation will just remove the cancer from the lining of the colon. If after examining the cancer cells they are found to be high grade your surgeon may recommend a second operation.

STOMA BAG At first it can be quite frightening to know you have got to have a stoma but trained stoma or colorectal nurses will usually discuss it with you before your operation. It will take time to get used to it but will get easier with time and practice. It would be helpful to have a close friend with you, in case you have a problem when you get home.

Make sure you have a good supply of bags and cleaning material at all times. If you get your stoma bag from your chemist, make sure to order them in good time if they do not routinely stock them. You can get small bags if you want to go swimming. Some have better draining facilites, others better filters to release air, some have softer fabric - but on the whole, they are all unprepossessing. You need a new one every couple of days. The Colostomy Association Helpline 0800 328 4257 or 0800 587 6744 will have details of local stockists which may be better for supplies.

If you are aged between 16 and 60, make sure your doctor signs a free prescription form.
It can be a big change in your life to have a stoma and you may find it very embarrassing.

Macmillan CancerLine can send you full details about coping with a colostomy or ileostomy and specialist nurses will discuss it with you on 0808 808 0121. You are not alone. It is estimated that 110,000 people are wearing a stoma bag at any one time. They were invented in 1944. Most people who wear a stoma bag say that in their experience the stoma bag is not noticeable and that you can carry on most activities including walking, cycling, driving, most sports and sex. It is advisable that you do not drink fizzy drinks including champagne; otherwise you may find that the bag will blow up like a balloon later on!

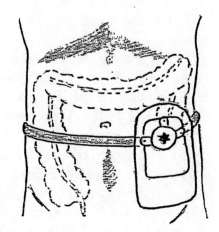

Stoma Bag

Rectal Cancer
Surgery

An anterior resection is usually used to remove tumours close to the colon and you will end up with having a similar operation to that of the colon operation.

An abdomino perineal resection is mainly used for cancer tumours in the lower end of the rectum. As the whole of the rectum and anus is removed, two operations will be performed and there will be an abdominal wound and a second wound where the anus has been closed. After this operation a permanent stoma bag will be needed.

A local or a transanal resection operation can be carried out for early stage anal cancers using an endoscope or, without an endoscope if the cancer tumour is close to the anus. If it is found to be high grade cancer a second operation will have to be carried out.

Total mesorectal excision (TME) operation involves removing the whole of the rectum including surrounding fatty tissues which contain the lymph nodes. Research has shown that a TME operation, which takes 3 to 5 hours, is a better operation than other types, reducing the risk of cancer recurring.

Chemotherapy this may be suggested if the cancer has spread to other parts of the body such as the lining of the rectum or the liver.

Erbitux is one of a class of smart cancer drugs that target tumours without damaging healthy tissues and with minimum side-effects. Erbitux used in combination with another bowel cancer drug, irinotecan, has been successful in shrinking serious cases of bowel cancer. But its high cost may result in some doctors being prevented from using the drug.

Many bowel cancer patients will now be offered a course of tablets called Xeloda (capecitabine), which is an oral form of chemotherapy for those patients who have undergone bowel cancer surgery, or it will help to shrink tumours in cases of advanced bowel cancer where patients cannot be operated on. It is claimed that Xeloda is 14% more effective in delaying or reducing the return of tumours, than current standard intravenous chemotherapy and less toxic.

Taking Xeloda will mean 20 fewer hospital visits during the patients' six months course of treatment. Hospital visits are only needed once every three weeks for blood checks and to discuss any side-effects. See chapter on Chemotherapy in Part Two.

Radiotherapy may sometimes be used to try and shrink the cancer tumours before surgery and afterwards to prevent the cancer returning. See further details under Radiotherapy.

After Surgery

If you have a major operation, you will probably be ready to go home after 10 days. But if you have keyhole surgery, you will be home within a few days.

After surgery you may have diarrhoea. Make sure you drink plenty of water. You need to experiment to find out which food suits you best. Drinking devil's claw tea may help to regulate your bowels. You may also find that your bowels pass more wind than before and cause pain. Drinking peppermint water and taking charcoal tablets may help.

It may take a long time for your body to adjust if a large part of your large bowel has been removed. Taking OxyTech tablets and/or drinking devil's claw tea can be very helpful.

Sex life after large bowel surgery the side-effects will depend upon the extent of your surgery as well as your treatment.

Most people return to a normal sex life particularly after any stoma has been removed. In men nerves responsible for erection will probably be damaged. In women the vagina may be reconstructed so that sexual adjustment must be made. Both men and women however, find that with patience and understanding, they can make changes in their sex lives that allow them to find pleasure in less conventional ways. I recommend **Macmillan CancerLine's** leaflets on 'Sexuality and Cancer'.

How to ensure a high success rate and reduce the likelihood of the cancer returning

It is most important that you take care of the BIG FOUR - avoid Geopathic Stress, destroy any microbes, mainly micro parasites, take adequate Q10 and ensure a high acid alkaline balance in your blood.

Take the necessary vitamins, minerals etc. as modern food no longer provides enough to prevent you suffering from malnutrition. Take at least 20 mcg daily of Vitamin D which is vital.

Also take enough exercise. Ideally exercise daily on a rebounder to vitalise your lymph system and help dispose of toxins from your body. Two minutes on a rebounder will double the number of white blood cells for one hour.

About 90% of people who get cancer have a thyroid gland which is out of balance. Using a MagneTech for one to two minutes daily direct will revitalise it. Do the same on the thymus, which matures your T-cells and say 20 minutes on your solar plexus where 70% of your immune system is located. Most importantly, use the MagneTech daily for 20 minutes directly on the problem area to heal it and any scar tissue.

You have got to take charge of your own health.

Case histories

The Geopathic Stress lines through a famous footballer's bed who died of bowel cancer a few years ago. At the time his cancer was diagnosed, the BIG FOUR registered as following:

Geopathic Stress	80%	(normal is 0%)
Micro Parasites	83%	(normal is 5% or less)
Q10	95%	(normal is 100%)
Acid Balance	5.2pH	(normal is 7.4pH)

Further cases

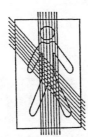

Retired Engineer
Geopathic Stress	84%
Micro Parasites	61%
Q10	81%
Acid Balance	4.6pH

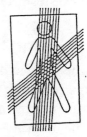

Retired Dental Nurse
Geopathic Stress	73%
Micro Parasites	82%
Q10	64%
Acid Balance	5.2pH

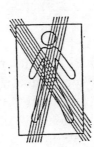

Tour Guide
Geopathic Stress	72%
Micro Parasites	84%
Q10	77%
Acid Balance	4.5pH

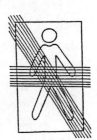

Kate
Geopathic Stress	67%
Micro Parasites	82%
Q10	73%
Acid Balance	4.4pH

BRAIN AND SPINAL CORD CANCER

Being told you have brain cancer must be terrifying, just the thought of tampering with your brain because of its role as the centre for controlling thought, emotions and feeling. The incidence of tumour of the brain, spinal cord and the rest of the central nervous system is less than 2% of all cases of cancer, but with the aid of computer assisted diagnostic methods, new surgical techniques, improved drugs and in combination with modern complementary remedies, the future treatments of brain tumours is now very much brighter.

SUMMARY

Your brain and spinal cord

The brain and spinal cord form the central nervous system, which controls much of what we do - walking, talking, breathing, digesting food, seeing, hearing, touching, tasting, smelling, thinking and memory.

The brain contains 10 million working cells. Brain tissues do not regenerate, but the brain is a remarkably adaptable organ, as one part of the brain can take over the function of a disabled or missing part.

The brain is a soft, greyish-white, spongy mass of nerves and supporting tissues enclosed inside the protective bony, three thin layers of tissue called meninges. Surrounding, cushioning and protecting the brain and spinal cord is a liquid produced by the brain called *cerebrospinal fluid.* This fluid brings nourishment from the blood to the brain and takes away waste matter. There is very little space inside the brain for expansion. While other parts of the body can contain large cancerous growths without initial detection, even a small growth inside the shell can cause serious problems.

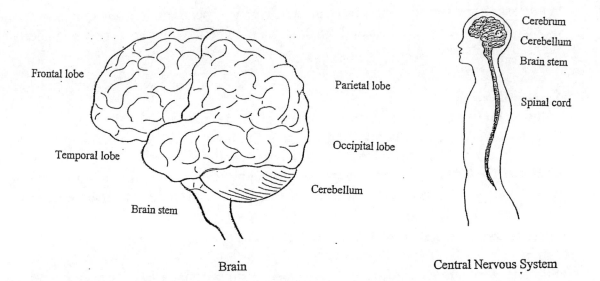

Brain   Central Nervous System

The brain has three major parts:

Cerebrum which is the largest part of the brain and fills most of the upper skull. It controls muscles, speech, emotions, thinking and learning.

Cerebellum is under the cerebrum at the back of the brain. It controls balance, and complex actions like walking and talking.

Brain stem connects the brain with the spinal cord. It controls hunger and thirst and most of the basic body functions such as blood pressure, body temperature and breathing.

Symptoms

In all types of brain tumours, except in pineal and pituitary gland tumours, the shortage of space for expansion inside the skull, may cause *raised intracranial pressure* due to a blockage in the *ventricles* (fluid which fills space in the brain), which leads to a build up of *cerebrospinal fluid* (CSF). This is the fluid which surrounds and protects the brain and spinal cord.

These may be some of the following symptoms:

- Headaches, vomiting, seizures, drowsiness, dizziness (vertigo) and ringing or buzzing in the ear.
- Loss of feeling in arms or legs, loss of smell (anosmia).
- Difficulty in swallowing (dysphasia) or with speech (dysarthria), one side muscle weakness (hemiparesis).
- Change in vision, speech, personality or memory.
- May affect nerves going to the face.
- Mental sluggishness or drowsiness.
- Uncoordinated, clumsy movement when walking (ataxic gait).

Research

Less than 5,000 people are diagnosed with brain tumours in the UK each year, of which about 350 are children. Most cases are cancer which has spread (metastasised), to the brain from other parts of the body, most commonly from cancers of the lungs, breast, kidneys and skin.

Diagnosis

In all cases of brain and spinal cord cancer, CT or MRI scans and, if possible, biopsy are carried out. In cases of pineal and pituitary gland tumours, other tests may be undertaken (see full details in Part Two).

Treatment

Will depend on your general health and the size, grade and position of the tumour. Steroid drugs may be used to reduce swelling around the tumour. If there is a build up of CSF fluid, a tube (shunt) may be inserted to draw off any excess fluid. Where possible, surgery is used to remove the tumour without damaging surrounding brain tissue. If this is not possible, radiotherapy and/or chemotherapy is often used. See latest Cyberknife treatment (page 33).

Benign and Malignant Brain Tumours

Benign

This consists of non-cancerous cells which have distinct boundaries. They can usually be removed by surgery and are not likely to return. Because the skull cannot expand to make room for the extra growth, benign brain tumours can be dangerous by pressing on sensitive areas of the brain so they may be treated as though they are malignant, even though they contain no cancer cells.

Malignant

Because malignant brain tumours are likely to grow rapidly, they are life-threatening. They may interfere with vital functions and press on or invade the surrounding tissues. A malignant brain tumour may spread to other locations in the brain or spinal cord, but seldom spreads outside the brain and spinal cord. If the tumour remains compact and does not spread, it is said to be *encapsulated.*

Types of Brain Tumours

Most brain tumours are named after the type of cells from which they developed.

Acoustic Neuroma

These are benign tumours which begin in the Schwann cells that produce the myelin which protects the hearing (acoustic) nerve in the cerebrum. It is usually a slow growing tumour on one or both sides of the brain. This type of cancer may also develop on other nerves such as the trigeminal, facial or vigal. Twice as many women get this type of cancer as men.

Symptoms The most common symptom is loss of hearing, sometimes buzzing or ringing in the ears, a feeling of fullness and pain in the ear. It can also cause numbness of half of the face. Large tumours may lead to problems in walking, e.g. walking awkwardly, stumbling and having difficulty in keeping your balance. Tumours may also affect speech, sight and can lead to headaches.

Diagnosis Your hearing will first be tested and sometimes your sense of balance. CT or MRI scans and a biopsy will also be carried out.

Treatment As acoustic neuronal tumours are often slow growing and small, no treatment may be necessary for a long time, in which case regular scans will be carried out to check for growth of the tumour.

If it is decided to treat the tumour, surgery is usually the best option. This may sometimes affect your hearing and damage facial nerves, causing problems with your eyes. Radiotherapy may be given instead of surgery.

CNS Lymphoma

The central nervous system is made up of the brain, the spinal cord and a network of nerves throughout the body.

Lymphoma is a general term for a group of cancers that develop in the lymph system which is part of the body's immune system (see details under lymphoma). CNS lymphoma is most often in the cerebrum of the brain, where it has mainly spread from high grade Non Hodgkin's Lymphoma elsewhere in the body.

Symptoms Any of those described before.

Diagnosis As above plus Lumbar puncture.

Treatment As described before.

Glioma

About half of all primary brain tumours in adults are gliomas. These tumours begin in the glia tissues, which are in the supporting tissues of the brain. Glioma is divided into the following types:

Astrocytoma is the most common type of glioma and develops from star shaped cells called *an astrocyte*. In adults, they mainly grow in the cerebrum. *Low grade astrocytoma* is a relative slow growing tumour that usually does not grow with the tissues around it. *Anaptastic astrocytoma* (Grade 3) grows more rapidly. *Glioblastoma multiform* (Grade 4) is the most malignant type and usually spreads quite quickly to other parts of the brain. It is a difficult tumour to treat and may come back after the first treatment (recurrence).

Symptoms Any of those described before

Diagnosis As described above.

Treatment As described before.

Brain stem glioma cancer occurs in the lower, stem like part of the brain where it is connected to the spinal cord and controls many vital functions. Tumours in this area are not subject to biopsy, generally cannot be removed and are treated with radiotherapy.

Ependyma is a very rare type of glioma in adults. It develops from the *epidermal cells* which line the ventricles (fluid filled space in the brain) and central canal of the spinal cord).

Symptoms, diagnoses and treatment as described before.

Oligodendroglioma develops in cells called *oligodendrocytes* which produce the fatty covering that protects nerves. This type of tumour is normally found in the frontal or temporal lobes of the cerebrum. This cancer is divided into *well differentiated tumours* (Grade 1 and 2) which are slow growing and *fast growing anaplastic oligodendroglioma*.

Symptoms, diagnosis and treatment as described before.

Mixed Glioma is a brain tumour in which two or three types of cell types - astrocytoma, ependyma or oligodendroglioma are involved.

Medullablastoma tumours are usually found in the lower part of the brain. They arise from developing nerve cells that normally do not remain in the body after birth. This cancer develops in the cerebellum in a part of the brain called the *posterior fosse*, but may spread to other parts of the brain. Very rarely it can spread to other parts of the brain or spinal cord through the CSF fluid.

Symptoms, diagnosis and treatment as described before, but diagnosis may include lumbar puncture and a myelogram to see if the cancer has spread to the spinal cord.

Meningioma is a common tumour and accounts for 20% of adult primary brain tumours and usually develops in women between the age of 30 and 50. A meningioma is a tumour of the *meninges* which are the protective membranes around the brain and spinal cord. Most meningoma tumours are benign. Because they grow very slowly, the brain may initially be able to adjust to their presence, but gradually it can lead to a build up of *cerebrospinal fluid* (CSF) or swelling around the tumour itself.

Symptoms - Headaches, sickness, visual problems, changes in behaviour and personality and epileptic fits. Meningiomas can grow in different parts of the brain causing symptoms related to that part of the brain. A tumour in the *frontal lobe* may cause change in personality and mood. There may also be paralysis on one side of the body (*hemi paresis*). A tumour in the *parietal lobe* of the brain may affect writing etc. and paralysis on one side. Tumours in the *temporal lobe* of the brain may cause memory loss and problems with co-ordination.

Diagnosis As described before plus an angiogram.

Treatment As described before. Where possible, surgery is the main treatment and, in many cases, the tumour can be removed completely with no complications as it is normally easily accessible. If the position of a tumour makes it impossible or too risky to remove surgically, radiotherapy may be used. Chemotherapy is very seldom used for meningioma.

Pineal Tumours

These tumours occur in or around the pineal gland, a tiny organ near the centre of the brain. The tumour may be slow growing *(pineacytoma)* or fast growing *(pineablastoma)*. Only 1% of these tumours are in the pineal region.

The most common pineal tumour is *germinoma* which develops from germ cells (cells in a very early stage of development). Other types of pineal tumours include *astrocytomas, teratomas and meningiomas.*

Diagnosis In addition to the usual tests, blood tests may be carried out for hormone levels, particularly as the pineal gland is affected. Lumbar puncture-this last test cannot be carried out if there is raised intracranial pressure so it will probably be done later on in your treatment.

Treatment Surgery is often difficult as the pineal region is at the centre of the brain. However, if possible, surgery is the first form of treatment to remove as much of the pineal tumour without damaging the surrounding brain tissue. Radiotherapy and chemotherapy are often used for germinoma tumours. Radiotherapy is sometimes given after surgery to destroy any remaining cancer cells or if there are signs that the cancer has spread to the spine.

Pituitary Gland Tumours

The pituitary gland is a small oval shaped gland at the base of the brain below the optic nerve (the nerve which leads to and from the eye). Nearly 10% of brain tumours are pituitary tumours and are mostly found in young or middle aged adults. They are nearly all benign and do not spread. Sometimes called *adenomas*, the pituitary gland produces hormones which control and regulate the other glands in the body. The pituitary gland has two parts:

Anterior (at the front), produce hormones which control and stimulate growth, the adrenal glands, thyroid glands, the production of breast milk after childbirth and the ovaries of women and the testes in men.

Posterior (at the back), produce hormones which stimulate the contraction of the womb during childbirth and the production of milk for breast feeding. It also controls the hormones which reduces the amount of urine produced by the kidneys.

<u>Symptoms</u> may put pressure on the optic nerve which can cause headaches and sight problems. Also it can change the normal hormone levels, leading to problems with the above glands etc. It can also lead to cessation of monthly periods and a reduction of the amount of breast milk. In men it may include impotence - loss of ability to have an erection. Infertility may affect both women and men. Often pituitary tumours may be discovered during tests for infertility. The tumour can cause excess growth hormones, causing enlargement of the hands and feet. The overproduction of hormones in the anterior part of the pituitary gland can produce *moon face*, weight gain, depression and an increase in facial hair in women.

<u>Diagnosis</u> Apart from CT and MRI scans, eye tests will be carried out to detect any pressure on the optic nerve and to test your range of vision.

<u>Treatment</u> The most common treatment is surgery where the aim is to remove the tumour leaving as much of the pituitary gland behind. To reach the pituitary gland, usually a small hole is cut on the inside of the roof of the nose or a small opening is made under the upper lip. Recovery after surgery is much quicker than from other brain tumour operations. In some cases the whole gland needs to be removed, in which case hormone replacement will have to be taken from then on.

Secondary Brain Tumours

The majority of malignant brain tumours are cancer cells, which have broken away from the *primary tumours* elsewhere in the body and travelled through the blood or the lymphatic system to the brain. The most likely types to spread to the brain are cancer of the lung, breast, large bowel, kidney and skin. When the cells from a biopsy are examined under a microscope, secondary cancer cells may look like cancer cells from the primary tumour i.e. like breast cancer rather than brain cells for example:

When there is more than one tumour in the brain, it is most likely that they are secondary cancer tumours as primary brain tumours usually remain and enlarge in one place.

If there is a history of cancer elsewhere in the body, it is normally a secondary brain tumour. Other secondary tumours may be found elsewhere in the body when the body is scanned.

<u>Symptoms, diagnosis and treatment</u> as described before.

Spinal Cord Tumours

The spinal cord starts at the bottom of the brain stem and runs down the centre of the spine almost to its base. It connects the brain to most of the body's nerves, carrying both incoming and outgoing messages. The spinal cord is protected by the bones in the spinal column (vertebrae). It is covered by three membranes (meninges) and has fluid to cushion it.

The most common type of primary spinal cord tumours are those similar to those in the brain, but the most common cancers in the spinal cord have metastasised from other parts of the body.

<u>Symptoms</u> This depends on where the tumour is located. If the symptom is pain, it is usually worse when you cough or strain. Tumours may reduce the flow of communication between the brain and the body, similar to spinal cord injuries. Some symptoms may mimic other diseases like multiple sclerosis, cervical disc disease or sciatica, making diagnosis difficult.

<u>Diagnosis</u> CT or MRI scan and analysing the spinal fluid.

<u>Treatment</u> The most common treatment is surgery. If the tumour cannot completely be removed, radiotherapy and or chemotherapy may be used.

How to ensure a high success rate and reduce the likelihood of the cancer returning

It is most important that you take care of the BIG FOUR - avoid Geopathic Stress, destroy any microbes, mainly micro parasites, take adequate Q10 and ensure a high acid alkaline balance in your blood.

Take the necessary vitamins, minerals etc. as modern food no longer provides enough to prevent you suffering from malnutrition. Take at least 20 mcg daily of Vitamin D which is vital.

Also take enough exercise. Ideally exercise daily on a rebounder to vitalise your lymph system and help dispose of toxins from your body. Two minutes on a rebounder will double the number of white blood cells for one hour.

About 90% of people who get cancer have a thyroid gland which is out of balance. Using a MagneTech for one to two minutes daily direct will revitalise it. Do the same on the thymus, which matures your T-cells and say 20 minutes on your solar plexus where 70% of your immune system is located. Most importantly, use the MagneTech daily for 20 minutes directly on the problem area to heal it and any scar tissue.

You have got to take charge of your own health.

Case Histories

John, world champion rally car driver, was given three weeks to live with a cancerous brain tumour. As he was in a private North London hospital, the doctors allowed two high powered fast spinning magnetic apparatus to be used direct where the tumours were on his head for 20 minutes each day. We lost contact with John, but we know he lived for another two years. John's bed was also moved out of Geopathic Stress.

At the time John was diagnosed with a brain tumour.

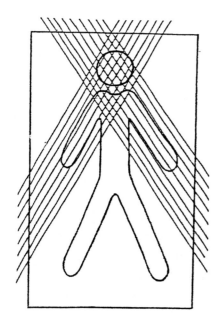

		(normal is)
Geopathic Stress	82%	(0%)
Micro Parasites	80%	(5% or less)
Q10	67%	(100%)
Acid Alkaline Balance	5.2pH	(7.4pH)
Vitamin D	16ng/lm	(35 ng/lm)

Geopathic Stress Lines under John's bed

KIDNEY CANCER (Renal cancer)

Kidney cancer is sometimes difficult to diagnose as you may have no specific symptoms and early detection may only be done as a result of having an abdominal ultrasound. Orthodox treatment is reasonably effective, particularly in conjunction with complementary treatment.

SUMMARY
- Symptoms
- Research
- Who is most likely to get kidney cancer?
- Your kidney
- Diagnosis
- Types of cancer
- Treatment
- How to ensure a higher success rate and reduce the likelihood of the cancer returning

Symptoms
A pain in the side that does not go away. Blood in urine. Feeling a lump or mass in the kidney region. Weight loss. Fatigue, Anaemia (deficiency of red cells or haemoglobin in the blood resulting in pallor or weariness). Recurring fevers. General feeling of poor health. Most people with any of the above symptoms will not have cancer of the kidneys. Sometimes cancer of the kidneys will be diagnosed following a scan carried out for a different reason.

Research
About 6,500 people in the UK are diagnosed with kidney cancer each year. The five year average survival rate, taking age into account, is about 45% both for men and women, unless a change of life-style is carried out which can make a vast difference to survival rate. Kidney tumours are getting more common. Since 1975, the incidence has doubled in both men and women over 65. This could have something to do with increased levels of obesity, but I firmly believe it is because Geopathic Stress has become many times stronger during this period.

Who is most likely to get kidney cancer?

- Smokers
- People who are overweight
- Long-term dialysis users
- Women treated with radiation for disorders of the uterus
- People who have worked with asbestos
- Affects more men than women and occurs most commonly in middle-age and older people

Your kidney

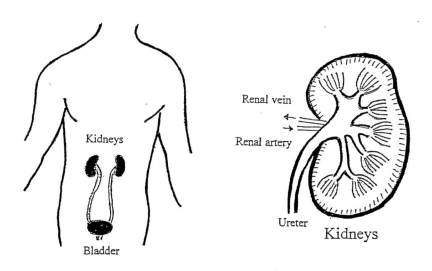

The kidneys are two bean-shape organs behind the abdomen. There is one on each side of the spine just below the liver and spleen. Weighing about 150g each, they are about 11 cm long and 5 cm thick. An adrenal gland is located on top of each kidney. The kidneys are encased in a membrane called a capsule. Inside each kidney are tiny tubules that filter and clean the blood, extracting the waste products and urine. The kidneys return to the circulating blood those substances that are necessary for normal chemical balance. Around 1800 litres of blood are pumped through the kidneys each day. The kidneys also make important hormones, such as erythropoietin (EPO) which helps regulate the formation of new red blood cells in the bone marrow. Overall, the role of the kidneys is to monitor the body's internal environment, keeping fluids and chemicals in balance. The centre part of each kidney is hollow and receives the body fluids. The urine, a sterile solution of varying concentration, leaves the kidneys and passes down the urether, a long tube, into the bladder.

Types of kidney cancer

The most common kidney cancer (about 90%) is **renal cell cancer (RCC)** or sometimes called **renal adenocarcinoma.**

A rare type of kidney cancer is **transitional cell cancer** which affects the renal pelvis. It is similar to cancer that occurs in the bladder and is often treated like bladder cancer. In children, mainly under 4, the most common kind of kidney cancer is called Wilm's tumour. Its treatment is different from adult cancer (see chapter on children's cancer).

Diagnosis

- Complete history and physical examination
- Blood and urine test
- IVU or VP (intravenous pologram). A dye is injected into a vein in your arm which travels through your blood stream to your kidneys. An X-ray screen can detect the dye passing through your kidney and can pick up any abnormalities.
- CT (computerised tomography) scan builds up a three-dimensional picture of the inside of your body.
- Ultrasound scan. Biopsy. A needle is inserted through your skin and muscle into your kidney guided while having a CT scan. The sample is examined under a microscope.
- MRI. Magnetic Resonance Imaging - sometimes a dye is injected into a vein in the arm to show a clearer image of the kidney.
- Angiogram - inserting a fine soft tube into the kidney and injecting a contrasting fluid, which shows any tumours on a TV image intensifier or rapid sequence X-ray picture.

Staging

The stage of cancer is a term used to describe the cancer size and whether it has spread beyond its original site. Knowing the extent of the cancer and grade helps the doctor to decide on the most appropriate treatment.

The commonly used stage system for cancer of the kidneys is:

Stage 1 The tumour is found only within the kidney and is less than 7 cm in size. It has not spread to nearby tissues, lymph nodes or other organs.

Stage 2 The tumour is larger than 7 cm in size, but has not spread beyond the outer layer (capsule) of the kidney.

Stage 3 The tumour has begun to spread outside the kidneys. It may have spread into the main blood vessels that are close to the kidneys (the renal vein or the inferior vena cava); the lymph nodes around the kidney; or into the fat that surrounds the kidneys. The adrenal gland, which is on top of the kidneys, may also be affected.

Stage 4 The tumour has spread either to nearby organs, such as the bowel or to parts of the body further away from the kidney, such as the lungs or the brain.

Grading

Grading refers to the appearance of the cancer cells under the microscope. The grading gives an idea of how quickly the cancer may develop. Grading systems usually use three grades:

1. Low-grade the cancer cells look very like the normal cells of the kidney. They are usually slow-growing and are less likely to spread.
2. Moderate-grade the cancer cells look abnormal.
3. High-grade the cancer cells look very abnormal. They are likely to grow more quickly and are more likely to spread.

Treatment
Surgery
Nephrectomy - Removal of the affected kidney and the surrounding tissue. Removal of a kidney is a big operation and the patient needs to be reasonably fit, so surgery may not be possible for everyone.

Partial nephrectomy entails only removing part of the kidney surrounding the tumour, if the tumour is small.

Patients who have open surgery have to stay in hospital for around ten days and may need 12 weeks to recover. With **keyhole** or **laparoscopic** surgery, patients can be in and out of hospital in less than two days and the patient is left with a much smaller wound. (One surgeon who carries out a keyhole operation is Neil Barber, Consultant Urologist at Frimley Park Hospital, Surrey).

Robotic Surgery now enables very accurate keyhole surgery to be carried out (see full details under surgery Part Two).

Cryosurgery
Cryosurgery, or Targeted Cryo-ablation of the kidney (TCAK) involves inserting under ultrasound guidance, a number of probes into the kidney. A gas (e.g. Argon) is passed down these probes under pressure and, at the tips, it is allowed to expand and flow back out through the other channels of the probes.

This rapid expansion of the gas at the tips causes a significant cooling effect, known as the Joule-Thompson effect. An ice ball is formed which destroys the tissues and tumour in close proximity at the tips. By suitable positioning of these probes the whole tumour or kidney is treated. The process often also involves the use of a second gas (e.g. helium) to actively thaw the area. Several freeze/thaw cycles may be carried out. Additional probes are used to measure the temperature to ensure adequate control.

Cryosurgery is often suitable for those with localised tumours, where the cancer is contained within the liver and when radiotherapy has failed but the cancer is still in the kidney.

Trans-rectal ultrasound is used for insertion and guidance of the five to eight needles. This is done under general or spinal anaesthetic and lasts about 1-2 hours. You will normally be in hospital for 2-3 days after treatment, but with a catheter in place for a couple of weeks.

It is a relatively non-invasive technique with minimal blood loss. There is a short recovery time and the operation can be repeated if not totally successful.

Immunotherapy or Biological therapy
This treatment stimulates the immune system to fight the cancer itself by using substances found naturally in the body, which can be synthesised in the laboratory and used in large quantities to treat cancer and prevent it returning after surgery.

Immunotherapy is proven to be especially effective against kidney cancer that has either spread to other parts of the body or is at high risk of returning.

The treatment has been around for over a decade, but is still in its trial phases because results are mixed and unpredictable.

The type of treatment is called interferon alpha-Za. It is injected by yourself or a friend into your stomach or at the top of the leg three times a week. A free home nurse support service is usually at hand to help new patients with their first few injections. Ask your doctor about the side-effects expected. Often taking a paracetamol tablet after injecting yourself and rest, will reduce most of the side-effects.

Hormonal Treatment

The hormone progesterone may help to control cancer cells that have spread beyond the kidney and in some cases may shrink the cancer. Progesterone is taken daily in tablet form. Any side effects are usually mild.

Radiotherapy

Radiotherapy is only helpful in relatively small numbers of people with kidney cancer.

Chemotherapy

Chemotherapy has not shown to be helpful in treating kidney cancer.

Magnetic Therapy

Very powerful magnetic therapy produced by spinning, strong magnets has been used for two decades for treating cancer with no side-effects. I do not know of any cases where this therapy has been used to treat kidney cancer, but there are no reasons why strong magnetic therapy should not help in kidney cancer cases. I know of cancer cases where strong magnet therapy has been a great help in treating cancer tumours in the pancreas, lungs, throat, spine and leg bone.

How to ensure a high success rate and reduce the likelihood of the cancer returning

It is most important that you take care of the BIG FOUR - avoid Geopathic Stress, destroy any microbes, mainly micro parasites, take adequate Q10 and ensure a high acid alkaline balance in your blood.

Take the necessary vitamins, minerals etc. as modern food no longer provides enough to prevent you suffering from malnutrition. Take at least 20 mcg daily of Vitamin D which is vital.

Also take enough exercise. Ideally exercise daily on a rebounder to vitalise your lymph system and help dispose of toxins from your body. Two minutes on a rebounder will double the number of white blood cells for one hour.

About 90% of people who get cancer have a thyroid gland which is out of balance. Using a MagneTech for one to two minutes daily direct will revitalise it. Do the same on the thymus, which matures your T-cells and say 20 minutes on your solar plexus where 70% of your immune system is located. Most importantly, use the MagneTech daily for 20 minutes directly on the problem area to heal it and any scar tissue.

You have got to take charge of your own health.

LEUKAEMIA

Many think of Leukaemia as a children's disease, but in fact fewer than ten per cent who get leukaemia are children. See separate chapter under 'Children's Cancer' for childhood leukaemia.

The survival rate from leukaemia has increased dramatically over the last thirty years and even more if complementary treatment and change of lifestyle are carried out at the same time, including taking account of the BIG FOUR.

SUMMARY
- **Leukaemia**
- **Symptoms**
- **Research**
- **Who is most likely to get leukaemia?**
- **Diagnosis**
- **Treatment**
- **More details on blood cells**
- **How to ensure a higher success rate and reduce the likelihood of the cancer returning**

Leukaemia

Leukaemia is a cancer of the white blood cells. All blood cells are produced in the bone marrow. Bone marrow is the spongy substance at the core of the main bones in the body - the spine, pelvis, upper arms, legs, ribs and skull.

Bone marrow (more details at the end of this chapter) contains and produces:
- Red blood cells which carry oxygen around the body.
- White blood cells which help fight infection.
- Platelets which help the blood clot and control bleeding.

There are two different types of white cells - lymphocytes and myeloid cells. These white blood cells work together to fight infection. Normally, white blood cells repair and reproduce themselves in an orderly and controlled way. In leukaemia, the process spirals out of control and the cells continue to divide but do not mature.

These immature dividing cells fill up the bone marrow and stop it from making healthy bone marrow and blood cells. As the leukaemia cells are not mature, they cannot work properly. This leads to an increased risk of infection because the bone marrow cannot make enough healthy white blood cells.

There are four main types of leukaemia:
Acute lymphoblast (ALL)
Acute myeloid (AML)
Chronic lymphoblast (CLL)
Chronic myeloid (CML)

ALL are cancers of the immature lymphocytes called lymphoblasts or blast cells. There are two different types of lymphocytes - T-cells and B-cells (see further details in chapter on immune system). Often the leukaemia occurs at a very early stage in the immature lymphocytes, before they have developed as far a becoming either T-cells or B-cells. However, if the cells have developed this far before becoming leukaemia, the type of leukaemia may be known as T-cell or B-cell leukaemia.

AML is an overproduction of immature myeloid white blood cells (blast cells). Cells which have started to show some of the features of myeloid cells and are said to show some *differentiation.* Cells which do not show signs of becoming a particular type of white blood cell are known as *undifferentiated.*

There are different sub-types of AML depending upon exactly which type of cell has become leukaemia, at what stage of development *(maturation)* the cells are and whether the cells are *differentiated.* Knowing the sub-type of AML is important as it helps decide on the best treatment.

Symptoms
As the leukaemia cells multiply in the bone marrow, the production of normal blood cells is reduced. You may therefore become tired and lethargic due to anaemia, which is caused by lack of red blood cells. Tendency to bleed or bruise easily, shortness of breath, bone or joint pains, frequent infections, abdominal pain or swelling. The spleen is quite often enlarged, which may cause some discomfort in the upper left part of the abdomen, particularly when you bend over or exercise or it may give you a feeling of fullness in your stomach soon after eating a relatively small meal. Sometimes tiny red dots or purple spots on the skin. Also swollen lymph glands. Marked sweating, particularly at night. You may lose some weight with or without a loss of appetite. If the central nervous system is affected, headaches, blurred vision, confusion and unexplained fever may occur.

Research
About 6,800 new leukaemia cases are diagnosed each year in the UK, with over 4,000 deaths. Leukaemia is more common in people over 50 with more men diagnosed than women.

Who is most likely to get leukaemia?
- Some patients who have had radiotherapy and chemotherapy, thereby weakening their immune system.
- People who have long term exposure to certain chemicals and drugs, such as benzene, chlorambucil and chemotherapy drugs.
- I have not come across a case of leukaemia where the person was not sleeping in a Geopathic Stress place, with the Geopathic Stress lines nearly always covering the whole bed. In most cases, the person was low in Q10, high in micro parasites and had a low acid/alkaline balance.
- Unhealthy diet and lack of exercise can also be a contributing factor.

Diagnosis

Blood tests usually show low numbers of normal white blood cells and abnormal leukaemia cells. A sample of bone marrow is needed to confirm the diagnosis. A lumbar puncture is carried out to see if the spinal fluid has any leukaemia cells. A chest X-ray is also done, which will show if there are any enlarged glands in the chest. Other tests may be necessary depending on the symptoms. These tests will help to identify the precise type of leukaemia.

Treatment

The main treatment for leukaemia is usually a combination of chemotherapy drugs. The aim is to destroy the leukaemia cell, so the bone marrow can work normally again.

The initial treatment nearly always involves two courses (or cycles) of chemotherapy drugs. A bone marrow test is taken at the end of the treatment to check if you are in remission i.e.there is no evidence of leukaemia.

If there are no signs of leukaemia cells in the blood or bone marrow, further chemotherapy treatment is given to be on the safe side and to prevent the cancer returning.

If the initial cycles of chemotherapy treatment did not succeed in destroying the leukaemia cells, or if there is a relapse (1 in 5 have a relapse), even stronger chemotherapy and often a bone marrow transplant is needed. This may involve up to three months in isolation in hospital. 1 in 4 members of a family will be a suitable donor for bone marrow. The bone marrow is usually extracted from the donor's hip bone and injected into the patient's spine, so the patient's blood can start producing cancer free blood.

More details on blood cells

There are three major types of cells in the blood. Red blood cells (erythrocytes), white blood cells (leukocytes) and platelets (thrombocytes). All of these cells are produced by the stem cells in the bone marrow. Most blood cells mature in the bone marrow, but some also mature in the thymus, spleen, lymph nodes and tonsils. After maturing, the adult cells slowly seep into the blood vessels and become part of the blood.

Red blood cells carry oxygen from the lungs to the other cells in your body and bring back waste products or carbon dioxide. A lack of red blood cells makes it difficult for cells to absorb oxygen. This condition is called anaemia and results in weakness, lack of energy, dizziness, headache and irritability. Red blood cell counts are part of the blood counts monitored in blood tests.

White blood cells are the main components of the immune system. Their primary role is to fight infection. There is normally only about one white blood cell for every five hundred red blood cells. If an infection enters your body, the number may increase dramatically. If the white blood cells count is abnormally low, your chance of fighting an infection is very much reduced.

See separate chapter on immune system.

Platelets are essential in the clotting process. Checking the platelet count is part of the testing procedure for those who are suspected of having or who have leukaemia. An abnormally low platelet count (called thrombocytopenia) may result in excessive bleeding from wounds or in mucous membranes, skin or other tissues.

How to ensure a high success rate and reduce the likelihood of the cancer returning

It is most important that you take care of the BIG FOUR - avoid Geopathic Stress, destroy any microbes, mainly micro parasites, take adequate Q10 and ensure a high acid alkaline balance in your blood.

Take the necessary vitamins, minerals etc. as modern food no longer provides enough to prevent you suffering from malnutrition. Take at least 20 mcg daily of Vitamin D which is vital.

Also take enough exercise. Ideally exercise daily on a rebounder to vitalise your lymph system and help dispose of toxins from your body. Two minutes on a rebounder will double the number of white blood cells for one hour.

About 90% of people who get cancer have a thyroid gland which is out of balance. Using a MagneTech for one to two minutes daily direct will revitalise it. Do the same on the thymus, which matures your T-cells and say 20 minutes on your solar plexus where 70% of your immune system is located. Also use the MagneTech daily for 20 minutes under your feet to revitalise your body through your body's meridians.

You have got to take charge of your own health.

LIVER CANCER

Cancer originating in the liver is rare in the UK but secondary liver cancer is very common. Usually the tumour has spread from the lungs, the breast, the prostate gland, the large intestine (colon) or the womb (uterus). Several orthodox treatments are successful particularly if complimentary remedies are incorporated at the same time.

SUMMARY
- **Symptoms**
- **Research**
- **Who is most likely to get liver cancer?**
- **Your liver**
- **Diagnosis**
- **Treatments**
- **How to ensure a higher success rate and reduce the likelihood of the cancer returning**

Symptoms
Discomfort in the upper abdomen on the right side, which becomes more acute with deep breathing. A hard lump just below the rib cage on the right side. Abdominal swelling. Pain around the right shoulder blade. Feeling full or bloated. Episodes of unexplained fever and nausea. Jaundice, which means that the skin and eyes look yellowish and urine is dark.

Research
Primary liver cancer is rare in the UK but comparatively common in the tropics, where it is believed to be due to two factors - chronic hepatitis B infection and ingestion of food such as nuts and grains contaminated with the fungus aspergillus flavus, which produces the poison aflatoxin. The great majority of people who develop primary liver cancer have liver cirrhosis (chronic liver disease marked by degeneration of cells, inflammation and thickening of tissue) most are males, many of them alcoholics.

Who is most likely to get liver cancer?
- People who have cancer elsewhere in the body which has spread as secondary cancer to the liver (at present thousands of bowel cancer patients die each year in the UK of liver cancer).
- Men (twice as likely as women) over 60.
- People who have a chronic infection from hepatitis B or C.
- People who have cirrhosis of the liver.

- Alcoholics.
- People who have been exposed to aflatoxin.
- People who have one or more of the above and who are Geopathic Stressed, high in micro parasites, low in Q10 and have very acidic blood.

Your liver

Your liver is the largest organ in your body and lies behind the ribs to the right side of your stomach. Your liver has two parts, a large right lobe and a small left lobe. Your liver performs many complex functions. It breaks down worn-out red blood cells and converts them into bile, regulates the level of many hormones, stores sugar and regulates the amount which circulates in the blood. It controls the metabolism of cholesterol and stores vitamins A, D, E and K. It also converts the lower co-enzyme Q in food into Q10 which is the sparking-plug for every cell in the body.

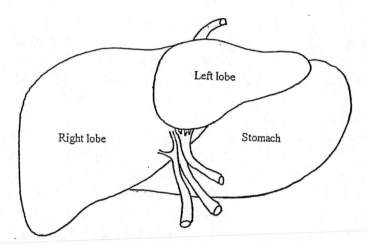

Diagnosis

There are many tests to diagnose liver cancer.

- Complete history and physical examination.
- Blood and urine test.
- IVU or VP (intravenous pologram). A dye is injected into a vein in your arm which travels through the blood stream to your liver. An X-ray screen can detect the dye passing through your liver and can pick up any abnormalities.
- CT (computerised tomography) scan builds up a three-dimensional picture of the inside of your body.
- Ultrasound scan.
- Biopsy. A needle is inserted through your skin and muscle, into your liver guided while having a CT scan. The sample is examined under a microscope.
- MRI (magnetic resonance imaging) - sometimes a dye is injected into a vein in the arm to show a clearer image of the liver.
- Angiogram - inserting a fine soft tube into the liver and injecting a contrasting fluid, which shows any tumours on a TV image intensifier or rapid sequence X-ray picture.
- AFP Blood tests such as alpha fetoprotein and liver function tests are also carried.

Treatment

Surgery

If you have localised liver cancer you may have a hepatectomy, an operation which can remove up to two thirds of your liver. Your liver is the only organ which grows back to full size. This is a major operation and it can take a long time to recover.

The biggest problem with liver surgery is blood loss which can be so great that the patient cannot be transfused quickly enough. However the recently developed **Habib Resection Device** delivers strong radio waves into the tissue surrounding a tumour via a series of electrodes. The heat they deliver dries and seals off blood vessels within 40 seconds and the surgeon can then safely remove a tumour without having to worry about stemming major blood loss and having to transfuse huge amounts of blood. In normal liver surgery as much as 20 pints of blood can be lost, but with Professor Nagy Habib's, (Head of Liver Services at Hammersmith Hospital, London) ground breaking machine, barely a thimbleful of the patient's blood is lost. The hand-held machine only costs about £1,600 and has now benefited more than 100 patients in the USA and the UK. Often patients are home about five days after surgery.

Radio Frequency Ablation (RFA)

If the position of the tumour makes surgery impossible, for example, if it involves removing too much of the liver or if it is on an artery or vein, also if the patient cannot cope with surgery, the idea is to attack the tumour with high radio frequency ablation.

A CT scan is taken to establish the size and shape of the tumour.

First a fine needle is inserted into the tumour using ultrasound for accurate guidance. Through the needle, alcohol is injected into the liver reducing the blood flow to the area. After removing the needle, an electrode is inserted. Radio frequency waves (like those used in microwave ovens) are passed through the electrode into the tumour heating it to 60°C, in effect cooking it. Throughout the cooking procedure, chilled saline solution is flushed through the electrodes to stop them becoming too hot and to ensure the tumour is 'cooked' evenly. It also ensures the radio frequency penetrates deeper and can treat a large area. Treating an area of 3 cm takes about 12 minutes. If the tumour is bigger the electrodes can be moved slightly to 'cook' the neighbouring area. This procedure can be carried out quickly with the minimum of fuss. No general anaesthetic is needed and you can go home the same day or following morning.

A few days afterwards you return to the hospital for an examination. Some harmless dye is injected into your veins, which is carried to your liver. You then have a CT scan. Treated tissue does not take up the dye because all the cells have been destroyed, but the living tumours do. If the tumour looks dark grey it is cooked. It if looks light it is still raw and you may need another treatment.

You will be asked to return for more CT scans just to make sure the cancer does not come back. It if does the area can be treated again.

This treatment has been carried out successfully in the USA and Europe for many years and for several years at St. Bartholomew's Hospital in Smithfields in London and at The Royal London Hospital in Whitechapel.

I believe RFA will eventually take over from surgery as it is far less traumatic and recovery is quick.

Laser

Other ways of using heat includes using laser (an intense beam of light).

Percutaneous ethanol injections

Using a small needle, your doctor will put alcohol (ethanol) directly into your liver to kill the cancer cells. This may need to be done once or twice a week over a period, either as an outpatient or in hospital. You may have a fever and pain after having this injection.

Chemotherapy direct into the liver

Chemotherapy drugs are delivered directly into the liver. Another option is to have a small pump implanted to give you continuous chemotherapy.

Cryosurgery

Cryosurgery, or targeted cyro-ablation of the liver (TCAL) involves inserting, under ultrasound guidance, a number of probes into the liver. A gas (e.g. Argon) is passed down these probes under pressure and, at the tips, it is allowed to expand and flow back out through the other channels of the probes.

This rapid expansion of the gas at the tips causes a significant cooling effect, known as the Joule-Thompson effect. An ice ball is formed which destroys the tissues and tumour in close proximity at the tips. By suitable positioning of these probes, the whole tumour or liver is treated. The process often also involves the use of a second gas (e.g. helium) to actively thaw the area. Several freeze/thaw cycles may be used. Additional probes are used to measure the temperature to ensure adequate control.

Cryosurgery is often suitable for those with localised tumours where the cancer is contained within the liver and when radiotherapy has failed, but the cancer is still in the liver.

Trans-rectal ultrasound is used for insertion and guidance of the five to eight needles. This is carried out under general or spinal anaesthetic and lasts about 1-2 hours. You will normally be in hospital for 2-3 days after treatment, but with a catheter in place for a couple of weeks.

It is a relatively non-invasive technique with minimal blood loss. There is a short recovery time and the operation can be repeated if not totally successful.

How to ensure a high success rate and reduce the likelihood of the cancer returning

It is most important that you take care of the BIG FOUR - avoid Geopathic Stress, destroy any microbes, mainly micro parasites, take adequate Q10 and ensure a high acid alkaline balance in your blood.

Take the necessary vitamins, minerals etc. as modern food no longer provides enough to prevent you suffering from malnutrition. Take at least 20 mcg daily of Vitamin D which is vital.

Also take enough exercise. Ideally exercise daily on a rebounder to vitalise your lymph system and help dispose of toxins from your body. Two minutes on a rebounder will double the number of white blood cells for one hour.

About 90% of people who get cancer have a thyroid gland which is out of balance. Using a MagneTech for one to two minutes daily direct will revitalise it. Do the same on the thymus, which matures your T-cells and say 20 minutes on your solar plexus where 70% of your immune system is located. Most importantly, use the MagneTech daily for 20 minutes directly on the problem area to heal it and any scar tissue.

You have got to take charge of your own health.

LUNG CANCER

The UK is ranked eleventh in Europe in percentage of people with lung cancer alive after diagnosed, due to the length of time to be diagnosed, scanned and treated. Most people diagnosed have been smokers, but survival rates can be improved with powerful complementary remedies, which have no adverse side-effects.

SUMMARY

Symptoms
Research
Who is most likely to get lung cancer?
Tobacco and smoking
Your Lungs
Diagnosis
Types of Lung Cancer
Treatment
How to ensure higher success rate and reduce the likelihood of the cancer returning
New suggested treatment
Case Histories

Symptoms

Wheezing, 'smoker's cough' persisting for months or years. Increased, sometimes blood-stained, sputum [1]. Persistent ache in the chest. Congestion in lungs. Enlarged lymph nodes in neck, loss of the voice due to affecting the nerves to the voice box (larynx), weight loss.

Research

Over 38,000 people will be diagnosed with lung cancer in the UK each year. More people die of lung cancer than of any other cancer, with the second lowest 5 year survival rate. Over 90% will die within one year. In Japan people smoke 3 times as many cigarettes as the UK, but unfortunately lung cancer is much higher in the UK, so smoking is not the only cause.

Who is most likely to get Lung Cancer?

80% of sufferers are smokers.
Marijuana and crack-cocaine smokers.
People between 50 and 70 years of age.
Workers in toxic environments.
People whose lungs have been scarred due to lung infection, tuberculosis and other chronic lung disease.
People deficient in Vitamin A and D.
People who are affected by the BIG FOUR.

[1] Sputum = a mixture of saliva and mucus coughed up

Tobacco & Smoking

About 30% of cancer deaths can be attributed to tobacco smoke. Smoking has been linked to cancers of the lungs, head and neck, mouth, throat, vocal cords, bladder, kidneys, stomach, cervix and pancreas as well as leukaemia.

Research has shown than women are more vulnerable to lung cancer than men and tend to be diagnosed at a younger age - even though they had smoked fewer cigarettes - possibly because nicotine triggers a gene which drives cancer growth.

Over 2000 chemical compounds are generated by tobacco smoke and many of them are poisonous. During smoking the following is released.

> Carbon monoxide, reducing the oxygen to organs such as the brain, lungs and heart.
> Tar leading to cancer-causing chemicals
> Nicotine, an alkaloid found in tobacco, is not only addictive but also acts as a cancer promoter making it easier for cancer cells of all types to spread throughout the body.

In addition, smoking tends to reduce levels of Vitamin C and several other antioxidants. If it is impossible for you to stop, you may consider smoking American spirit cigarettes, which contain only tobacco, not the hundreds of chemicals that are put into ordinary cigarettes - and therefore does you about 80% less harm. Alternatively smoke Barlites 'electronic smoking' device which it is claimed tastes like real cigarettes, but has no tobacco, can be smoked anywhere and saves you 75% on the cost of real cigarettes.

Passive Smoking

Whilst it should not be ruled out completely, I believe the dangers of passive smoking were exaggerated to get anti-smoking legislation passed through Parliament. Of course you should not smoke near other people, particularly near children, the unwell and the elderly. Most non-smokers find it unpleasant; babies and young children's lungs cannot cope with smokers fumes and asthmatics condition is further impaired in a smoked-filled environment, but if you are Geopathically stressed you could be seriously affected.

Your Lungs

The main organ of the *respiratory system*. The two lungs in your chest, supply the body with the oxygen needed for *aerobic* metabolism and eliminate the waste product carbon dioxide.

When you breathe in, air passes from your nose or mouth through the windpipe (*trachea*) into one of the two airways (*bronchi*), which enter the lungs. These airways divide to form smaller tubes, at the end of which are millions of tiny sacs. It is here that the oxygen is absorbed from the air and passed into the bloodstream, to be circulated around your body. Your lungs are surrounded by a protective lining that consists of two membranes called the *pleura*.

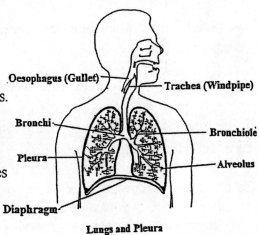

Lungs and Pleura

Diagnosis

It is often very difficult to diagnose cancer in its early stages. The most common tests are chest X-Rays, CAT (computer tomography) scan, MRI (magnetic resonance imagining) scan, biopsy or bronchoscopy (a narrow, flexible, fibre-optic tube which is introduced through the mouth and guided into the lungs. A light is shone down the tube allowing the surgeon to inspect a portion of the bronchus), pulmonary function tests, sputum analysis, blood tests and physical examinations. Sometimes a biopsy of lung tissue is taken for analysis.

If it is suspected the cancer has spread, further tests such as a colonoscopy, an examination of small intestine and liver biopsy. A revolutionary new photo dynamic therapy puts a camera into the lungs along with a blue light that can detect tumours. The blue light slows up the tumours, turning them red/mauve, while surrounding healthy tissues are grey/blue. See further details below under 'Treatment'.

Types of Lung Cancer

Cancer can develop in the lungs in two ways. Primary, when cancer starts in the lungs or secondary or metastasis, where the cancer has spread from another part of the body through the bloodstream or the lymphatic system.

There are a number of different types of tumour which may cause lung cancer, the most common responsible for more than half of all cases, arises in the cells lining of the bronchi., the medium-sized air passage is called *bronchial carcinoma*. 10% of cases arise in the mucous glands of the air passage and is called *adenocarcinoma*. Most of the remainder of tumours belong to no specified type.

Treatment

Treatment may very much depend where the cancer is and whether it has spread to other parts of the body. In about 20% of cases, if the tumour is located in one lobe or in one lung, surgery to remove the lobe or lung may be the best solution. Chemotherapy is sometimes used first to shrink the tumour to make an operation possible.

Photo Dynamic Laser Treatment (PDT) (see page 45)

This 'pioneering' laser treatment is painless and destroys the cancer tumours in a very short time. This treatment is often carried out on an outpatients basis or requiring a short stay in hospital. PDT removes the need for surgery, chemotherapy and radiotherapy.

See details on using a nebuliser to breathe in vapourised 100% stabilised allicin liquid (see page 216).

A new drug 'Tacera' – taken in tablet form has shown to be quite effective.

How to ensure a high success rate and reduce the likelihood of the cancer returning

It is most important that you take care of the BIG FOUR - avoid Geopathic Stress, destroy any microbes, mainly micro parasites, take adequate Q10 and ensure a high acid alkaline balance in your blood.
Take the necessary vitamins, minerals etc. as modern food no longer provides enough to

prevent you suffering from malnutrition. Take at least 20 mcg daily of Vitamin D which is vital.

Also take enough exercise. Ideally exercise daily on a rebounder to vitalise your lymph system and help dispose of toxins from your body. Two minutes on a rebounder will double the number of white blood cells for one hour.

About 90% of people who get cancer have a thyroid gland which is out of balance. Using a MagneTech for one to two minutes daily direct will revitalise it. Do the same on the thymus, which matures your T-cells and say 20 minutes on your solar plexus where 70% of your immune system is located. Most importantly, use the MagneTech daily for 20 minutes directly on the problem area to heal it and any scar tissue.

You have got to take charge of your own health.

New suggested treatment

Dr Tom Ballard, Seattle, USA successfully treated Upper Respiratory Infection (URI) and pneumonia with nebulised allicin liquid with dramatic results.

As allicin has had a good effect on cancer tumours, why not inhale the allicin vapour through a nebuliser?

Recommended treatment Start by filling the nebuliser's receptacle with 2 ml of sterile saline and 2 ml of allicin liquid. Gradually increase the proportion of allicin liquid and less sterile saline. You might cough a little when you start inhaling.

Switch nebuliser on. Breathe in vapour from nebuliser, hold breath to a count of 10 (about 7 seconds), then breathe out to a count of 10. Start all over again by breathing in nebuliser vapour. Carry on this procedure for about 10 minutes, if you are mixing allicin liquid half and half with sterile saline. As you increase the proportion of allicin liquid, use the nebuliser less until you are using allicin liquid neat, when you only need to use the nebuliser for 5 minutes a time. Do this three times a day.

As mentioned before, also use two MagneTechs (powerful rotating magnetic apparatus) side by side on lungs or front and back near lungs for about 30-40 minutes per day.

As neither using allicin liquid or powerful rotating magnetic apparatus has shown any side-effects over many years, is it not worth trying these treatments, when conservative treatment has shown such poor results?

Case Histories

Geopathic Stress Lines
through John's bed

When John came to see me, he looked very pale - John had lung cancer. I found he slept in a very Geopathically Stressed place (see sketch opposite). Together we worked out how he could sleep in a Geopathically Stress-free place in his bedroom. John moved his bed. The next time I saw him, a few days later, he looked less pale and said he was sleeping so much better.

Malcolm, from Kent, (mentioned in the first chapter and under bone cancer), was diagnosed apart from his bone cancer, with secondary cancer in his lungs. He used two powerful rotating magnetic apparatus on his lungs each day and took allicin extract from garlic in liquid form. The lung cancer reduced by a 'massive amount' (Malcolm's words), thereby enabling an operation to remove the remainder of the cancer cells.

LYMPHOMA –
HODGKIN'S DISEASE AND NON HODGKIN'S LYMPHOMA

Lymphoma is a general term for a group of cancers that develop in the lymph system as part of the body's immune system. Lymphoma can start almost anywhere in the body - in a single lymph node or in a group of lymph nodes and can spread to any part of the body including the liver, bone marrow and spleen. There is a very high cure rate for early stage lymphomas and even higher if complementary remedies are incorporated during and after treatment.

SUMMARY
- Hodgkin's Disease and non-Hodgkin's Lymphoma.
- Symptoms
- Research
- Your lymph system
- Hodgkin's Disease
- Non-Hodgkin's Lymphoma
- Case history
- How to ensure a high success rate and reduce the likelihood of the cancer returning

Hodgkin's disease and non-Hodgkin's lymphoma

Although these two cancers are both lymph system diseases with some similarities, they differ widely in cell origin, how they spread and how they are treated. In diagnosing lymphoma the doctor will need to know the number and location of the affected lymph nodes, the type of lymphoma and whether the disease has spread to the bone marrow or organs outside the lymphatic system. Identifying the exact type of lymphoma requires that you are tested carefully before a diagnosis is made.

Hodgkin's disease is often recognised by the presence of large irregular cells in the lymph tissues called Reed Sternberg cells. The disease tends to follow a more predictable pattern of spread, which is generally more limited than that of the non-Hodgkin's lymphomas.

Non-Hodgkin's lymphoma (NHL) All other lymphomas are grouped together and called non-Hodgkin's lymphoma. By contrast, NHL cancer can begin in organs like the liver and bone rather than in the lymph nodes. NHL is the most common lymphoma in adults.

Symptoms
- Painful swelling in the neck, armpit or groin of lymph nodes which lasts more than six weeks and does not respond to antibiotics.
- Fever, night sweats, fatigue and weight loss.
- Itching and reddened patches on the skin.
- In cases of NHL - nausea and vomiting or abdominal pain.

Research

Lymphoma accounts for over 10,000 cancer cases diagnosed each year in the UK. Hodgkin's disease was first identified in 1832 by Thomas Hodgkin. Before 1970, most people with lymphoma died within two years of diagnosis. Today, lymphoma has a five year survival rate of over 50%.

Your lymph system

The lymph system is made up of a network of thin tubes that branch into the tissues throughout the body. The tubes carry lymph to all parts of your body. This fluid seeps out of the blood vessels. Lymph is a colourless watery fluid that contains infection fighting white blood cells called lymphocytes. Situated along this network are small glands called lymph nodes. They vary greatly in size. Some are as small as a pinhead and others are the shape and size of butter beans. They also vary in number from person to person and in different parts of the body. In your armpit, for example, there will be about 30-50 small nodes. The lymph nodes act as filters to remove infection from the draining body fluid and are packed with lymphocytes. Lymph nodes are mainly in the neck, armpits and groin. Other parts of the lymphatic system includes the spleen, thymus and bone marrow (see elsewhere how these organ functions). If the spleen is removed, its normal functions are taken over by other body tissue.

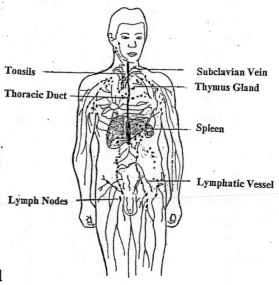

If the lymph nodes trap an infection or cancer, they will usually swell. With infection, the swollen nodes are usually hot, painful and tender to touch. With cancer cells, however, the nodes are often painless and do not cause any discomfort when touched. Any painless swollen nodes should be checked by your doctor, although the swelling is likely to be caused by something other than cancer.

When a lymph node swells as a result of cancer, it is because the cancer cells, trapped by its filter system continue to divide and produce new cells within the node. The cancer may have started in the lymphatic system, in which case it is called a lymphoma. Or the cancer cells may have spread from a cancer in another part of the body, such as breast, prostate or bowel.

Diagnosis

In order to diagnose lymphoma and determine whether it is Hodgkin's or Non-Hodgkin's cancer, a biopsy has to be carried out to remove part of all of a swollen lymph gland, so the cells can be examined in the laboratory. Further tests such as X-rays, Lymphgram, CT and MRI scans, blood and urine tests may be required to find out the exact size and position of the lymphoma and whether it has spread. If a blood test suggests that the bone marrow is affected by the cancer, a bone marrow biopsy may be taken.

'Staging' from 1 to 4 is the term used to describe the size and position of the cancer and whether it has spread.

Stage 1 One group of lymph nodes are affected and the lymphoma is only on one side of the diaphragm (the sheet of muscle under the lungs that controls breathing).

Stage 2 Two or more groups of lymph nodes are affected and the lymphoma is only on one side of the diaphragm.

Stage 3 There are lymphoma cells in lymph nodes above and below the diaphragm. The spleen may be affected.

Stage 4 The lymphoma has spread beyond lymph nodes, for example, to the liver, lungs or bone.

Treatment

Lymphoma is normally treated with chemotherapy and radiotherapy. For very localised disease, when the cancer has not spread beyond its original site, radiotherapy alone may be used.

Case History

16 years old Peter from Bournemouth, *started feeling very unwell, losing appetite etc. At hospital he was diagnosed with Hodgkin's disease and diabetes. Peter's mother, Maria, as a qualified nurse, had seen the terrible side-effects from chemotherapy, which the hospital recommended for Peter. So she and her husband signed a hospital disclaimer form, taking full responsibility for their son's health and Peter was discharged.*

Peter's parents had heard about Geopathic Stress and found Peter's bed had two very strong Geopathic Stress lines running through it.

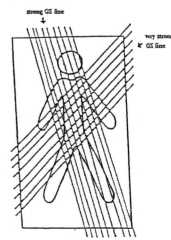

They made Peter a vegetarian and gave him lots of vitamins, minerals and herbs to boost his pancreas.

This is almost 20 years ago and Peter is not only in excellent health, but no longer diabetic.

P.S. Peter's mother, Maria, slept in a Geopathic Stress bed when she was pregnant, which I have found in all cases of children and grown-ups getting lymphoma which includes Hodgkin's Disease, Non-Hodgkin's lymphoma and Multiple Myeloma and also leukaemia.

Peter's bed

How to ensure a high success rate and reduce the likelihood of the cancer returning

It is most important that you take care of the BIG FOUR - avoid Geopathic Stress, destroy any microbes, mainly micro parasites, take adequate Q10 and ensure a high acid alkaline balance in your blood.

Take the necessary vitamins, minerals etc. as modern food no longer provides enough to prevent you suffering from malnutrition. Take at least 20 mcg daily of Vitamin D which is vital.

Also take enough exercise. Ideally exercise daily on a rebounder to vitalise your lymph system and help dispose of toxins from your body. Two minutes on a rebounder will double the number of white blood cells for one hour.

About 90% of people who get cancer have a thyroid gland which is out of balance. Using a MagneTech for one to two minutes daily direct will revitalise it. Do the same on the thymus, which matures your T-cells and say 20 minutes on your solar plexus where 70% of your immune system is located. Most importantly, use the MagneTech daily for 20 minutes directly on the problem area to heal it and any scar tissue.

You have got to take charge of your own health.

MELANOMA (SKIN) CANCER

> Most skin cancers are very visible so they are easier to identify earlier than many other cancers. Therefore they can be treated at an early stage giving a higher success rate of survival. The main cause of skin cancer is no doubt the sun, but the BIG FOUR are also present in most cases, so they must be dealt with to ensure as near as possible a 100% survival rate, but also to prevent skin cancer in the first place.

SUMMARY

- **Symptoms**
- **Research**
- **Diagnosis**
- **Types of Skin Cancer**
- **Treatment**
- **Prevention**
- **How to ensure a higher success rate and reduce the likelihood of the cancer returning**
- **Case Histories**

Symptoms

Changes in a mole or other lesions on the skin including bleeding, itching, pain, size, texture, softening, ulcerating shape-especially increasing irregularity of outline and changes in colour such as darkening or different shades of brown, green, pink or red; a new growth or sore which does not heal within four weeks. Those moles which become nodular (knotty) are the most malignant as they tend to penetrate deeply.

To summarise, watch out for moles that change size, colour, shape or that itch or bleed.

Research

About one in 300 to 400 moles General Practitioners are asked to look at are cancerous and only one cancer in 100 is malignant melanoma. About 7000 cases are diagnosed each year in the UK, mainly in the middle aged and elderly. Some 4000 women and 3000 men are diagnosed each year. Only half of all skin cancers develop from pre-existing moles and occur mainly in very light skin types. Melanoma is rare in very dark skin types but when it does develop, it tends to occur under finger nails or toenails or on the palms or soles.

Nearly everyone has pigmented moles but only one mole in a million becomes malignant. Hairy moles hardly ever turn into malignant melanomas.

Malignant melanoma are more common on a man's head, neck and back (often due to the fact that men take their shirts off for recreational sport), while women's often occur on legs and arms.

Warts do not turn into cancer.

Diagnosis

Your doctor must decide from the symptoms above if you have skin cancer. Approximately 54% of melanoma is diagnosed by doctors by looking at the skin. If your doctor thinks your mole looks suspicious he/she will arrange for further investigation and if necessary a biopsy which involves cutting out any skin that looks unusual and examining it for cancer.

If a melanoma is confirmed more biopsies may follow to confirm the extent of the cancer. Normally results from a biopsy take 2 to 3 weeks, which can be stressful and worrying for the patient and unsightly, as a biopsy may leave marks on, for example, the face or skin that are visible.

A new scanning technique SIAscopy [1] may make the whole diagnostic process less liable to human error and less traumatic. With this new technique a hand held scanner is placed in contact with the skin and directs separate infrared, green and blue light on it.
Blood, the dark skin pigment and the skin protein collagen, all absorb and reflect different wavelengths of light in different ways. This information is transmitted to a computer and a diagnosis is carried out in seconds. SIAscopy is the only skin-imaging technology that can penetrate as far as 2 mm below the surface of the skin. It increases diagnostic accuracy up to 95% and is known to be the most accurate method of deciding whether a mole should be removed or not without the need for an incision.

Types of Skin Cancer
Non-melanoma (skin) cancer
A less serious but much more common type of skin cancer is:

Basal Cell Cancer (BCC)
It usually occurs on the area of the skin which has been over exposed to the sun. Often it will appear as a small raised bump, which has a smooth pearly appearance. Another type looks like a scar and feels firm. Basal cell cancer is very slow growing and seldom spreads to other parts of the body.

Squamous Cell Cancer
This type of skin cancer rarely spreads. Squamous cancer cells are flat and grow faster than Basal cell cancer. This type of cancer is much more common in men than women and is related to the accumulated amount of sun exposure and the degree of skin pigmentation.

Malignant Melanoma Skin Cancer
Is the most serious type of cancer and frequently occurs in white women and men over the age of 40 with fair skin, red or blond hair, lots of moles on their body and skin that freckles and burns easily.

---

[1] The NHS Hospitals which can provide SIAscopic scanning include Addenbrook's Hospital Cambridge, Bedford Hospital, Norfolk and Norwich University Hospital and Solihull Hospital. Patients must be referred for diagnosis and treatment by their GP. Private clinics using the system include the Anelca Clinic in Central London, the Burghley Park Clinic, Swindon and LifeScan UK, Guildford. Private consultations start at about £200. For up to date information, contact Astron Clinic, Cambridge.

Women are most often diagnosed with melanoma on the arms and legs and men on the trunk, head and neck. Often the first sign is a change in the size, shape or colour of an existing mole. It may also appear as a new, abnormal lump in normal skin or as a new, ugly-looking mole.

Eye Tumours (Intraocular melanoma)

Melanoma can also affect the choroids of the eye, the layer under the retina (see Chapter on 'Other Types of Cancer').

Treatment

Melanomas can be **surgically** removed with a wide area of normal-seeming tissue around them and skin grafting may then be necessary. **Cryosurgery,** using extreme cold to freeze-off the lesions is sometimes considered. **Radiotherapy** can also be used in areas such as the eyelids, nose or ears which are hard to treat with surgery. **SIAscopy** may also be used in conjunction with surgery to ensure all cancer has been removed. A new successful treatment for BCC is **Photo Dynamic Therapy (PDT)**. First a cream, containing special chemicals, which attracts the abnormally growing cancer cells, making them sensitive to light. The cream is covered by a light-blocking dressing. The next day, the patient lies down with protective glasses and the dressing is removed. A laser is shone on the cancer. This triggers a chemical reaction, which enables the light sensitive chemicals, to enter the cancer and kill it. Generally, the procedure is repeated a week later.

If the cancer has spread or metastasized to other parts of the body, then other treatments such as radiotherapy or chemotherapy may be involved.

Prevention

Needless to say, you should have respect for the sun. Wear a hat and T-shirt, especially when the sun is extremely hot in the UK or abroad (clothes must not be too thin otherwise almost all the sun's UV (ultra violet) radiation penetrates right through). Only stay in the summer mid-day sun for 15 minutes to generate adequate vitamin D and do not forget to apply sunscreen every two hours. (See details regarding essential Vitamin D in Part Four).

How to ensure a high success rate and reduce the likelihood of the cancer returning

It is most important that you take care of the BIG FOUR - avoid Geopathic Stress, destroy any microbes, mainly micro parasites, take adequate Q10 and ensure a high acid alkaline balance in your blood.

Take the necessary vitamins, minerals etc. as modern food no longer provides enough to prevent you suffering from malnutrition. Take at least 20 mcg daily of Vitamin D which is vital.

Also take enough exercise. Ideally exercise daily on a rebounder to vitalise your lymph system and help dispose of toxins from your body. Two minutes on a rebounder will double the number of white blood cells for one hour.

About 90% of people who get cancer have a thyroid gland which is out of balance. Using a MagneTech for one to two minutes daily direct will revitalise it. Do the same on the thymus, which matures your T-cells and say 20 minutes on your solar plexus where 70% of your immune system is located. Most importantly, use the MagneTech daily for 20 minutes directly on the problem area to heal it and any scar tissue.

You have got to take charge of your own health.

Case Histories

Allicin gel and capsules

"A while ago I went to my GP and was told that I had a patch of skin cancer (BCC) and an appointment was made at the Dermatology Clinic in order to have it removed. My daughter sought alternative advice and 100% stabilised allicin was recommended for me to use. I was sceptical at first, but decided to give it a go. I took four 450 mg allicin capsules a day and applied allicin gel direct on the skin cancer patch several times a day. Imagine my delight when, I went for my appointment at the Dermatology Clinic 5 weeks later, to be told that I no longer required surgery, as the skin cancer had disappeared!

'Vincent' UK July 2009 - The BIG FOUR were also dealt with.

Sun Beds

Jenny M, a 23 year old nursery nurse, was diagnosed with skin cancer on her chest. It was claimed the cancer was due to her having used sun beds

*She used a sun bed two to three times a week, often staying under the super strength ultra violet lamps for nine minutes at a time. After six months she spotted a red rash on her chest and cut down her sessions. As the rash was still present after two years a friend convinced her to visit her GP and skin cancer was diagnosed. She was **successfully** treated.*

I have found she was sleeping in a very Geopathic Stressed place and her body contained a large amount of micro parasites which thrive on the extra heat from the ultra violet lamps.

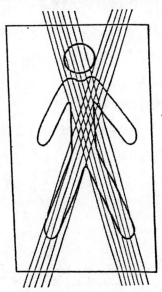

Geopathic Stress lines through Jenny M's Bed when she was diagnosed with skin cancer

I firmly believe you very seldom get cancer from using sun beds, unless you are also Geopathic Stressed.

MOUTH AND NECK CANCERS

These types of cancers can often be detected early for example in the mouth, by yourself, your doctor or dentist and in the throat by the feeling of a lump or a change in voice. Early detection and modern treatments mean that these cancers can be cured in most cases.

It is hoped that you will have the Photo Dynamic Laser Therapy (PDT) for your cancer, which takes less than one hour and requires only a short stay in hospital and you will not need surgery, including any reconstruction surgery, radiotherapy and chemotherapy. PDT treatment involves injecting a light sensitive drug and later using a laser which destroys the cancer tumours. (See Part Two for full details). It is, however, vital to incorporate complementary remedies.

Cancer of the mouth and neck is diagnosed almost twice as often in men than women. This is mainly thought to be due to men smoking cigarettes and drinking alcohol more. As smoking and drinking alcohol has increased among women, more women are being diagnosed with mouth and throat cancer fifteen to twenty years after starting. About 8,000 people are diagnosed with mouth and neck cancer and about 3,000 die each year in the UK. This cancer is rare in people in their thirties and younger.

SUMMARY
- Mouth cancer (oral cavity area)
- Larynx cancer (voice box) and Pharynx (Throat) (see separate chapter on Thyroid cancer)
- Case History - throat cancer
- Nasal and Sinus cancers
- How to ensure a higher success rate and reduce the likelihood of the cancer returning

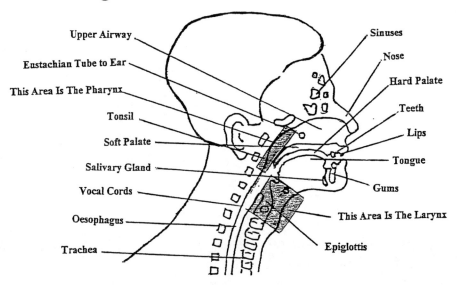

MOUTH CANCER

'Oral cancer' is the term given to cancer arising in the area of the mouth and oral cavity including the lip, the tongue, the hard palate, the floor of the mouth, the lining of the cheeks, the small area behind the wisdom teeth, the tonsils and the gums.

- **Symptoms**
- **Your mouth**
- **Who is most likely to get cancer of the mouth?**
- **Diagnosis**
- **Treatment**

Symptoms

Often oral cancer causes the same symptoms as other problems that occur in the mouth, like sores or ulcers. However with cancer they do not heal and are often painless. It is, therefore, important to see your doctor/dentist if they do not heal within two to three weeks. Sometime oral cancer can also cause difficulty in swallowing, problems with speaking clearly, pain in the cheek or side of the face, pain in the ear or side of the head, a lump that you can feel in the neck, episodes of choking or episodes of bleeding. Any symptoms like these should be assessed by your doctor even though cancer is not the only possible cause.

Your mouth

As shown on the diagram on the previous page, your mouth is basically a box-like cavity with lips at the front and the oesophagus (gullet) and larynx (throat) at the back.

Who is most likely to get cancer of the mouth?

- Usually people over 45
- Cigarette smokers
- People with fair skin that have been exposed to strong sunlight, may get mouth cancer, especially lip cancer.

Diagnosis

Initially your doctor will check the inside of your mouth. Examination may include looking at the back of the throat using a *nasopharyngoscope* which is a flexible fibre optic instrument introduced through the nose. This examination is uncomfortable, but not painful. If there are any suspicious areas, your doctor may suggest a *biopsy*, so a small sample of tissue can be sent for a laboratory test. In addition, any combination of the following endoscopies may be recommended; a *gastroscope* to examine any or the entire gullet (oesophagus) and the stomach, a *bronchoscope* to examine the airways and upper part of the lungs.
Usually a *CT scan* of the head or a *MRI scan* is taken to see exactly where and how deep the tumour is. In a few cases, a special X-ray or bone scan may be needed. Blood tests are also taken and sometimes lung function tests are required.

Treatment

Photo Dynamic Laser Therapy (PDT) It is hoped that you can have this treatment.

Surgery The nature of the operation will vary considerably depending on the site and the extent of the tumour. Larger tumours may have an effect on function and/or appearance. If other structures are involved a large amount of tissue may need to be removed. For example if the tumour is in the gums, some teeth will need to be removed. Sometimes samples of lymph nodes in the neck may be taken. Reconstructive surgery may sometimes be needed.

Radiotherapy Because the external beam of radiotherapy can be directed to virtually any part of the mouth, it is ideal if the tumour is in an inaccessible area which would otherwise need major surgery. Sometimes brachytherapy is also carried out. (See Part Two under radiotherapy).

Chemotherapy is not usually recommended for treating oral cancer.

PHARYNX (THROAT) and LARYNX (VOICE BOX) CANCER

SUMMARY
- **Symptoms**
- **Your neck**
- **Diagnosis**
- **How throat cancer is spread**
- **Treatment and how to learn to talk if your voice box is removed**

Symptoms
Hoarseness of the voice, lump seen or felt on the side of the neck. Later on it may cause some discomfort. Sometimes involving the ears. Bleeding, resulting in coughing up or spitting blood.

Your neck
As the diagram on the previous page indicates, the larynx is in the region of the vocal cords. The pharynx region is higher up behind the mouth.

Diagnosis
Usually the doctor starts the examination of the throat area with a **nasoendoscope**, which is a flexible fibre optic instrument introduced through the nose. This examination is uncomfortable, but not painful. Sometimes a **light and mirror system** is used to see the back of the throat. Often an **EUA** (examination under anaesthetic) is also carried out, during which an **EUA biopsy** may be taken. **Microlaryngoscopy** may sometimes be used under general anaesthetic, which enables the vocal cords to be magnified and seen with a microscope system.

In many cases a CT scan will be carried out to assess the extent of the tumours and to establish if there are any enlarged lymph nodes in the area.

How throat cancer spreads?
It is thought that cancer of the vocal cord stays contained for sometime and does not spread

because there are few lymphatic vessels in the area. Cancer in the pharynx area further from the vocal cords may spread to local lymph nodes at an earlier stage.

Treatment

Radiotherapy is the first choice because it combines the chance of cure and preserving the voice.

Surgery may also be recommended, particularly if the cancer has reoccurred after radiotherapy. If the tumour is relatively small, it may be possible to remove it with **partial laryngectomy.**

Photo Dynamic Laser Therapy (PDT) It is hoped that you have this treatment.

Total laryngectomy this surgery involves the removal of the entire larynx including the vocal cords. After such an operation, you will need to learn to speak in a different way. During the operation an opening will be created in your trachea through to your oesophagus, so air from your lungs can be forced through to your mouth. The opening is called a *trachea-oesophageal fistula.* The fistula has a one-way valve system built in to prevent food from your mouth going down and into your lungs. The valve is usually changed and cleaned by the patient. By blocking the tracheotomy opening with your thumb or finger, you can use the air to make sounds without your vocal cords. This technique, which requires some training, is the most common method of restoring speech.

My wife Lena had a tracheostomy (sometimes called a stomy) fitted soon after her throat cancer was diagnosed, as the tumour was so large that she could suddenly not breathe. Before Lena learnt to speak quite well using the above method. She used to write hilarious notes to her doctors, hospital staff and visitors.

There are two other ways you can learn to communicate which also need some practice. *The Electrolarynx* is a small, hand-held device that creates vibrations when you hold it to your throat, under your jaw or even against your cheek. It creates vibrations that you can then change into clearly intelligible words by using your mouth.

Oesophageal Speech requires you to learn to expel air from your stomach (as a controlled belch and use the air for speech).

With any of these methods of speaking, you will no doubt see a speech therapist. If possible meet one or several patients who use the above method of speaking, so you can hear first hand what their voices sound like and what problems they have encountered.

Cancer can begin in other parts of the pharynx such as the back of the nasal passages or in the upper part of the throat. It is important that you understand from your specialist where the problem is and the options that are available for treatment.

Case History

John, a farmer in Somerset, was diagnosed with throat cancer. He moved his bed into a Geopathic Stress-free place and used a MagneTech (powerful high speed magnetic apparatus) daily for a month. He had no other treatment during this period. When he returned to hospital to have his larynx (voice box) checked, the doctor informed him that there was no need for surgery, as he no longer had any cancer tumour. (August 2006).

It must be emphasised that we all react differently to any treatment, so strong magnetic therapy may not be successful for everybody.

NASAL AREA CANCER

The nasal area is divided into two parts, nasopharynx (above the airway to the mouth behind the tonsils) and the nasal cavity. Cancer in these two areas are treated differently, so it is important for you to know exactly what kind of cancer you have so you can understand what treatment will be involved.

SUMMARY

- **Symptoms**
- **Your nasal area**
- **Diagnosis**
- **Treatment**

Symptoms

Nasopharynx cancer - most common symptoms are painless, enlarged lymph nodes in the neck. Other symptoms include trouble in breathing or speaking, frequent headaches, a lump in the nose or neck, pain or ringing in the ear (tinnitus) or hearing problems.

Sinus and nasal cavity cancer - Infection, pain or blocked sinus which does not clear. Swelling around the eyes, lump or sore in your nose that does not heal, headache, numbness in your cheek, upper lip, upper teeth or side of your nose, double vision.

The above symptoms do not mean that you have cancer in the nasal area, but it is wise to see your doctor if they last more than two to three weeks.

Your nasal area

As shown on the diagram on the first page of the chapter, this area includes your nose and a very complex structure that lies within the facial cavity and extends to your ear and neck. It reaches from the back of your nose and upper throat to just below the base of the skull and just above the soft palate. The sinuses are small cavities or tunnels around or near your nose. They help to filter, warm and humidify the air you breathe. Your sinuses also help to give your speech resonance. Two openings on the side of the nasopharynx lead into the ear. The nasal cavity and sinuses are lined with mucosa, a mucous producing tissue.

Diagnosis

Nasopharyngeal cancer Your doctor will usually first physically examine your throat, feel for any swollen lymph nodes in your neck and examine your throat with a long-handled mirror. A nasoscope, a thin lighted tube, will be used to check the nose for abnormal areas. Hearing and nerve functions will also be examined. CT and MRI scans and blood tests will be taken. A biopsy will be taken to determine any cancer.

Nasal cavity and sinuses cancer A nasoscope will be used to check the nasal cavity. Also CT and MRI scan, blood test and biopsy as above. About 70 to 75% of cancer in this area is squamous cell cancer. Adenocaricinoma that arises from gland cells account for about 10 to 15% of these cancers. The balance is malignant lymphomas and melanoma cancer.

Treatment

Photo Dynamic Laser Therapy (PDT) It is hoped that you can have this treatment. (See page 33).

Radiotherapy both external and brachytherapy (see Part Two under radiotherapy).

Surgery is usually reserved for later treatment.

Chemotherapy together with radiotherapy has sometime proved very successful.

How to ensure a high success rate and reduce the likelihood of the cancer returning in all cases of mouth and neck cancers.

It is most important that you take care of the BIG FOUR - avoid Geopathic Stress, destroy any microbes, mainly micro parasites, take adequate Q10 and ensure a high acid alkaline balance in your blood.

Take the necessary vitamins, minerals etc. as modern food no longer provides enough to prevent you suffering from malnutrition. Take at least 20 mcg daily of Vitamin D which is vital.

Also take enough exercise. Ideally exercise daily on a rebounder to vitalise your lymph system and help dispose of toxins from your body. Two minutes on a rebounder will double the number of white blood cells for one hour.

About 90% of people who get cancer have a thyroid gland which is out of balance. Using a MagneTech for one to two minutes daily direct will revitalise it. Do the same on the thymus, which matures your T-cells and say 20 minutes on your solar plexus where 70% of your immune system is located. Most importantly, use the MagneTech daily for 20 minutes directly on the problem area to heal it and any scar tissue.

You have got to take charge of your own health.

OESOPHAGEAL CANCER

> One of the reasons for the low survival rates in cases of oesophageal cancer is that many of the patients (40% in a Scottish audit study) have several co-existing medical conditions, which preclude them from certain orthodox treatments. It is, therefore, vital that complementary remedies are incorporated in the treatment program.

SUMMARY
- **Symptoms**
- **Research**
- **Who is most likely to get cancer of the oesophagus?**
- **Your oesophagus**
- **Diagnosis**
- **Orthodox treatment**
- **After surgery**
- **Barrett's Oesophagus and symptoms**
- **How to ensure a higher success rate and prevent the likelihood of the cancer returning**
- **Case History**

Symptoms
The most common symptom is difficulty in swallowing. Food may seem not to pass in the usual way, feeling as though it sticks behind the breastbone. There may be a sensation of pressure, burning or pain in the chest, hoarseness, cough, fever, choking or coughing up blood. Later there is difficulty in drinking liquid. Eventually, there will be considerable weight loss.

Research
More men (about 4,500), than women (about 2,800), are diagnosed with oesophageal cancer each year in the UK. It occurs most often between the age of 50 and 80, (the median age is 72). Apart from lung and pancreatic cancer, this cancer has the lowest five year survival rate. The patients who survive have nearly all become free from Geopathic Stress and ensured their immune system has been boosted.

Who is most likely to get cancer of the Oesophagus?
- Smokers.
- Frequent and or heavy alcohol drinkers.

- People who have had damage to the lining of the oesophagus.
- Men over 60.
- People who have had other head or neck cancer.
- People with Barrett's oesophagus (see below).
- People affected by THE BIG FOUR.

The Oesophagus

This is the gullet or swallowing muscular tube about 25cm (10 inches) long that carries the food from the mouth to the stomach. It lies just in front of the spine and behind the wind pipe (trachea).

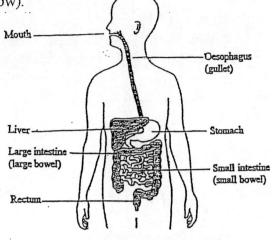

The Digestive System

Diagnosis

This will no doubt involve a barium meal X-ray. The barium liquid drink will coat the inside of your oesophagus. The X-ray will investigate if there has been a change in the shape of your oesophagus. Your doctor may also insert an illuminated tube into your oesophagus to collect cells and tissues that will be looked at under a microscope to establish if there are cancer cells.

If cancer cells are found, you will need further tests to see if the cancer has spread. This might include a bronchoscope to look at your lungs and a laryngoscope to look at your voice box. You may also have an endoscope ultrasound and scans such as MRI, CT or PET to determine the stage of your cancer.

Orthodox Treatment

By the time cancer of the oesophagus has been diagnosed, it has often spread to other parts of the body nearby. This will have a bearing on treatment and involve either surgery, radiotherapy or chemotherapy or a combination.

Surgery may involve the removal of the oesophagus (oesophagectomy).
Any remaining part of the oesophagus that is healthy is reconnected to the stomach. A plastic tube or part of the intestine is sometimes used to connect the two parts, so you can still swallow. Often a tube is inserted to keep the oesophagus open.

Photodynamic therapy (PDT) is the latest very successful method of destroying the cancer tumours in the oesophagus, without involving surgery (see under laser treatment in Part Two).

If you have other medical conditions that prevent you from having the full treatment necessary, I highly recommend using powerful rotating magnets direct on the cancer area.

This may reduce the cancer so much that only a much milder orthodox treatment is necessary.

After Surgery

To keep your lungs clear after the operation, you will be taught special breathing and coughing exercises. I would also recommend using a nebuliser, using stabilised allicin drops with or without sterile saline in the receptacle to revitalise your lungs. See more details under lung cancer. Using strong rotating magnets on the lung will also help your breathing.

If you have problems with swallowing, try to eat several small meals and snacks during the day and or nutritional drinks. Drinking liquids through a straw may be easier. If you cannot swallow, you may have food in liquid form via a tube from your mouth to your stomach or directly into your stomach.

Barrett's Oesophagus

This often occurs in people who suffer persistent heartburn, caused by the stomach contents 'splashing' back up into the oesophagus.

The stomach produces acid to help to digest food and is lined by tissue that is resistant to acid, but the oesophagus is not. Normally a valve at the bottom of the oesophagus prevents acid from splashing up into the gullet. However some people have a weak valve which allows the acid to flow backwards into the oesophagus.

This causes the cells lining the lower part of the oesophagus either to change or be replaced with cells that could become cancerous. Although most cases appear to remain benign, the medical profession say a large majority of patients with oesophagus cancer, begin with Barrett's Syndrome.
Fair-skinned men are more susceptible to Barrett's oesophagus than fair-skinned women.

Symptoms of Barrett's Oesophagus

Some people have no symptoms at all and Barrett's oesophagus is discovered during tests for other medical conditions. Common symptoms include heartburn, digestion problems, nausea, vomiting, difficulty in swallowing food and/or pain.

How to ensure a high success rate and reduce the likelihood of the cancer returning

It is most important that you take care of the BIG FOUR - avoid Geopathic Stress, destroy any microbes, mainly micro parasites, take adequate Q10 and ensure a high acid alkaline balance in your blood.
Take the necessary vitamins, minerals etc. as modern food no longer provides enough to prevent you suffering from malnutrition. Take at least 20 mcg daily of Vitamin D which is vital.
Also take enough exercise. Ideally exercise daily on a rebounder to vitalise your lymph system and help dispose of toxins from your body. Two minutes on a rebounder will double the number of white blood cells for one hour.
About 90% of people who get cancer have a thyroid gland which is out of balance. Using a

MagneTech for one to two minutes daily direct will revitalise it. Do the same on the thymus, which matures your T-cells and say 20 minutes on your solar plexus where 70% of your immune system is located. Most importantly, use the MagneTech daily for 20 minutes directly on the problem area to heal it and any scar tissue.

You have got to take charge of your own health.

Case History

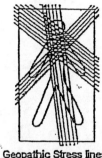

Catherine M in the Midlands was diagnosed with a cancer tumour in the oesophagus. A major operation was carried out on 27 August, but due to severe complications, the tumour was not removed. In October, Catherine was offered 15 weeks chemotherapy, which she refused.

In November, Catherine was told she was sleeping in a very Geopathic Stressed place. Her husband moved her bed into a stress free place and within days she could swallow liquid food and slept better.

Geopathic Stress lines through the bed where Catherine originally slept.

After a few weeks, Catherine could eat solid food and was no longer lying or sitting down most of the day. She started to go for walks, which she had not done for several months.

By Christmas, Catherine was looking much better, putting on weight, much happier in herself and very busy cooking etc.

After speaking to the hospital in October, Catherine did not think 'she would see Christmas'.

PANCREATIC CANCER

Even though pancreatic cancer is one of the less common cancers, if you are diagnosed, you have the least chance of surviving more than five years than from any other cancer (below 3%).
However, the latest Photo Dynamic Laser Therapy (PDT) and strong magnetic therapy, are probably the most successful treatments. It is also vital to incorporate complementary remedies.

Summary

- Symptoms
- Research
- Your Pancreas
- Cause of Pancreatic Cancer
- How Pancreatic Cancer can spread
- Diagnosis
- Treatment
- How to ensure a higher success rate and reduce the likelihood of the cancer returning
- Case History

Symptoms

Pain in upper abdomen and near centre of back. Unexplained weight loss and loss of appetite. Intolerance to fatty foods. Enlargement of abdominal, liver and spleen. Jaundice – yellowing of the skin. Often tumours in the pancreas are in an advanced state before being spotted because the disease can be virtually symptom-free to begin with.

Research

About 7000 people in the UK die of pancreatic cancer each year. It is the fifth most common cause of cancer deaths. The number of terminal cases has scarcely changed over the last 30 years.

Your Pancreas

The pancreas produces digestive enzymes which pass into the first part of the small intestine (duodenum). The pancreas also monitors the concentration of glucose in the blood and secretes appropriate amounts of the hormone insulin and glycogen to lower or raise the amount of sugar, as necessary.

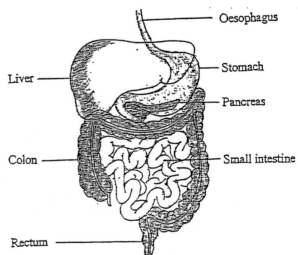

Causes of Pancreatic Cancer

In most cases this type of cancer affects people aged between 60 and 80 when often the pancreas has been damaged by smoking, heavy drinking and being Geopathic Stressed for a long time. Diabetics are also more likely to be affected.

How Pancreatic Cancer can spread

It may spread to adjacent structures including the bile duct and the duodenum, to lymph nodes in the area (for example near the stomach or the small intestine) and across the peritoneal cavity to the colon, small intestine, spleen or other structures including the liver or the lungs.

Diagnosis

The first test is a CT scan and ultrasound. Sometimes an MRI scan is performed and a test using an endoscope, whereby a thin tube is inserted through the mouth into the stomach and then into the duodenum from which the opening of the pancreas can be seen. A dye can be injected into the pancreatic duct, so an X-ray can show certain kinds of problems. This test is called an endoscopic retrograde cholangio-pancreatography (ERCP).

Treatment

The main problem with the pancreas is its location. There are lots of major organs close by - the stomach, colon, liver, kidneys and spinal cord which all have their own blood supply.

Surgery If the cancer is removable, major surgery can involve the removal of the head of the pancreas together with parts of the duodenum and the bile duct. This is a very complicated operation.

Photo Dynamic Laser Therapy (PDT) It is hoped that you can have this treatment (see page 45).

Radiotherapy Standard radiotherapy is fairly ineffective as surrounding organs are also eradicated, so this limits the dose of radiation. In about 30% of pancreatic cancer cases, the tumour has not spread and the latest **Cyberknife** can be used, whereby a movable robotic arm is attached to a miniaturized radiotherapy machine guided by sophisticated software. The machine fires hundreds of pencil-thin beams of radiation from thousands of angles around the tumour. (See further details about Cyberknife under radiotherapy in Part Two).

Chemotherapy may help to shrink the tumour before surgery or cyberknife.

Magnetic Therapy See Powerful Magnetic Healing under Part Five and case history below.

Most doctors admit, in advance cases of pancreatic cancer, the best advice is to alleviate the symptoms and maintain quality of life for as long as possible. Radiotherapy can help to control pain.

If the entire pancreas has been removed by surgery or if it has been affected by some other treatment, daily insulin injections will be needed to replace the insulin the pancreas normally produces.

Case History

Tony (Cornwall) was diagnosed with a cancerous tumour on his pancreas and in his liver. His hospital doctor could not recommend a treatment and gave him less than three months to live. Luckily his brother John knew about the danger of Geopathic Stress. Dealing with it had made a vast difference to the health of his milking cows. A safe place was found for Tony to sleep and sit immediately. Tony used two MagneTechs (the strong high speed magnet apparatus), which he used either side of his body where the pancreas is, for forty minutes twice a day. Tony also started taking daily, 300mg Q10, 350mg Vitamin E, 200mcg Selenium & Zinc and 3g Vitamin C.

Tony went back to the hospital two weeks later. A nurse could no longer feel the tumour on his pancreas and the doctor gave him seven years to live! When Tony first went to the hospital, he could only walk 50 yards with discomfort. After using the magnetic apparatus he could walk two miles without getting tired.

How to ensure a high success rate and reduce the likelihood of the cancer returning

It is most important that you take care of the BIG FOUR - avoid Geopathic Stress, destroy any microbes, mainly micro parasites, take adequate Q10 and ensure a high acid alkaline balance in your blood.

Take the necessary vitamins, minerals etc. as modern food no longer provides enough to prevent you suffering from malnutrition. Take at least 20 mcg daily of Vitamin D which is vital.

Also take enough exercise. Ideally exercise daily on a rebounder to vitalise your lymph system and help dispose of toxins from your body. Two minutes on a rebounder will double the number of white blood cells for one hour.

About 90% of people who get cancer have a thyroid gland which is out of balance. Using a MagneTech for one to two minutes daily direct will revitalise it. Do the same on the thymus, which matures your T-cells and say 20 minutes on your solar plexus where 70% of your immune system is located. Most importantly, use the MagneTech daily for 20 minutes directly on the problem area to heal it and any scar tissue.

You have got to take charge of your own health.

STOMACH CANCER

As there may be no obvious symptoms, cancer of the stomach can be quite advanced before it is diagnosed.
Even if part or the whole of the stomach is removed people can lead quite normal lives. It is however vital to incorporate complementary remedies for more success.

SUMMARY

- Symptoms
- Research
- Who is most likely to get stomach cancer?
- Your stomach
- How stomach cancer tends to spread
- Diagnosis
- Main types of stomach cancer
- Treatment
- How to ensure a higher success rate and reduce the likelihood of cancer returning

Symptoms

Early detection can be difficult because symptoms in the early stages are very slight like e.g. non-specific indigestion, a sense of discomfort or vague pain. Fullness, bloating or burping. Slight nausea, heartburn, indigestion or loss of appetite - these are all symptoms which are easy to ignore. However see your GP if they persist, even intermittently, for two weeks or more.

Later signs can include - dark stools, which may signal blood in the stools. Vomiting, sometimes bloody. Rapid weight loss. Severe abdominal pain. Weakness and fatigue (these symptoms may also indicate the presence of a stomach ulcer).

Research

Over 9,000 cases of stomach cancer are diagnosed in the UK each year. This number has reduced dramatically over the past 60 years. It is believed this is due to a better diet including more vegetables and fruit and an improvement in standards of food preparation and preservation.

Who is most likely to get stomach cancer?

- People over 55
- Men are one and half times more likely to get it than women
- Black people
- People with peptic ulcers

- People who have a low intake of fruit and vegetables
- Cigarette smokers
- People with *Helicobacter pylori* - the bacteria that causes some ulcers and inflammation
- People who have had stomach surgery
- People affected by the BIG FOUR

Your stomach

The stomach lies under the ribs in the left upper part of the abdomen, crossing over to the right below the liver. It hangs completely free in the abdominal cavity. The upper part of the stomach connects to the oesophagus and the lower part connects to the small intestine.

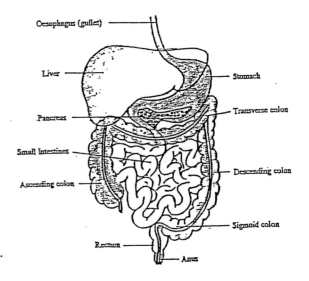

Your digestion system

The stomach acid, hydrochloric acid and the digestive juices (enzymes) pepsin, work together to process your food in a churning action. These chemicals also protect against infection and many organisms are destroyed by the acids. This strong acid and the pepsin is secreted by cells in the lining of the stomach.

The onward passage of partially digested food is controlled by the muscular ring (the pylorus) at the lower outlet of the stomach. Large lumps of food tend to cause the pylorus to close, so that they are retained longer in the stomach for further chemical action.
The average stomach can hold about 1.5 litres. The stomach empties into the duodenum which is the first part of the small intestine.

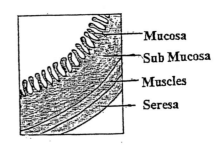

Layers of the stomach wall

The lining of the stomach consists of four layers. The inner layer, the *mucosa* contains the glands that secrete the acid and the pepsin. The *mucosa* is supported by the next layer, the *sub mucosa*. Outside that is the layer that contains the *muscles* needed for the mixing and churning action of the stomach. The outermost layer is a thin smooth layer called the *serosa*.

How stomach cancer tends to spread

The cancer begins in the mucosal lining of the stomach. As the cancer grows, it penetrates more deeply into the stomach layers and then to the outside of the stomach wall. If it does, it may spread to nearby organs such as the pancreas or spleen.

The cancer may also spread to the lymph nodes nearby or to distant lymph nodes, for example in the neck. The cancer may also spread across the abdominal cavity to other parts of the abdomen, which may cause ascites, which is the fluid that accumulates in the peritoneal cavity, causing the abdomen to swell.

Stomach cancer may also cause secondary cancer tumours on the ovaries in women or near the rectum or the navel or may spread through the bloodstream to the liver.

Diagnosis

Biopsy is usually the first test carried out with a *gastroscopy*, where a thin tube with a telescopic system is passed down the gullet into the stomach to inspect it and take specimens of anything that appears suspicious. Sometimes a special X-ray of your stomach will be taken after you have drunk a white liquid (barium meal) which will show up on the x-ray. If cancer is found, laboratory tests such as red and white blood cell counts and plasma tumour markers will be taken. Further tests may be recommended to establish if the cancer has spread elsewhere. These tests may include ultrasound, CT or MRI scan.

Main types of stomach cancer

Adenocarcinoma is the cancer which arises from the mucosa layer in the stomach. The main ones are:

- *superficial spreading* is a thin spread layer over the mucosa. If the growth is small, it is called *early* stomach cancer.
- cancer ulcer is formed like a sharply defined ulcer; however, they are not caused by and have nothing to do with ordinary stomach ulcers.
- *polypoid* grow with a stalk area and a branched head. This type of cancer is the least aggressive.
- *infiltration* is the most common type of stomach cancer. Sometimes this cancer grows in a diffuse way throughout the whole wall of the stomach. This is a more aggressive cancer with *linilis plastica* and is the most aggressive.
- malignant tumours which may originate in the stomach like *lymphomas* (cancer of the lymphocytes) and *sarcomas* (cancer of connective tissue). See separate chapter for these types of cancers.

Treatment

Surgery is the most important treatment. *Partial gastrectomy* is when part of the stomach is removed and with *total gastrectomy* the whole stomach is removed. After a partial gastrectomy, the part of the stomach which remains is connected to the small intestine. After a total gastrectomy, the oesophagus will be connected direct to the small intestine.

If the cancer has spread to other structures nearby, part of the pancreas, liver or spleen may need to be removed at the same time.

As in all cancer surgery, the actual extent of the operation may differ from what was planned depending on what the surgeon finds during the operation.

Photo Dynamic Laser Treatment (PDT) (see page 45)

This 'pioneering' laser treatment is painless and destroys the cancer tumours in a very short time. This treatment is often carried out on an outpatients basis or requiring a short stay in hospital. PDT removes the need for surgery, chemotherapy and radiotherapy.

See details on using a nebuliser to breathe in vaporised 100% stabilised allicin liquid (see page 216).

Radiotherapy may be used to relive symptoms, reduce bleeding or shrink a tumour blocking the stomach.

Chemotherapy is not too successful in treating stomach cancer, but new drugs are being developed all the time and you may agree to participate in a clinical trial.

Other treatments may be used in certain circumstances for example laser or injecting into blood vessels if there is bleeding.

After partial or total gastrectomy, you will initially be given liquids by mouth, then soft and finally solid food. You may temporarily have problems eating certain foods and a diet low in sugar and high in fat and proteins may be suggested, with the addition of dry foods and fluids between meals. It is usually more comfortable to eat little and often.

How to ensure a high success rate and reduce the likelihood of the cancer returning

It is most important that you take care of the BIG FOUR - avoid Geopathic Stress, destroy any microbes, mainly micro parasites, take adequate Q10 and ensure a high acid alkaline balance in your blood.

Take the necessary vitamins, minerals etc. as modern food no longer provides enough to prevent you suffering from malnutrition. Take at least 20 mcg daily of Vitamin D which is vital.

Also take enough exercise. Ideally exercise daily on a rebounder to vitalise your lymph system and help dispose of toxins from your body. Two minutes on a rebounder will double the number of white blood cells for one hour.

About 90% of people who get cancer have a thyroid gland which is out of balance. Using a MagneTech for one to two minutes daily direct will revitalise it. Do the same on the thymus, which matures your T-cells and say 20 minutes on your solar plexus where 70% of your immune system is located. Most importantly, use the MagneTech daily for 20 minutes directly on the problem area to heal it and any scar tissue.

You have got to take charge of your own health.

THYROID CANCER

Cancer of the thyroid is not common and is curable in most cases. You can live without the thyroid and take tablets. It is, however, vital to incorporate complementary remedies.

SUMMARY

- **Symptoms**
- **Research**
- **Who is most likely to get thyroid cancer?**
- **Your thyroid**
- **Types of thyroid cancer**
- **Diagnosis**
- **Treatment**
- **How to ensure a higher success and reduce the likelihood of cancer returning**

Symptoms

A hard irregular lump that does not seem to move. Softer, mobile and more than one lump and slow growing indicate a benign tumour. Usually the cancerous lump is not painful or tender (if the lump causes pain, it probably is not thyroid cancer). There may also be enlargement of one or more nearby lymph nodes either above or below the thyroid nodule.

Research

Thyroid cancer is the most common cancer in the head and neck area and can occur at any age, even in teenagers. However in 75% of cases of lumps or nodules in the thyroid they are not cancerous. Less than 1,000 people are diagnosed with thyroid cancer each year in the UK.

Who is most likely to get thyroid cancer?

- People who have had radiation treatment on the head or neck earlier in life. Sometimes 20 years or even longer.
- Twice as often found in women as in men and more often in fair-skinned people than in black people.

Your thyroid

The thyroid is a ductless gland located in the front of the throat below the Adam's apple and just above the breastbone. It is U-shaped and has two lobes, one on each side of the windpipe. Your thyroid produces two iodine containing hormones, thyroxine and tri-iodothyroinine. These act directly on almost all cells in your body to control the rate at which they break down and build up chemical substances (metabolism). The thyroid is controlled by the pituitary gland in your brain. There is a feed back mechanism by which the level of thyroid-stimulating hormone (TSH) in the blood also controls the pituitary, reducing its output of TSH if necessary.

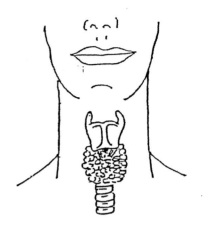

Types of thyroid cancer

There are four types of thyroid cancer. The three most common types begin in the thyroid cells that produce thyroxine and are named by their appearance under the microscope i.e. *papillary, follicular and anaplastic.* The latter is more common in later adulthood, is more aggressive with a high tendency to spread.

Medullary carcinoma of the thyroid is more unusual. It begins in other cells inside the thyroid and is sometimes associated with problems in other glands in the body.

Diagnosis

Your doctor must first of all get the full details of the lump from you and examine your neck carefully. If there is cancer then a *thyroid scan* uses an isotope that behaves in the same way as iodine and shows whether the nodule is actively taking up the isotope and/or *ultrasound* to show whether the nodule is a cyst, which are seldom cancerous and need only to be kept under observation.

If the above tests have indicated cancer, a *fine-needle biopsy* is carried out with a thin needle under local anaesthetic. If there is still evidence or suspicion of cancer, this will be followed by either a surgical biopsy or a more extensive operation. To assess the extent of the tumour and whether lymph nodes are involved, a *CT scan* of the neck may be recommended.

Treatment

Surgery As thyroid cancer is often slow growing, particularly in younger people, surgery is recommended. Part or the whole thyroid may need to be removed. Skin in the neck area heals very well and scars often become invisible after a time. If the entire thyroid has been removed or if the amount remaining is insufficient to produce enough thyroxine for your body, you will need to take thyroxine tablets for the rest of your life which **must** be taken every day, but have no side-effects. You need to be monitored on a regular basis to check the thyroxine dose is correct. If the dosage is too low, you may gain weight, feel tired and be affected by the cold weather more.

Radioactive Iodine In most cases this is recommended to kill any remaining cancer cells. Because of the safety measures associated with all radioactive substances, it is to be done carefully in hospital over a few days in an isolation room so other patients do not get radiation. Nursing staff will only stay in your room for short periods of time and will take special precaution when disposing of your urine etc... Visitors may be allowed in for short periods of time (no children or pregnant women) or they can talk to your through an intercom.

The treatment is not painful.

External radiotherapy May also be recommended.

Chemotherapy This is not too successful in treating thyroid cancer, but new drugs are being developed all the time and you may agree to participate in a clinical trial.

How to ensure a high success rate and reduce the likelihood of the cancer returning

It is most important that you take care of the BIG FOUR - avoid Geopathic Stress, destroy any microbes, mainly micro parasites, take adequate Q10 and ensure a high acid alkaline balance in your blood.

Take the necessary vitamins, minerals etc. as modern food no longer provides enough to prevent you suffering from malnutrition. Take at least 20 mcg daily of Vitamin D which is vital.

Also take enough exercise. Ideally exercise daily on a rebounder to vitalise your lymph system and help dispose of toxins from your body. Two minutes on a rebounder will double the number of white blood cells for one hour.

Using a MagneTech for four to five minutes daily direct on the thyroid to revitalise it and heal any operational scars. One minute on the thymus, which matures your T-cells and say 20 minutes on your solar plexus where 70% of your immune system is located and on your reflexology points under your feet.

You have got to take charge of your own health.

OTHER CANCERS

> **Previous chapters give details of about 93% of the most common cancers. Here are outlines of some other cancers. A combination of various orthodox treatments are used to treat all these cancers. I suggest you contact Macmillan Cancer Support (see Part Eight) and obtain further details on any of the cancers below.**

Adrenal Glands

This cancer can affect one or both glands. There is one adrenal gland on top of each kidney.

Eyes (Retinoblastoma)

This type of cancer can affect various parts of the eyes (see under childhood cancer).

Gallbladder Cancer

This is rare and seldom occurs unless there is a history of gallstones.
It is four times as common in women than men. The cancer may cause jaundice and tenderness in the upper right abdomen but is sometimes symptomless. It is diagnosed by ultrasound scanning. The cancer is treated by removing as much of the tumour as possible. Sometimes the cancer has invaded the liver.

Unknown Primary Tumours

This is when secondary cancer cells, which have broken away from the primary tumours, have been diagnosed but where the original cancer has not been diagnosed due to (a) The secondary cancer has grown and spread very quickly, while the primary cancer is still too small to be diagnosed, (b) The primary cancer has been hiding behind the secondary cancer or (c) Your immune system may have destroyed the primary tumours, but not the secondary cancer.

Ureter and Renal Pelvis

This cancer occurs at the exit of the kidneys. About 300 people are diagnosed per year - it affects more women than men.

How to ensure a high success rate and reduce the likelihood of the cancer returning

It is most important that you take care of the BIG FOUR - avoid Geopathic Stress, destroy any microbes, mainly micro parasites, take adequate Q10 and ensure a high acid alkaline balance in your blood.
Take the necessary vitamins, minerals etc.as modern food no longer provides enough to prevent you suffering from malnutrition. Take at least 20 mcg daily of Vitamin D which is vital. Also take enough exercise. Ideally exercise daily on a rebounder to vitalise your lymph system and help dispose of toxins from your body. Two minutes on a rebounder will double the number of white blood cells for one hour.
About 90% of people who get cancer have a thyroid gland which is out of balance. Using a MagneTech for one to two minutes direct daily will revitalise it. Do the same on the thymus, which matures your T-cells and say 20 minutes on your solar plexus where 70% of your immune system is located. Most importantly, use the MagneTech daily for 20 minutes directly on the problem area to heal it and any scar tissue.
You have got to take charge of your own health.

ANIMAL CANCER and how to keep your pets healthy

It is estimated over 400,000[1] in total of dogs and cats die of cancer each year in the UK. This has soared over the last 20 years due to weaker immune systems. The main reason for this has been caused by environment pollutions and stress, more inbreeding, inappropriate diets, pesticides and fertilisers in gardens and fields and excessive vaccinations. It is very important you consider both conventional and complementary therapy to ensure the best outcome. Diet and change of sleeping place may also have to be considered. There is so much which can be done so never consider cancer as a death sentence to your pet.

Symptoms

It is important you watch out for any changes in your animal's health, especially as they get older.

If you notice any of the signs listed below you should take your animal to your veterinary surgeon as soon as possible. The earlier the cancer is detected the better the chance that your animal will fully recover.

The most common signs of cancer reported by The American Veterinary Cancer Society are:

- Abnormal swelling that persists or continues to grow
- Loss of appetite
- Bleeding or discharge from any opening
- Persistent lameness or stiffness
- Reluctance to exercise or lack of stamina
- Sores that do not heal

[1] According to research carried out by the well-respected Morris Animal Foundation in the USA, 25% in total of dogs and cats die of cancer. There are 10 million dogs and 7.7 million cats in the UK. No similar research has been done in the UK, so using the same percentage and estimating the average life of dogs and cats is 10 years, about 460,000 in total die of cancer each year in the UK.

- Weight loss
- Offensive odour
- Difficulty eating or swallowing
- Difficulty in breathing
- Straining to urinate or defecate

Research
Dogs and Cats
Again according to research carried out by the well-respected Morris Animal Foundation in the USA, it is estimated 47% of non accidental deaths in dogs are caused by cancer and 32% in cases of cats. Golden Retrievers and Rottweilers are at higher risks of cancer because their popularity results in much inbreeding. Likewise Siamese cats have a higher risk among cats. Grey and white horses, white cows and white rabbits are more likely to get skin cancer as they are less protected from the sun. White bulldogs are forbidden to be bred in many countries.

Incidences of cancer are higher in dogs and cats than humans but lower in horses and cows, while cancer in birds is rare.

Dogs, for instance, have a higher rate of skin, breast and bone cancer than humans, who have a higher rate of lung cancer due to smoking.

Dogs and cats metabolism is much quicker than in humans (they also breathe seven times more per minute). Therefore, cancer can develop at a faster rate, but likewise animals can often respond quicker to treatment and can achieve remission sooner.

What is the most likely cause of domestic animal cancer?
Cancerous cells crop up on a daily basis, but are routinely destroyed and eliminated by a healthy immune system.

Parasites love Geopathic Stress and play a major part in weakening the immune system. These are not just visible skin mites or intestinal tape worms, but microscopic parasites. Animals can so easily pick up parasites outdoors from other animals, bird droppings etc. Like in humans, I have found micro-parasites in all cases of animal cancer. The contents inside a 450 mg 100% stabilised allicin garlic capsule per day in animal food, will normally kill the parasites. If your animal is high in micro-parasites, or for horses, large dogs etc. use one to two times 5 ml stabilising allicin liquid. Check correct quantity and results with muscle test.

Q10 is lacking in all cancer cases in humans and animals. The liver is nearly always weak in cancer cases. This prevents the liver effectively converting Q10 from food. As Q10 is not only a very powerful antioxidant, but also one of the ingredients which gives each cell its energy, so lack of Q10 weakens the immune system. The livers ability to produce Q10 diminishes with age and increases the likelihood of getting cancer.

Chemicals In food and liquids, pesticides and fertilisers in the garden and fields plus what comes through the food chain, is having its effect on our animals' health.

Other causes Things which could also affect your animal's health include over vaccination, electro pollution, cat litter trays, inappropriate diet, chemicals in the home etc. This will be dealt with later.

Geopathic Stress It is seldom animals get cancer unless they sleep and rest in a Geopathic Stress place. During sleep the brain does the body's 'housekeeping' including creating 80%

of your new cells, giving the right signals for the body to operate properly, to create and absorb the correct level of vitamins, minerals, trace elements etc. together with adjusting the hormone balance. Geopathic Stress will interfere with this process and leave the immune system weak. The immune system will become much stronger again when Geopathic Stress does not affect your animal's system. Cats unfortunately are their own worse enemy - they love Geopathic Stress!

When it comes to small animals, who are normally in cages most of the time, like hamsters, ferrets, guinea pigs, rabbits, mice, rats etc., it is vital the cage is not in a Geopathic Stress place.

Dr. E. Jenny of West Germany conducted experiments over many years with a total of 24,000 mice, studying their behaviour in Geopathic Stress places. The mice persistently attempted to escape from their boxes, showed weight loss, were more susceptible to cancer tumours, had smaller litters and a higher death rate of young than their control group, which were kept in places free of Geopathic Stress.

The American Noble Prize winner, Melvin Goldwin, who studied, among other things, the effect of carcinogenic tar on the skin of hamsters, found that the hamsters did not develop cancer, as anticipated, until they were kept in Geopathic Stress places.

Types of cancer and specific treatment
Dogs
The most common cancer in dogs is:

Breast Cancer (Mammary tumours) is most common in female dogs over six years old. If not spayed, a female dog has a 25% chance of getting mammary tumours. Most successful if spayed within 3 months of birth. Most mammary tumours (about 50% are malignant, some are benign) are painless mobile masses near one or more of the teats. Malignant breast cancer tends to spread to nearby lymph nodes. It can also spread to the lymph nodes near the groin, causing a painful inflammation. Breast cancer can sometimes spread to the lungs.
Orthodox Treatment Surgery offers moderate success for malignant tumours of less than 2cm (3/4in). Chemotherapy is certainly not going to give your dog a better quality of life as part of palliative care and is very expensive.
Nose and mouth cancer This usually appears as brown or black nodules, sometimes with a crusted surface. This type of malignant melanoma often grows fast and spreads locally and to other parts of the body.
Orthodox Treatment: mainly involves surgery to remove the melanoma and a wide surrounding area. It may also involve radiotherapy.
Skin Cancer (melanoma) in appearance like above. Often the growth is a relatively harmless skin disorder, but it is very important to see a vet for a correct diagnosis.
Orthodox treatment. Usually removed by surgery.
Lymphatic cancer tumours Lymphomas and lymph sarcoma are cancers that develop from lymphatic tissues, which are mainly located in the lymph nodes. They are also present in certain organs and other body structures including liver, spleen, intestines and bone marrow.
Orthodox treatment In most dogs the cancer has become widespread by the time of diagnosis. Surgery is used to remove the affected lymph nodes. Chemotherapy is often very effective in small dogs, but not so successful in larger dogs.

Other types of dog cancer

Abdominal Cancer Tumours are quite common but difficult to diagnose. Later they cause abdominal enlargement and weight loss.

Orthodox Treatment Surgery may sometimes be possible.

Bone Tumours are most common in medium to large size dogs and can quickly spread from the affected bone to the lungs.

Orthodox treatment: Surgery or immunotherapy may sometimes be suggested.

Osteosarcomas mainly occur in the long bone of the legs in mature dogs but can also occur in the jaw and in the ribs. If in the leg, it is often diagnosed by being painful when pressed, in dogs that have developed lameness, without any suspected injury to the leg.

Orthodox Treatment: Most common treatment is amputations of one joint above the affected area, if the lungs are free of cancer and the vet feels your dog will not have too much difficulty walking on three legs. (See case history using strong magnetic therapy).

Brain Tumours

Orthodox Treatment: Surgery may sometimes be possible.

Lung Cancer is seldom primary cancer, but secondary cancer spread either from bone tumour or soft tissue cancer.

Orthodox Treatment If cancer has been discovered elsewhere in the body, the chest is usually X-rayed to determine if the cancer has spread to the lungs.

Prostate An enlarged prostate in an unneutered dog over six years old is mainly due to an enlargement of the prostate gland. However, an enlarged prostate gland in a neutered dog is most likely to be cancer due to a tumour.

Orthodox Treatment: Surgical removal of part of the prostate gland is the only treatment, but can lead to urinary incontinence.

Testicular Cancer Typical occurrence in dogs over seven years old with one or both testicles undescended. They have a 50% chance of developing a testicle tumour.

Orthodox Treatment: Surgical removal of testicle/s is simple and effective.

Cats

Most of the cancers described regarding dogs are also in cats with the same orthodox treatment. The exemption is as follows:

Feline Breast Tumours This is not so common in cats and generally only in older female cats.   Spayed at an early age reduces the risk.

Head, Nose and Neck Cancer Is less common in cats.

Lymph sarcoma Mainly occurs in cats around eight to ten years.

Skin Cancer Melanomas is more common in cats than dogs.

Osteosarcomas Seldom occurs in cats.

Testicular Tumours Are rare in cats.

Feline Leukaemia (cancer of the white blood cells) Is the most common cancer in cats and kills more cats than anything except accidents. It can affect all body organs including skin, liver, spleen, intestines and more. Many cats are vaccinated against this cancer.

Orthodox Treatment Chemotherapy can control the tumours temporarily, on average four months, before the tumour returns.

Diagnosis

Many tumours just under the skin and in the lymph nodes can be felt from the outside during routine examinations by you. Other tumours can be detected by your vet during routine physical examinations or may be suspected from your animal's symptoms.

If cancer is suspected your vet may take an X-ray or ultrasound scans (sonograms). A MRIS (Magnetic Resonance Imaging Scan) or CAT (Computer Aided Tomography) scans can also be carried out in certain surgeries.

Even after these scans, it may be difficult for your vet to make a conclusive diagnosis without a biopsy for subsequent examination under a microscope.

Sometimes blood tests may be necessary to diagnose cancer in the spleen or liver or to check for leukaemia.

Treatment - Orthodox

Domestic animals can more or less get the same type of cancer as humans. The main difference between the treatments is one of cost and ethics. Less aggressive chemotherapy and radiotherapy treatments may be used, so as not to cause unnecessary side effects. However this may not be strong enough to eliminate the cancer. Also many owners, not insured, may be unable to afford these expensive orthodox therapies. So you may decide to concentrate on your animal's quality of life, including pain relief, even if this means a shorter life expectancy.

Orthodox treatment may buy the time necessary to allow the slow-acting natural therapies to take effect and benefit your animal's immune system.

If you also choose to use complementary therapy, it is advisable to get your vet's support. But stand your ground, when it comes to Geopathic Stress, parasites and Q10, which will always make the orthodox treatment more effective.

Surgery This is the most often used and most effective treatment by removing the tumour and surrounding healthy tissues and local lymph nodes.

Radiotherapy If it has not been possible to remove the cancerous mass completely or if surgery is not possible, localised radiotherapy can be carried out at specialised surgeries.

Chemotherapy Certain types of lymphomas and leukaemia respond well to chemotherapy, which will kill fast multiplying cancer. For other types of cancer, chemotherapy is unlikely to increase life expectancy. Chemotherapy drugs are generally cellular poison, which can be very toxic, and itself cause cancer as confirmed by The World Health Organisation. Chemotherapy also poses a risk to vets, nurses, pharmacists and others who handle the drugs.
They are all advised to wear gloves so, what is it doing to the inside of your beloved pet? Sometimes 80% of the active ingredient in the chemotherapy drug goes straight through pet's system.

Immunotherapy This treatment stimulates an animal's immune system, so it can attack the tumour.

Remember to shift your focus from 'cure' to daily remission and quality of life.

Treatment - Complementary

About 20% of dogs and cats live longer than one year after having only orthodox treatment. One veterinary clinic found on average cancer returned six and a half months after surgery. It is therefore vital, as with humans, you incorporate complementary remedies at the same time.

The law regarding complimentary treatment for animals broadly states that you can treat your own animals yourself, but only vets can treat other peoples animals. An animal health practitioner, who is not a vet, should only treat your pet if that person has been given the go ahead by a vet. Just a phone call is enough. But do tell your vet about any treatment your animal is having.

With or without orthodox treatment, very good results have been achieved by boosting your animal's immune system, by ensuring it is not sleeping in a Geopathic Stress place during the night and day, eliminating parasites with stabilised allicin garlic capsules or liquid (chemotherapy will, of course, do this!), increase Vitamin C, D and Q10, good diet, exercise and the use of strong high spinning magnetic apparatus direct on the cancer area and on the thyroid and thymus.

Acupuncture Used by vets or practitioners trained in Acupunture for animals can be a help in stimulating the body to release endorphins, which is a natural painkiller and prostaglandin, which reduces pain and inflammation by suppressing cortisone.

Bach Flower Remedies

Doctor Edward Bach (1880-1936) discovered 38 flowers that are ideal for use in healing negative emotional states in humans. The remedies are prepared from the flowers of wild plants, bushes and trees in pure spring water. Right from the beginning Dr. Bach used the remedies on animals with remarkable success. The Rescue Remedy - for emergencies and crisis situations - is a combination of 5 of the 38 remedies selected by Dr. Bach for all kinds of emergency situations, including before and during cancer treatment also for animals. They have no harmful side effects, are non toxic and do not influence or are not influenced by drugs. If the wrong Bach flower remedy is given, it has no side-effects. The Rescue Remedy and the other Bach flower remedies can be bought over the counter (see Page 237). Dosage: In case of Rescue Remedy, no matter what size your animal is, add two drops to a 30ml bottle of water. From this 'treatment bottle' give four drops at a time, at least four times a day. Put the remedy into the bowl each time you change the water, otherwise apply the dosage directly into the mouth from a dropper or syringe. If using a glass dropper, make sure your animal does not swallow or break the glass dropper.

Healing This is a very powerful therapy which most people can carry out themselves to the benefit of their beloved animal. At the same time you too will benefit from the calming effect that healing brings.

Make your animal comfortable and get yourself into a state of peace. Hold the palms of your hands above or on your animal near the health problem. On your pet's eyes.

Focus on the problem and send lots of love. Your beloved pet will feel the warmth of your healing heat even if you may not feel it yourself. Often you can see the pleasant reaction. Heal on a daily basis for a few minutes or longer.

Remember healing need not have any religious connections.

Herbs Buy a good book on healing animals with herbs. The before mentioned 100% stabilised allicin is not only the best way to kill micro parasites, but is also a very powerful immune booster.

Homeopathy Many vets now use homeopathy in conjunction with orthodox treatment. Two leading experts in alternative veterinary medicine, Doctors P.J. Bradfoot and Rick Palmquist, define Homeopathy as "the branch of medicine which seeks to identify the toxins in the body, helps to mobilise the natural defence mechanisms and free the body from toxic debris. The working principles of this form of biological medicine use the body's own self regulating mechanisms to bring about a true healing".

Magnetic Therapy Has proved over many years to be a very powerful way of treating cancer in humans and animals without causing any side effects. It is important that very powerful high rotating permanent magnets are used. This type of magnetic therapy can be used at home on a daily direct on the problem area. The treatment can be used in conjunction with orthodox treatment and any other complimentary treatment (see Page 232).

Over the counter Do not assume medicine which is available to humans without a doctor's prescription is suitable to animals - check with your vet.

Whatever treatment is decided upon, it is most important to eliminate or reduce the causes of the cancer in the first place to prevent the cancer returning.

How to prevent cancer in the first place
Apart from preventing Geopathic Stress and parasites, taking account of the following will help you to have a happy and healthy animal for many years.

Affection and love There is no doubt animals who are well cared for with lots of love and affection will be much healthier, as it has a direct influence on your pet's immune system. By stroking and cuddling your pet you boost your animal's thymus, which matures the body's T-cells, so they can fight more effectively any intruder (viruses, bacteria, parasites etc.).

Cat Litter Trays
Scoop-able litter trays have the advantage that the clay (quartz silica) contains sodium benlonite, expands the litter over 15 times when wet, which makes it easier to remove the wet lumps without replacing the whole tray's contents. This is why the litter must not be flushed down the toilet.

Unfortunately, when your cat digests the clay while cleaning its feet, it expands and forms a solid mass in the animal's intestines. This draws fluid out of its body causing dehydration and urinal tract problems.

Also when your cat inhales the silica dust it may not only be carcinogenic, but could cause the nasty lung disease, pneumonoultramicroscapicsilicovolcanoconiosis. (Longest word in

English!) This inhaled silica dust could also be the cause for the steady rise in asthma in cats.

Why not use your shredded paper or use safe biodegradable toilet flushable litter tray contents instead.

Chemicals outdoors

<u>Insecticides</u> - including poison for ants, fleas etc. contain different active ingredients, which can accumulate in your pet's body and can be carcinogenic.

<u>Antifreeze</u> (ethylene glycol) is very dangerous. It could, by mistake, be in puddles when used during cold weather, which your pet may drink. The poison affects kidney function.

<u>Pesticides, herbicides and fertilisers</u> used in the garden can greatly affect your pet's health. Do no go for a walk or let your cat onto your nearest golf course. An eighteen hole golf course can use over 20 tons of dry and liquid chemicals per year. Some people apply chemicals four times a year to their lawns, so the choice is beautiful lawns or healthy pets. Tests have been carried out which show an increase in cancer in relation to the amount of chemicals used in gardens.

Indoor chemicals - which are a danger to your animals include: bleach, detergents, stain remover, furniture spray, polish which can give your wooden furniture a very dangerous formaldchyde coating, (use natural oils or beeswax), artificial colours and fragrances, benzene found in many detergents and even cleaning products. Naphthalene, a cousin to Benzene is often an ingredient in carpet cleaning and deodorizers (see details under human breast cancer, how dangerous deodorizers can be to women).

Why not make your own chemical free products or make your own cleansing products with items such as baking soda, lemon juice, oregano, vinegar and other safe inexpensive substitutes.

<u>Rodenticides</u> intended to kill rats, mice etc are some of the deadliest substances for other animals. Even if the poison is kept in safe containers, dogs and cats can easily be poisoned by eating a rodent that has consumed the poison.

<u>Paint</u> When painting your home inside, keep your animals outside or at a friend's house.

Drinking Water - if your animal does not drink enough, its body cannot function properly. A dog should drink one ounce (28ml) of water per pound (0.455kg) of body weight per day. If your dog drinks three or more times this amount, it may have diabetes or kidney failure. A cat can go without food for a day and lose up to 40% of its normal body weight, but a water loss of up to 15% can be fatal. If a cat stops eating, it must drink more water to offset the decrease in food intake.

<u>Tap Water</u> - In my opinion water straight out of the tap is the best. It is alive, checked daily and contains good minerals etc.

<u>Chlorine</u> - this can only exist under pressure. So long as the water stands for 1 hour before being drunk, the chlorine has evaporated.

<u>Ozonated</u> - water is very clean and is very good for the whole animal's body. (See Page 225).

<u>Geopathic Stress</u> - I have heard many cases where domestic animals will not drink water in a Geopathic Stressed house, but rely on water outside - often polluted.

<u>Bowl</u> - apparently, cats drink more water from a ceramic dish. A heavy one cannot be easily moved and should be cleaned with boiling water.

Exercise - one of the primary advantages of exercise, as in humans, is to increase your animal's oxygen supply and help move its lymph through its channels (which has no pump) and thereby detoxify and eliminate toxins from its body. Exercise reduces stress, anxiety and depression by releasing the feel good hormones from the brain. Only 20% of dogs get enough exercise.

If your animal is having orthodox treatment, do not overdo the exercise.

Flea and Tick Medication - if you decide to use sprays, pills or injections to destroy fleas and ticks on your animals, it is important you contact your vet for advice, in case your pet develops unusual behaviour or becomes unwell.

You should bear the following in mind:
- Cats are more sensitive to anti flea and tick products than dogs. So ensure you do not use products on cats, which are specified for dogs. Organophosphate insecticides for example could even cause death in cats.
- Never use anti flea and tick medication on very young, ill or elderly pets, or if you're pet is pregnant.
- Do not use flea shampoos, sprays or other products near your animal's eyes, ears or genitalia.
- If you are decontaminating your home for fleas etc., make sure you remove your cat/s in particular from your home.
- Not all 'natural' products are entirely safe.
- Why not try an alternative to toxic products, like: herbal flea powder and collar, natural shampoos. Add brewer's yeast and garlic to your animal's diet. Sprays or powders containing pyrethrins or natural pyrethrums are less toxic.
- Ensure you have a good filter, like a Hepa filter, on your vacuum cleaner and use special anti flea mineral salt on your carpets.
- Ensure your pets have a strong immune system, which has the ability to fight off the fleas etc., themselves in the first place. So no Geopathic Stress, no parasites and good nutrition. When your pets have a strong immune system, the fleas and ticks find your pet's blood less appetizing and move onto an animal with a weaker immune system, which gives off a particular odour that makes its blood tastier.

Medicine The increased use of pharmaceutical drugs will weaken the immune system. Use safe and non invasive medicine and treatments.

Overweight Over one third of Britain's dogs and cats are overweight, even though there is no evidence that fat pets are more likely to get cancer. But if they do, they are more difficult to treat. If your pet is overweight reduce its food slowly, particularly with cats, as a quick fast can be dangerous.

Spay Or Neuter Can cut down the risk of cancer in both dogs and cats. Spaying a female eliminates the possibility of uterine or ovarian cancer and drastically reduces the risk of breast cancer, particularly if the pet is spayed before her first cycle. Dogs go into heat at the earliest at five months. Cats around five to six months.

Neutering a male eliminates the possibility of testicular cancer. Disease of the prostate, is sometimes avoided in dogs by neutering. Prostate cancer is quite rare in cats.

Supplements Even though processed pet food manufacturers claim they add adequate vitamins and minerals into their animal food, most are destroyed during processing. Also, your own homemade food may not contain adequate vitamins etc. as vegetables and meat have almost 50% less nutrients than they did 50 years ago, so ensure your pets have additional supplements as follows:

Vitamin A particularly important for cats that cannot produce their own Vitamin A.
Vitamin C acts as a cellular antioxidant, thereby may protect against cancer. It boosts the immune system by detoxing and protects against various carcinogenic chemicals digested. Even though dogs and cats produce their own Vitamin C, stressed (including Geopathic Stress), an illness or an infection will reduce their natural supply. Age will also reduce the production of Vitamin C. If ill the recommended daily dose for cats and small dogs are 0.5g - 1.5g, medium size dogs 1.5g - 3g, large dogs 3-6g, and giant dogs 6-7g.
Vitamin D longhaired dogs and cats do not absorb enough Vitamin D from the sun during the winter. Diet accounts for very little of the Vitamin D that makes its way into the bloodstream. See full details in Part Four, why this is one of the most vital supplements. Recommend a 20 mcg (800 iv) capsule in oil, cut open and squished into your pet's food during the winter months.
Vitamin E will boost the immune system and is very good for your pet's heart.
Q10 Like in humans, Q10 is a vital supplement to help prevent cancer. Q10 is the sparking plug in every cell and your pet may not produce enough from its food if its' liver is below par or as your pet gets older. See full details in chapter on Q10 regarding humans (P.18). Recommend a 30mg capsule in soya oil cut open and squished into your pet's food.
Magnesium to ensure your pet's calcium can be used effectively. Recommend 200mg per day.
Calcium suggest a ground-up medium size eggshell.
Selenium the UK has one of the lowest levels of Selenium in the world. In human trials, thousands of people who took 200mg over seven years had a 50% drop in cancer death rate compared to the placebo group. So, another essential trace element to give your pet. Recommended dose 50-100micrograms (not milligrams) daily.
Beta-Carctene converts to Vitamin A if the body needs it. Many studies in humans have shown additional intake of Beta-Carclena have reduced the risk of cancer.
Allicin from garlic to prevent viruses, bacteria, fungi and parasites. This will also boost the immune system. Recommend one 180 mg capsule per day. Open the capsule and spread contents into your pet's food (See details on allicin in Part One).
Seaweed is the most nutritious plant in the world and contains over 100 vitamins, minerals and trace elements in a natural form. The best seaweed comes from the North Atlantic and is still growing when it is harvested and frozen within 24 hours. It should be in a granule form free from dust for animals. Seaweed makes dogs more healthy, positive, coat more shiny and co-operative (20% of dogs have behaviour problems). Seaweed gives cats extra energy and makes their fur glossy.

Other useful supplements are Omega 3, lecithin and Omega 6 .

Summary The most important supplements to give your pet are vitamin D, Q10, allicin and seaweed.

Give Pills to cats Cats very often will not allow something strange put into their food, such as medicine or supplements. So to get your cat to swallow a tablet or capsule do the following:

Put some butter (or other spread) on your middle longest finger and press the tablet or capsule on to it. Squeeze your thumb and middle finger hard on either side of your cats mouth, so your cat has to open its' mouth. Then pop your finger with the pill or capsule down your cat's throat.

Vaccinations Many vets now believe the number of vaccinations carried out today is doing more harm than good to our dogs and cats. Unfortunately, it represents a large part of a veterinary surgery's income. Without vaccinations, many vets would have financial difficulty as it can represent over 50% of their income.
No long-term comparative studies have been carried out to evaluate if vaccinations are necessary or effective for dogs or cats. Unfortunately, many vets refuse unvaccinated pets for treatment.

Puppies and kittens must, of course, be vaccinated against distemper, hepatitis and parvovirus. Usually pets are given 2-4 doses at six weeks or older spread over two to four weeks. A booster vaccination is given at one year old. Obviously, they must be given shots for rabies in many countries outside the United Kingdom.

The most common vaccines given:

Dogs
- Canine Distemper virus - a dangerous viral infection.
- Hepatitis - a viral infection that mainly affects the liver.
- Parvovirus - a severe and often fatal virus affecting the lining of the intestinal tract.
- Leptospirosis - a bacterial infection affecting the liver.
- Parainfluenze - a virus that along with the hepatitis virus can cause upper respiratory infection.
- Coronquirus - is very similar to Parvovirus. It can be very severe, but has a different affect on the intestinal tract and is generally not fatal.
- Bordettela (kennel cough) cannot protect against all types of influenza. Many kennels insist on this vaccination before accepting your dog for boarding.

Almost 70% of dogs with behavioural problems, nervous or worrying dispositions or short attention span developed their difficulty within three months of a vaccination.
The American Animal Hospital Association recommends dogs should only have vaccinations for Distemper, Hepatitis and Parvovirus every three years.

Under present vaccinations schedule, which recommend five live vaccine boosters every year, by the time your dog is 10 years old it will have received at least 60 live vaccine viruses. This does not include other vaccinations for boarding or travelling. Is it any wonder your dear pets are suffering?

When vaccines work, it has been found they last on average for dogs:
Distemper 5-7 years, Parvovirus 7 years, Parainfluenze 3 years, and Kennel cough 7 years.

Cats
There is a dilemma when it comes to feline leukaemia vaccine, which is given to prevent one of the most common cancers in cats. Since the vaccine was introduced about twenty

years ago, the cases of feline fibro sarcoma have become common at an average age of eight. Before then it was very rare. If you still decide to go ahead with the feline leukaemia vaccine, insist that it is not given in the scruff of the neck or between the shoulder blades, but injected in the rear legs, so should the vaccine causes sarcoma cancer the affected limb can be amputated, if there is no other way of saving your cat's life.

Tilering This is a process whereby a blood sample is laboratory tested to determine your pet's immunity level, so you only give a booster if your animal needs it. Many pets are protected even five years after the last injection. Ensure the vaccine is given in different places i.e. neck, shoulder, hindquarter and keep a record where the vaccine was given. Often skin cancer can develop if an animal is continually injected in the same place.

Dogs and cats
In one survey 35 people were questioned, whose animals had cancer. It confirmed 90% of the animals had been vaccinated within two months of developing cancer.

Many people, including vets, do not connect the onset of arthritis and skin conditions with the vaccinations given a couple of months previously.

It is not advisable to give vaccine before anaesthetic in case of surgery. Vet Richard Pitcairn warns "Giving a vaccine to an animal with cancer is like pouring petrol on a fire".

Pregnant pets should not be vaccinated nor old or ill animals.

One must bear in mind; no vaccine for humans or animals gives 100% protection or is 100% safe. In all cases a weak immune system is to blame for failure.

A very healthy alternative to over vaccination is 100% stabilised allicin, Vitamin D, Q10, seaweed and homeopathic remedies, which can also prevent side effects from vaccination.

Nutrition

Healthy nutrition is a very important factor in keeping your animal healthy, so it maintains a strong immune system to prevent cancer in the first place and create a strong immune system if it has cancer treatment. Even though most processed pet food manufacturers claim the food contains all the supplements your pet needs, can you be certain? Cooked processed food destroys on average up to 75% of natural vitamins, so additional supplements are important. It has definitely been shown, when you give good quality seaweed in addition to even 'good quality' processed pet food, there is a noticeable improvement both mental and physical in the animal.

Like human processed food, processed pet food contains vast amounts of chemicals, such as preservatives, colouring agents, emulsifiers, lubricants, flavouring agents, solvents etc. Three common preservatives used to stablize fats and oils have shown to be carcinogens. Some even contain propylene glycol, a cousin of antifreeze, which destroys red blood cells.

Unless percentages of ingredients are mentioned on the packeting, 'beef dinner' may only contain 10% of beef and 'with cheese' 10% of cheese. Cats should mainly eat meat and fish. On the packeting of many well known makes of cat food, it only mentions it contains

14% in chunks of meat or fish. How much more meat or fish does it contain?

Mainly due to a modern demand for 'low maintenance' pets, 95% of our dogs and cats get their main nutrition from processed pet food - would you consider it healthy only to eat processed food from the Supermarket. Your pet would be far better off eating your left over food provided it incorporates other ingredients described before. Not vegetarian food for cats.

During the three day working week, due to strikes, during the Heath Government, pet food manufacturers had the first call on tins, as it was almost impossible to dump the 'unfit for human consumption' pet food!

Home Made Pet Diet

Dogs are related to wolves that eat a lot of vegetables. But one third to one half of the daily diet could be animal products preferably raw, such as beef, chicken, turkey, organic meat and some fish. One third should be made up of cooked grain such as oats or oatmeal, millet, barley and split, vegetables etc. can be used.

If you decide you want to feed your dog on cooked meat, some nutrients are reduced through cooking, but not completely destroyed. Some vitamins and minerals are made more available by light cooking. Ensure the cooking juices, where many vitamins and minerals end up, are served with the food.

If you are worried about giving your dog bones, they can be ground up beforehand. Some vets are worried your dog might get parasites from raw meat, so try and buy your dog meat from a reputable butcher. If your dog should get parasites from raw meat or from other animals, ensure you kill the parasites with 100% stabilised allicin. Also for your own sake prevent your dog spreading parasites to your family from their faeces and saliva. Don't let your dog lick your face.

To save time when making your own dog and cat food, make it once a week into several portions and store it in your freezer.

Sometimes other animal proteins may be substituted with some milk, raw egg yolks etc. Also raw vegetables and fruit. The food should also include polyunsaturated oils such as olive or sesame. Dogs should not be given cooked bones.

In one study about 10 years ago, the diet of over 100 dogs was changed from processed pet food to a natural diet. After six months the visits to the vets had dropped by 85%. The dogs had more energy, improved teeth and gums, glossier coats and skin. Also their weight and behaviour had improved. As mentioned elsewhere, because the dogs had an improved immune system, they had less fleas and ticks. All round they were healthier.

Cats are carnivores so mainly need meat and other animal products. Do not give them salt, sugar or milk, nor canned tuna, ham or pork. Do give them some treats now and again such as a soft boiled egg, cooked meat or poultry. Cats need Vitamin A as their bodies cannot produce this vitamin.

It is very important that your cat has a balanced diet, so you may decide to discuss a diet plan with a nutrionist.

Switching Over To A Homemade Diet

If you decide to switch over to a homemade diet, it will cost more and take time. It must be a well balanced diet. Keep your pet's teeth healthy by not making the food too soft. The change over for dogs should take about three weeks. To avoid most intestinal problems to start with, gradually increase the amount of homemade food with good quality processed food.

As you know, cats are fussier than dogs. Try and give your cat a spoonful of the homemade diet at first. Then try three or four meals of the new diet at first (remove after half an hour) and revert to two meals a day, after one week. You can try some cooked chicken, liver or a sardine to start off with as a bribe.

Some people decide to go half way and feed their dogs 50% dried food. Regarding cats, you may choose to mix homemade and processed food 50/50 or entirely high quality commercial food.

Chocolate and coco is dangerous for dogs and cats because two of the ingredients, theobromin and caffeine, are toxic to animals. Remember, plenty of fresh water each day. Tap water is alive due to spinning and tested daily, not like dead bottled water.

Medicine for dogs and cats

Due to the increase in environmental pollution, commercial pet food and unnecessary vaccinations, dogs and cats suffer a range of modern degenerative illnesses not seen 40 years ago. This will lower the immune system and prevent your pet fighting off cancer.

This has been a great opportunity for pharmaceutical companies to present a large range of new drugs. Most of the main drugs for humans have been adapted for pets. There are even new drugs to deal with the side effects of drugs.

Unfortunately more and more powerful combinations of drugs are being developed where previous ones have failed. Also drugs are often given in far too big dosages.

Here is a list of certain health problems pets have and the side-effects caused by common drugs given:

Anti-stress say before an operation
Can cause seizure. Use Bach Flower 'Rescue Remedy'.

Diabetic
Dosages must be very strictly administered as serious problems can be caused with even small overdoses.

Painkillers - typical drug used is Paracetamol
Can cause liver damage and is extremely likely if given to cats.

Parasites and fungals
As with humans, drugs are very much a hit or miss, as many drugs do not work. Many side-effects can be very disturbing for your pets. 100% stabilised allicin eliminates all microbes.

Respiratory and bacterial infections
Antibiotics are often given which can cause severe digestive problems, as it kills off the good bacteria in the colon. Penicillin can cause allergic reactions, even sudden death. If antibiotics are given, ensure probiotics are also given or tablets to introduce billions of good bacteria like Bio-Culture capsules from Pharma Nord.

Steroids - often used with chemotherapy

Side-effects can be many. Never stop this drug abruptly. After two weeks the steroid drugs should be cut down gradually.

<u>Thyroid</u> - under active

Use drugs with caution in pets with diabetes and with problems with the heart and adrenal glands. Like in humans strong magnetic therapy is a very powerful method of bringing the thyroid back into balance.

Alternatives to Pharmaceutical drugs

Many vets are now turning to non invasive and very effective alternative forms of medicine and treatment such as Acupuncture, Bach Flower, Kinesiology, Homeopathy, Strong Magnetic Therapy, Nutrition, 100% stabilised allicin garlic etc.

Or contact a Member of the British Homeopathic Veterinary Association near you for advice on Homeopathy and how to feed your companion animals.

Cancer case histories

Osteosarcoma *8 year old Dylan, a big black dog, was diagnosed with aggressive osteosarcoma on his front right leg. His vet's only solution was to amputate the leg. Two MagneTechs (high powered spinning magnets) were used on Dylan's leg each side of the tumour. Within one month, the tumour had cleared and the leg healed up.*

Prostate cancer *10 year old Clapper, a cross breed, had developed prostate cancer and had great difficulty passing water. Clapper was given three weeks to live as no surgery was recommended. Two high powered spinning magnetic apparatus were used for about 20 minutes daily directly on the front lower half of his body, within days he could urinate normally and was soon enjoying life as before.*

In both cases Geopathic Stress was involved and put right.

Summary

A successful treatment for cancer depends on three things:

1. <u>Your vets full support</u> Find a vet you feel comfortable with and who specialises in cancer. Take the opinion of a complementary therapist. Then make your decision regarding treatment with a positive attitude.

2. <u>Strengthen immune system</u> by keeping your pet out of Geopathic Stress and other environmental dangers. Give good nutritional food and supplements including seaweed and stabilised allicin garlic. Strong magnetic therapy will also improve the immune system.

3. <u>Full emotional support</u> and love from you. Make your pet's bed warm and comfortable.

Animals are excellent patients. Few complain or ever utter a sound. Their emotions are in their eyes.

You receive so much love from your pets, so by keeping them healthy, you help your own health. In several nursing homes, it was found medication to the residents was greatly reduced (by almost 70%) when animals were part of the environment.

Final Note

Remember what is best for your pet

If for example, your pet had cancer in its leg and your vet's treatment could give it an extra year or so of life, how could you explain to your pet that suffering from the cancer treatment was for a reason? That lying in a small cage, surgically maimed and hooked up to a drip for weeks, perhaps months, would be 'worth it'. Would it not be kinder to have your pet put to sleep and out of its misery, thereby giving it a loving and peaceful death? If your pet is not in too much pain, you may prefer to take it home, give it a nice warm bed, its favourite food, maybe some painkillers and lots of love during its short life.

PART FOUR

NUTRITION

CONTENTS

- **Nutrition** - cancer and malnutrition
- **Modern food** - lacking in nutrition
- **Free Radicals and Antioxidants**
- **Supplements** - to help cancer patients
    Vitamin A, B12, C, D, E, Folic Acid, Magnesium, Pycnogenol, Seaweed and Selenium
- **TOP** - It is not what you eat, it is mainly how you eat it
- **Other powerful supplements**
    Allicin, B17, Essiac and Pau D'Arco
- **Special diets - Gerson, Macrobiotic, Bristol Cancer Centre, Dries Cancer Diet and Grape Diet**
- **Green and white Tea**
- **Manuka Honey**
- **Salt** - what many people are short of
- **Water and Ozonated water**
- **Dairy Products** - why they increase the risk of cancer
- **Food Sweeteners**

NUTRITION

Many people who are diagnosed with cancer suffer from malnutrition, even if they have been on a healthy diet.

Geopathic Stress is the most 'anti-nutrient' on the planet. When you are asleep, your body is designed to repair and heal, as your brain is no longer busy with all your body's physical activities during the time you are awake. Seeing and hearing also occupies a large part of your brain's activities.

During sleep, your brain will do your body's 'housekeeping', including creating most of your new cells, adjusting hormone balances, revitalising heart, kidneys, liver etc. But as your body also has to fight Geopathic Stress, it has to reduce some of its activities, which it feels it can delay and put on the 'back burner', like not fully looking after your digestive system. This can result in you only absorbing 50% of the goodness from your food and thereby weakening your immune system. These body functions will usually return to normal very quickly once your body no longer has to fight Geopathic Stress.

Parasites partly live on your nutrients food. Lack of Q10 means your cells have less energy to process your food. Too acidic blood depletes your body's stock of vital minerals etc. which are needed to make your blood more alkaline.

Even when you have dealt with the BIG FOUR, a healthy diet with plenty of fresh vegetables and fruit will not be enough for you. You need some vital supplements modern food cannot provide.

MODERN FOOD

Agricultural land in the western world can now produce ten times as much food as a hundred years ago. To achieve this, as the soil becomes exhausted, nitrogen and fertilizers containing phosphorus are applied, but this deprives the soil even more of vital trace elements.

Over the last hundred years, we in the UK have mainly gone from physical jobs, to desk jobs. So instead of needing an average of 3,000 calories a day, we now only need 1800-2500. Vital vitamins, minerals and trace elements follow the intake of calories. As we need fewer calories, we absorb less vitamins etc. On top of this, we eat far more 'empty' calories e.g. sugar and fat. Even if we feel healthy, we need extra supplements all the time, such as multivitamins or even seaweed, which is the most nutritious plant in the world.

It is also very important to absorb enough Vitamin D either from the sun or in capsule form, so you can absorb calcium more effectively. (See page 208).

Remember, no particular food will prevent or cause cancer, whatever evidence the thousands of research projects round the world have claimed to prove, as they did not take into account the BIG FOUR.

FREE RADICALS AND ANTIOXIDANTS

Free radicals are energetically unstable and highly dangerous materials, which are constantly generated during the body's functions such as respiration, oxidative energy, metabolism and immune activity. Free radicals are also produced from UV radiation, smoke, pollution, heavy metals and rancid fatty acids etc. The harmful effects of free radicals are far reaching including the destruction of the immune system, which is meant to destroy any cancer cells the body is constantly producing.

One of the body's natural mechanisms of preventing and neutralising the damage caused by free radicals are its own antioxidants in vitamins A, B, C, E and the mineral selenium which all work individually and together in your body. These vitamins and minerals have shown in many research studies involving hundreds of thousands of people, to reduce the risk of cancer.

VITAMIN A AND BETA CAROTENE

Fat-soluble Vitamin A retinal has been found to help reduce the risk of cancer. It also protects the mucous membranes of the mouth, nose, and throat and reduces the risk of infection. It is vital for eye and retina functions, healthy skin, antioxidant and immune system booster.

While you can overdose on fat-soluble Vitamin A, **water soluble beta carotene,** is made into Vitamin A by your body, is non toxic and constitutes an extremely potent source of antioxidant.

Fat-soluble Vitamin A is mainly found in liver, fish, cabbage, potatoes and apples. Large doses of beta carotene are found in carrots, sweet potato and in lesser amounts in other vegetables. The lack of vitamin A is mainly caused by alcohol, coffee, smoking, heat and light.

Recommended daily doses for cancer patients:

Vitamin A retinal

Children 1,000-3,000 mcg (3,000-10,000 ius).

Toxicity may occur above 4,000-20,000 mcg per day long term or 25,000 mcg single doses.

Adults 2,250-6,000 mcg (7,500-20,000 ius) - if pregnant or trying to conceive, do not exceed 3,000 mcg (10,000 ius).

Toxicity may occur above 8,000-30,000 mcg per day long term or 300,000 mcg single doses.

Beta Carotene

Adult 3,000-30,000 mcg (10,000-100,000 ius).

VITAMIN B12

Water-soluble Vitamin B12 is necessary for the production of red blood cells and to help the blood carry oxygen to convert the calories into energy. B12 also increases resistance to diseases by helping your immune system create T- and B- cells. Your liver contains large quantities of B12, so it may take some time before any shortage is noticed. This shortage is not due to insufficient intake through your diet, but because your body has difficulty absorbing B12. This could be due to damage to the lower small intestine where the B12 is absorbed through the mucous membrane. This can also be caused by inflammation, major operations on the intestines or by certain drugs including some chemotherapy drugs. Folic acid needs B12 to be absorbed. Strict vegetarians may also need to take B12 as this vitamin may be lacking in their diet.

Vitamin B12 is mainly found in liver and kidneys. Smaller amounts are found in milk, eggs, cheeses, turkey, chicken, oysters, sardines, tuna and shrimps.

Lack of B12 is mainly due to alcohol, smoking and difficulty in absorbing vitamins.

Recommended daily dose for cancer patients.

Children 25-250 mcg (µn)   **Adult's** 500-1000 mcg (µn)

If difficulty in absorbing B12, you will need 10,000 mcg injection at regular intervals. Overdose not reported with oral dose.

VITAMIN C

Water-soluble Vitamin C is vital, due to its antioxidant and immune boosting functions (antiviral and anti-bacterial) and its ability to work together with Vitamin E at the cell membrane interface to produce a very powerful antioxidant. Vitamin C makes collagen keeping bones, skin and joints firm and strong. It helps make anti-stress hormones and turns food into energy.

A ten year study of 11,000 men and women by research at the University of California, found that women with the highest Vitamin C intake, had a 25% lower death rate from heart disease and 42% reduced death rate from cancer.

Vitamin C is found in large amounts in cabbage and in most other vegetables and fruit.

Lack of Vitamin C is mainly due to alcohol, smoking, pollution, stress and fried food.

Recommended daily dose for cancer patients. **Children** 500-1,000mg **Adults** 2,000-10,000mg

Mega-Dose Vitamin C

A ten year study of 11,000 men and women by research at the University of California, found that women with the highest Vitamin C intake, had a 25% lower death rate from heart disease and 42% reduced death rate from cancer.

It has been known for a long time, that giving large quantities of Vitamin C by intravenous infusion, has been a successful way of treating cancer.

There are a number of doctors in the UK who now offer Vitamin C intravenous infusions, but this can be expensive. Also you need strong veins, as several litres of liquid is put in, several times a week.

Fortunately, a new form of Vitamin C, called LypoSpheric has recently been launched. By encasing the Vitamin C in fat molecules, the product has been designed to deliver to the liver per sachet, the equivalent to a dose of 10g Vitamin C given intravenously. Cancer patients may take three to five sachets a day. (Children one to two sachets a day).

Increase dosage level slowly over a 7 day period. Squeeze the contents of the sachet into 1-2 ounces of water. Drink the whole mixture in one swallow. If you do not like the taste, substitute the water for cooled fruit or vegetable juice.

Recommend that you split the dosage between morning and early afternoon. Taking the product too late in the evening may cause a burst of energy, which could interfere with your normal sleep schedule. It is also recommended that you take the powder on an empty stomach, a few minutes prior to a meal, to ensure that the maximum and quickest entry of the LypoSpheric into the bloodstream. If you take it with a meal, it will take longer for the LypoSpheric to get into your bloodstream.

LypoSpheric can be taken while having cancer treatment, such as chemotherapy, radiotherapy, laser or hormone treatment.

Consult your doctor if you are on Warfarin.

For more information and to purchase LypoSpheric – contact www.lypospheric.co.uk

VITAMIN D - the sunshine Vitamin
There would be no life on earth without the sun.

Vitamin D deficiency is now known to be connected with most types of cancer.

Research in the USA estimates 10% of total cancer deaths are attributed to insufficient vitamin D. Applying the statistics to the UK, 15,000 cancer deaths could be caused by too low vitamin D levels in your body.

Vitamin D is mainly produced by your body from exposure to UVB rays from the sun. As many of us now have indoor jobs and cover ourselves with clothes and sunscreen when in the sun, due to the fear of skin cancer, (see below) we are not getting enough of this vital vitamin.

Vitamin D helps your body absorb calcium and phosphorus which is essential for bone and tooth growth. Lack of Vitamin D has also shown links with arthritis, autism, asthma, chronic pain, diabetes, heart attacks, infertility, multiple sclerosis, osteomalacia and lack of mental agility. T-cells which play a vital role in the immune system (see Part Seven) rely on Vitamin D to become active.

How vitamin D protect against cancer

Apoptosis   This is the normal process when cells die off naturally, to be replaced by new healthy cells. Cancer cells lose this ability, which causes them to grow uncontrollably. Vitamin D helps make cells that have turned cancerous die when they are supposed to.

Cell differentiation   Normal cells evolve and take on specialised jobs. Eventually normal cells differentiate until they can no longer divide and they stop growing when they have reached maturity. Cancer cells lose this ability and therefore do not stop growing. They can reproduce haphazardly and quickly. Vitamin D helps make cancer cells differentiate and force them to specialise into the type of cells within an organ they are suppose to become.

Cellular proliferation   This is the growth and division of cells. The genes that control cellular proliferation are affected by vitamin D. The ability of genes to affect proliferation is impaired if vitamin D levels are low.

Regulation cell growth   Is the formation and differentiation of blood vessels. Cancer cells create new blood vessels so the cancer can grow. Vitamin D influences the gene that control angiogenesis, blocking cancer cells from creating new blood vessels, so they cannot keep growing.

Reduction of metastases   Metastases are the ability of cancer cells to enter the bloodstream and

and travel to other parts of the body where they invade normal, healthy tissues. Animal studies have indicated that vitamin D may inhibit the ability of cancer cells to spread in this way.

Research Dr Joan M Lappe and her colleagues (Nebraska USA) created a randomized double blind placebo-controlled trial, meaning neither the random selected participant nor the researchers knew who was getting vitamin D or a placebo. This groundbreaking study was conducted on 403 postmenopausal women over a period of four years.

The research showed that women who received 20 mcg of vitamin D per day for four years, reduced their risk of developing cancer of any kind by 60%, compared to those women who received a placebo. (75% when disregarding the women who were found later to have had cancer before the trial).

Skin cancer (Melanoma) Many researchers wonder if the avoidance of the sun, because of the fear of skin cancer, (which you are unlikely to get if you take care of the BIG FOUR) is worth the increase risk of and mortality from internal cancers due to lack of vitamin D. You are 60 times more likely to suffer other more dangerous types of cancer than skin cancer.

Vitamin D levels Can be measured in regular blood tests, so when you next have a blood test, ask for your vitamin D level to be checked. Vitamin D levels should be about 35ng/ml (nonograms per millilitre). Sometimes expressed in nmol/l. To change ng/ml to nmol/l, you need to multiply ng/ml by 2.5). Many people when they are diagnosed can be as low as 12 ng/ml.

Ultraviolet (UV) light
There are two kinds of ultraviolet light from the sun.

UVA rays are long rays which do not produce vitamin D. They pass through glass, clothing and deep into your skin causing premature ageing and wrinkles.

UVB causes sunburn and produces vitamin D through your skin.

Sunshine to give you enough Vitamin D Scientists agree that by far the best way to boost the vitamin D nutrients if you are fair-skinned, is to expose your face and arms for 10 to 15 minutes per day to sunlight without sunscreen at the time when (UVB) radiation is at its strongest, at noon and early afternoon, between April and October. This also builds up a reserve for the winter. UVB rays cannot penetrate glass or clothing, so you do not produce vitamin D just by sitting near a window.

Skin colour The amount of vitamin D your body produces very much depends on your skin colour and your age. Melanin is the pigment in your skin that gives you colour and it absorbs the UVB rays, inhibiting vitamin D production. People with dark or black skin need intense sunlight to penetrate the skin in order to produce vitamin D - up to 10 times the amount of sun that fair-skinned people require. Suntanned skin also blocks UVB rays from creating vitamin D.

Age As we get older, we produce less of the vitamin D precursor in our skin and therefore produce less vitamin D when exposed to the sun. Elderly people need to be in the sun four times as long as a young person.

Research carried out by Dr Oscar France from Warwick Medical School (UK) found by studying 3,262 individuals, aged between 50 and 70 years old, that 94% were low in vitamin D.

Weight If you are overweight, you have trouble making enough vitamin D from the sun. Vitamin D is a fat-soluble vitamin, so fat cells absorb it, making it less available for use in tissues and organs throughout the body. If you are obese, you need twice the amount of sunshine.

Latitude Studies have confirmed that people living at high latitudes (north of 35 degrees latitude, including Europe and USA, north of Los Angeles) are at a higher risk of developing cancer.

Research indicates that 60% of people in the northern hemisphere are deficient of vitamin D - 90% in the winter.

Research has shown that people diagnosed with cancer (colon, breast and prostate) in the summer and autumn, have a better chance of survival than those diagnosed with cancer in the winter and spring.

Sun beds A team, Lund Universal in Sweden, followed 24,000 women over a period of 15 years and found those using a sun bed every few months lowered their cancer risk by 40%. On the other hand, the ultraviolet light which is produced by modern sun beds are 10 to 15 times more intense, so 20 minutes on a sun bed can be the equivalent to 300 hours in the midday summer sun.

Food Vitamin D is also found in salmon, tuna and other oily fish, eggs and some breakfast cereals, but diet accounts for very little of the vitamin D that makes its way into your bloodstream.

To obtain the equivalent of 15 minutes exposure in the middle of the day, you would have to eat almost 3 kilo (6.25 pounds) of salmon per day.

Is D a vitamin? Vitamin D is more correctly an enzyme, as it is produced by your body, not like other vitamins which come from your food.

Recommended Vitamin D doses if you have cancer.

Adult For every 10 ng/ml you are below normal (35ng/ml). I recommend you take 20 mcg (800IU) vitamin D per day during the winter.

If you are as low as 12 ng/ml, take 80 mcg per day for two weeks, then down to 20 to 40 mcg per day as a maintenance dose. For safety, some recommend the highest dose per day is 50 mcg, but doctors claim there is no toxicity risk from taking up to 250 mcg per day, which is what the body can absorb in 15 minutes in the midday sun without any harm.

Children 20 mcg per day.

Vitamin D3 (cholecalciferol) suspended in an oil based capsule, is the most easily absorbed form of vitamin D.

VITAMIN E

Fat-soluble Vitamin E not only works together with Vitamin C, but also Vitamin A, B-complex vitamins and selenium in producing antioxidants, which form a shield around the cell, protecting it against free radical attacks. Vitamin E regulates the function of Q10, both of which are very good for all heart problems.

Vitamin E is found in unrefined corn oils, peanuts, and various seeds such as sunflower, sesame, beans, peas, wheat germ and eggs. Also in sweet potato and oily fish like salmon, tuna and sardines.

Lack of Vitamin E is caused by pollution, contraceptive pills, excessive diet of refined or processed fats and oils and cooking at high temperatures especially frying.

Recommended daily doses for cancer patients.

Vitamin E containing d-alpha-tocopherol, nature's own type of Vitamin E (not synthetic d-alpha tocopherol).

Children 70-100 mg   **Adult** 100-1,000 mg

No toxicity reported below 2,000 mg daily long term and 35,000 mg short term use.

FOLIC ACID

Folic acid has an important role in forming new red blood cells in the bone marrow and acid sometime before and during pregnancy.

Folic acid is mainly found in cabbage, spinach, potatoes and other vegetables, whole grain bread, nuts, seeds, liver, kidneys and yeast.
Lack of folic acid is mainly due to alcohol, epilepsy drugs and age-related. Also women on the p-pill.
Recommended daily dose for cancer patients.
Children   2.5-25 mcg   **Adults**   5-100 mcg
Overdose not reported below 15,000 mg.

MAGNESIUM

Magnesium is needed for Vitamin D synthesis, which, as described before, is very important in fighting cancer.
Low Vitamin D levels also mean low calcium absorption, which together with magnesium is required to regulate lymphocytes. These transform into killer cells, which are able to attack cancer. Magnesium is crucial to a healthy liver, so it can detoxify all the dead cells from radiotherapy and chemotherapy, micro parasites, harmful bacteria and viruses.
The liver also needs to neutralise the lactic acid produced by cancer cells and performs a natural blood cleaning job.
Unfortunately western agricultural practises have depleted the soil of many minerals, vegetables and fruit have lost over half their contents of calcium and magnesium. This has resulted in approximately 40% of people in the UK being deficient in magnesium. The increased consumption of dairy products has depressed the magnesium levels in our bodies. Magnesium pushes sodium out of our cells and potassium in, thereby preventing toxicity and the threat of cancer.
Magnesium is good for your heart and blood pressure.
Magnesium is found in wheat germ, almonds, cashew and other nuts, green leafy vegetables particularly cabbage, brewers' yeast, buckwheat flour, garlic, raisins, green peas, potato skins, crab and brown rice. Most of the magnesium content is lost in refined food. Microwave ovens destroy magnesium.

Recommended daily dose for cancer patients.
Children   400-800 mg   **Adults**   400-800 mg
No toxicity reported below 1,000 mg.

PYCNOGENOL

Pycnogenol is a natural complex extract from the Pinus Pinaster tree only grown in the forest along the Bay of Biscay.

The active flavonoids in Pycnogenol work as a very powerful antioxidant that enables Vitamins C and E to be regenerated many times throughout the body.
Pycnogenol contains powerful biological active compounds which relax blood vessels thereby protecting and improving your cardiovascular and circulatory system. It reduces inflammation, psoriasis and other skin disorders and helps to keep your skin young and supple. Also acts as a relief from hay fever and allergies. Pycnogenol has shown to be effective in protection against thrombosis events (DVT) and superficial vein thrombosis (SVT) in moderate to high-risk people during long-haul flights. For this I recommend 200 mg taken two to three hours prior to flying, 200 mg six hours later in mid flight and 100 mg the day after flying.

Recommended daily dose for cancer patients.
__Children__ 40 mg   __Adults__ 80-120 mg

Only mega doses of over 11,000 mg per day can be toxic.

SEAWEED

Seaweed is the most nutritious plant in the world and contains all the vital vitamins, minerals, trace elements etc. in a natural form. Brown seaweed also contains the cancer fighting substance polysaccharides.

The incidents of breast cancer in the USA remains one of the highest in the world, while Japan until recently had the lowest. Average seaweed consumption per person in Japan is 50 times higher than in the USA.
Polysaccharides in seaweed are now known to have anti-cancer, anti-coagulant, anti-thrombosis, anti-inflammatory and anti-viral properties. Research by the Japanese biomedical group Takora Shuz, discovered in laboratory tests, polysaccharides literally caused cancer cells to self destruct.

The advantages of taking seaweed:
* contains all the micro nutrients missing from processed food and depleted soil. It contains over 100 vitamins, minerals, trace elements, amino acids and other valuable compounds including iron, which is lacking in many people including vegetarians.
* significant support to immunity and recovery prior to, and throughout, cancer treatment as well as after treatment.
* has just enough iodine to regulate the thyroid and metabolism on a continuous basis, which is particularly important for vegetarians.
* highly alkaline, so helps stabilise the blood acid alkaline balance.
* provides the entire range of antioxidants in an easily assimilated natural and balanced form it binds and removes toxic metals including mercury.
* regulates fatty acid metabolism and electrolyte imbalance.
* claimed to be one of the best detox aids.
* improves dry skin, lifeless hair, nails and circulation.
* also very beneficial for animals.
* 1000 mg of seaweed powder is equal to a large plateful of broccoli.

Seaweed is increasingly being used instead of salt in high quality bread, as most of the excess sodium we consume is said to come from our daily bread. Seaweed is also an antidote to excess sodium.

Seaweed should not be confused with common kelp mostly from industrial-scale harvesting to 'feed' the alginate industry for extracts used in a variety of manufacturing applications. Seaweed is three times more beneficial than kelp.

The best 100% pure wild brown seaweed grown in shallow water off the Lapland coast of Norway. It is harvested in the summer to obtain seaweed in its most active state. This seaweed is characterised by its density and slow growth because the strong Arctic storms effectively 'cull' the old seaweed each winter. It is hand harvested, air dried and immediately milled. Sheffield Hallam University confirmed that under normal use, this seaweed poses no risk to human health.

This seaweed is characterised by its' density and slow growth because the strong Arctic storms effectively 'cull' the old seaweed each winter. It is hand harvested, air dried and immediately milled. Sheffield Hallam University confirmed that under normal use, this seaweed poses no risk to human health.

Recommended daily dose for cancer patients.
Children   500 mg   **Adults**   1 to 2g per day
Up to 7g per day has been taken by adults for prolonged periods without any side- effects and with marked improvement in general health.

SELENIUM

Selenium is a trace element which, together with the above vitamins, is a very powerful anti-oxidant. It is also a good antibacterial, antiviral effective detoxifier of heavy metals.
Northern Europe's soil has one of the lowest amounts of selenium. During the ice age, about 10,000 years ago, the selenium rich soil was scraped away by glaciers, so agricultural land in the UK contains very little selenium. As a result, the average daily intake from food is only 31 mcg, whereas the WHO recommends 50-200 mcg.

Initial trials in the USA showed selenium reduced the chance of getting cancer by 50%. But then one must seriously take into account how many people who were initially Geopathically Stressed, later moved their bed into a good place.
Selenium is found in seafood like tuna, oysters, herrings, plaice, cod and salmon. Brazil nuts and kidneys are particularly high in selenium. Also wholemeal bread and eggs contain selenium.
Lack of selenium is mainly due to refined food and UK depleted agricultural soil.

Recommended daily dose for cancer patients.
The best selenium capsules are the ones that contain the most easily absorbed L-Seleno-methionine, together with Zinc and Vitamin A, B6, C and E.
Children   30-50 mcg   **Adults**   200-400 mcg
Toxicity may occur in extreme high doses of 2,500-3,000 mcg per day.

TOP

The three main 'vitamins' you need when you are eating:

T is for time. Give yourself time to eat. The French are not necessarily healthier because they drink wine, but it relaxes them, so they spend longer eating. The Scandinavians light candles with their meals, which makes them relax and therefore they have less digestive problems.
If you eat under stress, your stomach can close down for up to two hours, so you do not obtain any benefit from your food.

O is for oxygen. Eat slowly so you can breathe more whilst eating and additional oxygen enters your stomach, making your calories burn more efficiently and thereby your body absorbs the maximum benefit from your food. If you do not burn your calories properly, they will be stored as fat.

Your calories burn better if you take oxygen enriched capsules with your main meal.

It is of major importance to your overall wellbeing to replace your "friendly" bacteria (probiotics), destroyed by many medical drugs including chemotherapy and antibiotics. Often probiotic products (including yoghurts and fermented food) fail to reach the intestines as they are destroyed by the acid environment of the stomach.
Ensure you take probiotic capsules, which each contain up to 4 billion of the most important 'friendly' bacteria lactobacillus acidophilus and bifid bacterium lactis, which are alive at the time of taking and that the capsules are guaranteed not to dissolve before they reach your small intestines, where they are needed. Good probiotic capsules do not have to be kept in the fridge.

P is for pleasure. Take pleasure in everything you eat, then your stomach will digest it; even if you are eating something you know is a bit 'naughty' or you feel is a little unhealthy! Your stomach will cope as long as you take pleasure in eating it.

- You must feed your soul.
- It is not what you eat; it is mainly how you eat it.

SUMMARY
Recommended daily dose for adults with cancer:

Vitamin A retinal	2,250 - 6,000 mcg
or Beta Carotene	3,000 - 30,000 mcg
Vitamin B12	5 - 100 mcg
Vitamin C	1 - 10g
Vitamin D	20 - 40 mcg
Vitamin E	350 - 1,000 mg
Folic Acid	5 - 100 mcg
Magnesium	400 - 800 mg
Pyconogenol	80 - 120 mg
Selenium	200 - 400 mcg
Seaweed capsules	500 - 2,000 mg

If this is too much for you to take or too expensive, then at least take 100 mg Co-enzyme Q10, 1,000 mg Seaweed and 20 mcg Vitamin D.

OTHER POWERFUL SUPPLEMENTS

ALLICIN
100% stabilised allicin produces one of nature's most powerful anti-parasitic, antibiotic, anti-viral, anti-fungal and immune boosting compounds.

Allicin is created from two components, an enzyme called Allinase and an amino acid called Alliin, which are kept completely separate inside garlic. In nature allicin protects the garlic bulb from any attack by microbes in the soil. Allicin is also formed if the garlic's structure is ruptured - typically by cutting and crushing. **Garlic is the only vegetable that seldom rots.**

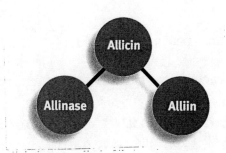

Chemists have discovered that the above highly reactive configuration gives allicin its remarkable antibiotic properties and, in particular, the potential to assist the immune system in a number of important ways including stimulating immune cells, killing pathogens and detoxifying carcinogens. Allicin is nature's antibiotic, antifungal and antiviral.

A patented process has now been developed to produce purified allicin liquid, making it the first health food supplement to provide a 100% allicin yield, the key active ingredient of fresh garlic.

Only garlic containing allicin is very alkaline and can therefore be readily absorbed by the body, penetrating cell walls and reacting with micro organisms.

Garlic is remarkable for the number of compounds it contains including 17 amino acids, at least 33 sulphur compounds, 8 minerals (germanium, calcium, copper, iron, potassium, magnesium, selenium and zinc) and vitamins A, B and C.

Of the more than two million packs of garlic supplements sold each year in the UK, very few contain allicin; therefore these products are mainly destroyed by the stomach's very strong acid.

How does Allicin work?

Because allicin is so "keen" in biochemical terms to react with micro-organisms, it is able to penetrate cell walls. In doing so it is then able to upset biochemical balance and impede activity. At low concentrations of allicin, the degree of interference may not be lethal, but sufficient to block the microbe's virulence. At slightly higher concentrations the effect could prove lethal for the micro-organism.

Allicin can:
- Boost your immune system to help protect you from infection.
- Give you a natural alternative to help fight microbes such as in viral, bacterial and fungal infections.
- Protect you against total infections such as tuberculosis and antibiotic resistant bacterial infection like MRSA, E-coli and C-difficile.
- Protect your body from further diseases and a wide range of environmental toxins.
- Prevent infection from returning and invading your body.
- Fight and protect you against parasites.

Allicin is like an exploding rocket that completely destroys microbes unlike using antibiotics, where a few microbes sometimes survive and multiply so the antibiotic is then ineffective. No microbes have been able to survive garlic since it started to be used over 6,000 years ago.

As mentioned in my first chapter, many people die of other illnesses after 'successful' cancer treatment, like pneumonia, septicaemia, heart attack etc. due to their immune system being further damaged by the often harsh cancer treatment.

Allicin has not only proved to be one of the best immune boosters, but is also very successful in destroying all types of micro parasites, very quickly.

Allicin will also deal with bacteria, viruses and fungus.

Pneumonia and upper respiratory infections

Dr Tom Ballard, Seattle, USA   16 November, 2007:

This winter I've treated patients with Upper Respiratory Infections (URI) with nebulised allicin and had dramatic results. One of those successes was with pneumonia.

Treatment:

A Standard nebuliser with sterile tubing is used. Five drops of stabilised allicin liquid and 10 drops of sterile saline placed in the receptacle. Patients inhale deeply into their lungs, hold for 30 seconds, and then slowly breathe out through their nose. Repeat until the solution is gone.

This technique exposes all the respiratory membranes to the allicin's anti-viral, fungal and bacterial affects.

Send patients home with the remains of the allicin liquid, instructing them to gargle five times a day using five drops in ¼ cup of warm, but not hot, water.

Outcomes:

I've treated eight severe URI patients on this protocol. They've all felt relief from the nebulisation and none have returned for further treatment.

The pneumonia patient came in complaining of malaise, lungs "heavy", mildly productive cough with yellow-greenish sputum, mild sore throat, and frontal headache. His throat and nasal mucosa were red and he had a slight amount of yellow nasal discharge. Moist rales in all lung fields.

After the allicin treatment I gave him a prescription for antibiotics and told him to collect it if he felt worse over the next few hours or was not better in 24 hours. I called him a few days later and he said that he felt great and never collected the antibiotic prescription.

Lung cancer

Recommended treatment. Fill a powerful nebuliser's receptacle with 2 ml of sterile saline[1] and 2 ml of allicin liquid. You might cough a little when you start inhaling, but carry on. Hopefully you will soon be able to take the allicin neat.

Switch nebuliser on. Breathe in vapour from nebuliser, hold breath to a count of 10 (about 7 seconds), then breathe out to a count of 10. Repeat by breathing in vapour from a nebuliser. Carry on this procedure for about 10 minutes if you are mixing allicin liquid half and half with sterile saline. Just 5 minutes if inhaling neat allicin.

Also use two powerful spinning magnets side by side on lungs front and back for about 20 minutes per day.

As neither using allicin liquid nor powerful spinning magnets over many years have shown any side effects, is it not worth trying this treatment, when conservative treatment has shown such poor results?

MRSA

The SUN newspaper reported on 12 June, 2008 that 52 patients with MRSA at University

Hospital East London had been successfully treated with allicin preparations. Many of the patients had wounds which refused to heal for several years, despite prolonged treatment with antibiotics. Dr Ron Cutler who led the trials, confirmed that he had patients who were due to have surgery to remove MRSA infected tissues, but after using allicin, their wounds had healed.

The bacterium Methicillin-Resistant Staphylococcus Aureus (MRSA) and several other strains of bacteria live in our gut, known as 'alert organisms'. In most cases, these bacteria cause no problem, but when they enter another body system such as the blood or urine, they may cause illness when they colonise. People carrying the bacteria in their nose, throat, and gut or on their skin, do not show symptoms. However, if the patient has a temperature and/or redness of a wound, this may indicate an infection. These bacteria are resistant to most conventional antibiotics.

Most patients with MRSA have been cleared of the bacteria by taking 2 x 5ml allicin liquid, twice a day with food, later reduced to 1 x 5ml twice a day.
Also spray allicin onto the affected areas. Afterwards apply allicin gel several times a day. Try and keep the wound unbandaged for as long as possible. Most patients found the MRSA infection had been resolved in 3-4 weeks.

John T, in Staffs, had contracted MRSA over 6 years ago in hospital, resulting in several long open wounds on this thigh, one 15 cm (6 inches) long and very deep. Within two weeks of taking allicin liquid, using the spray and applying the gel on the wound, all the smaller wounds had healed and the 15 cm (6 inches) wound had closed by 75%. The high power spinning magnetic apparatus was also used direct, which took the pain away within days.
Instead of using two crutches and the prospect of a leg amputation, John soon only used one crutch.

Deborah had two weeping MRSA wounds on her back for 2 years, during which time she had many courses of antibiotics and creams, but the many biopsies came back positive for MRSA. She had the wound dressed every day.
Deborah decided to use allicin, but her consultant and some district nurses were not happy about her decision.
After just a few weeks of spraying allicin liquid and applying allicin gel directly on the wounds and taking allicin orally, Deborah's wound had healed. The hospital confirmed her infection had cleared up and that she no longer needed a planned operation.

P.S. Ensure you are not sleeping in a Geopathic Stress place.

A whole range of other microbes have been successfully destroyed with allicin including Lyme disease, normally attributed to tick bites causing a bacterial spirochete called Borgdorferi. This disease can last for years if only treated with antibiotics.

VITAMIN B17

Vitamin B17 is a very powerful anti-cancer vitamin derived from seeds of all common fruit (except citrus).
Civilisations that eat a natural diet rich in B17, do not get cancer.

In 1952 Ernst Krebs, a biochemist from San Francisco, discovered the chemistry of cancer cells and the chemical properties of amygdaline now commonly known as Vitamin B17. He noticed that in theory **the B-17 should release poisonous cyanide at the cancer cell, but not at other cells.** Dr Krebs learned how to purify B-17 mainly from apricot kernels and developed a purified product as an anti-cancer drug under the name of **Laetrile.**

How does it work?
Its success depends on the marvels of enzymes. The enzyme beta-glycosidase is the only substance known that has the power to split the B-17 molecule and release the poisonous cyanide that is locked up inside. This enzyme is found in significant quantities in only one place, the malignant cells of humans and animals. The common body cells (somatic cells) are in no danger from the cyanide because they do not contain the enzyme beta-glycosidase and therefore no cyanide is formed at the somatic cells.

The enzyme rhodenase has the power to instantly convert poisonous cyanide into a substance that is harmless, even nourishing to somatic cells. Rhodenase is found in somatic cells, not malignant cells. So even if a small quantity of cyanide released at the cancer cell should spill over into a body cell, the enzyme rhodenase would immediately convert it before any harm could take place.

Dr Dean Burk was head of the cytochemistry section of the USA National Cancer Institute for many years. When he added B-17 to a cancer culture, he could see the cancer cells dying off like flies.

Gorillas in their natural habitat eat about 100 to 125 mg of Vitamin 17 every day. Like the populations of Hunzakuts, Abkhazians, the Eskimos, Hap, Indians and similar populations around the world, are free of cancer. The principle crop in Hunza is the apricot and the most prized food is the apricot seed. The Hunza eat 200 times as much B17 as we do in the UK.

As soon as you are diagnosed with cancer, eat large quantities of apricot seeds prior to any treatment, this will discourage the spread of the cancer and may even shrink the tumour.

The best way to eat the seed is to crunch in your mouth and massage the bits into a saliva paste. After chewing for a while - swallow. Do not swallow the seeds whole. If you do not like the taste, grind the seeds and use them as a spice for your food.

B17 Lactrile/Amygdalin Tablets
These tablets contain the active B17 ingredient derived from the apricot kernels. (Laetrile and Amygdalin refer to the same compound Vitamin B17). Take the tablets in conjunction with the apricot seeds.
Manufacturers recommend: as a nutritional supplement.
To prevent cancer: 2 to 4 100 mg tablets.
For cancer suffers: 4-6 500 mg tablets.

Apricot Seeds/Kernels
To prevent cancer: 1-2 seeds per day for life (less than 1g)
For cancer sufferers: 10-15 seeds per day (4-6g)

I recommend Phillip Day's book 'Cancer why we're still dying to know the truth', which tells the full story about B17 and how it has helped thousands fight cancer. The book and apricot kernels from the Himalayan mountains are available from Credence Publications www.credence.org.

ESSIAC

This non-toxic herbal formula was developed by Rene Caisse from a North American native recipe. Almost 70 years ago Caisse treated 30 terminal cancer patients with Essiac under the supervision of 5 doctors. After 18 months the doctors concluded Essiac had relieved pain, shrunk tumours and improved the survival odds of the patients. Caisse successfully treated thousands of cases of cancer before she died.

In 1937 the Royal Cancer Commission (Canada) came to the same conclusion that Caisse had, that Essiac (Caisse spelt backwards) was a cure for cancer. The Canadian Minister of Health and Welfare at the time of Caisse's death in 1978 burned all documents that had to do with Essiac, over 40 years of Caisse's administration! In 1938 Essiac came within three votes of being legalised by the Canadian Government as a remedy for terminal cancer patients but the pharmaceutical industry won again!

Caisse administered Essiac both orally and by injection. In cases where there was severe damage to life support organs, the patients died – but they lived for longer than the medical professionals had predicted and more significantly, they lived free of pain. Still others, listed as hopeless and terminal, but without severe damage to their support organs, were cured and lived 35-45 years (many are still living).

Luckily enough Dr Gary L Glum of Los Angeles [1] had managed to obtain the original formula of herbs to make Essiac teas and tinctures. The main ingredients used by Caisse were Sheep's sorrel (Rumex Acelosella) which she grew herself, Turkish rhubarb root (Rheum Palmatum), Burdock root (Arctium Lapps) and the inner bark of Slippery elm (Ulmus Fulva). Sheep's sorrel is the one claimed to destroy the cancer cells. The other three herbs are blood purifiers. Essiac has not been shown to have any side effects

Some of the benefits claimed for Essiac include strengthening of the immune system, removing toxins from the blood and therefore reducing the side effects of chemotherapy, radiotherapy and many drugs. Essiac increases energy levels and contributes to a feeling of well being which in turn influences the cancer patient's quality of life and potential for recovery. It normalises the thyroid gland and heals stomach ulcers.

Unfortunately since then our diet and our environment have become increasingly polluted, this has placed a growing burden on the body's immune and detoxification system making it more difficult to treat cancer. So to obtain the best results Essiac should be combined with other anti-cancer and cancer fighting remedies.

Anyone can take Essiac herbal remedies daily as a preventative treatment and to detoxify.

[1] **Full details of Rene Caisse and Essiac in his book 'Calling of an Angel'.**

PAU D'ARCO

Pau D'Arco has been known by the native Inca Indians of South America for over 1000 years and is called 'The Giver of Life'. This extract is also known by other names 'Lapacho Ipes' or 'Trumpet Bush' In 1968, the two Scottish Scientists A R Burnel an R H Thomson at Aberdeen University published their research on the contents of Pau D'Arco. They succeeded in identifying the very rare ingredient Lapachol. The American National Centre for Cancer Chemotherapy has proved Lapachol has a very strong healing effect on various cancers. Its molecular composition makes it uniquely suitable to induce strong biological activities against cancer.

Pau D'Arco was discovered over forty five years ago. It is told a Brazilian father of a young daughter with terminal cancer contacted a wise man of a local native tribe. He supplied some bark from a tree which grew in the Brazilian Rain Forest. The daughter was told to drink a tea made from the bark and she was healed in a short time.

Dr Orlando del Santi, who was a doctor in Santo Andre, heard about the daughter and decided to try the tea on his brother who had cancer. After his brother was declared free of cancer within a month, Brazilian doctors became very interested and from 1960 onwards many South American doctors have used Pau D'Arco to treat various cancers.

In a trial in California in 1997, nine patients with various types of cancer were given Pau D'Arco capsules to take with food. In three of the cases, the cancer disappeared completely and there were no side effects.

The American scientist Dr James Duke, who works for the United States Department of Agriculture, has investigated the toxicity of Pau D'Arco by the LD-50 test. This showed so little toxicity that it is almost 10 times less toxic than coffee.

SPECIAL DIETS

There are a number of dietary regimes which claim to benefit cancer patients. However, in all cases I have checked where a particular diet has shown fantastic results, the cancer patient has either by chance or knowingly moved their bed from a Geopathic Stress place into a Geopathic Stress free place. Also the various special diets have contained alkaline fruit and vegetables, thereby improving their acid alkaline balance. They have dealt with two of the BIG FOUR.

Gerson Regime is a low-fat, low animal protein, high carbohydrate dietary regime with particular emphasis on organic fruit, vegetables and whole grains which are high in potassium and low in sodium.

The Gerson regime consists of 12 glasses per day of freshly pressed vegetables (mainly carrot) and fruit juices, together with three daily meals of salads and vegetable soups. The regime also entails coffee enemas every three to four hours to stimulate the liver, which is your body's main detoxification organ. (In my opinion, a normal healthy diet and taking Bicarbonate of Soda (see Part One) is a far easier way to maintain a good acid alkaline balance).

Macrobiotic Diet aims to eliminate toxins accumulated by eating excessive greasy, animal, sweet, dairy foods and alcohol, with a balanced diet consisting of:

- 50-60% barley, millet, oats, corn, rye, wheat, buckwheat and brown rice.
- 25-30% vegetables, including cabbage which includes lots of Vitamin A, C and E. Folic acid, calcium, magnesium, phosphorus, iron and iodine. Also other vegetables such as kale, broccoli, cauliflower, greens, squash, carrots etc.
- the balance should consist of beans, seaweed, fish, seafood, soya products and drinking white or green tea.

Bristol Cancer Centre Diet encourages whole grains, cooked and raw vegetables, fruits and limited amounts of animal and dairy products.

Dries Cancer Diet mainly consists of a fresh fruit and raw vegetable orientated diet based on the bio-energetic properties of these foods. Jan Dries claimed he used this diet as a supplement to regular treatment, with very good results on over 600 cancer patients.

Hay diet plan

Already in 1911, Dr William Howard Hay realised the underlying cause of health problems was our body manufacturing and accumulating too much acid from the food we eat. (See Acid Alkaline balance in PART ONE).

This results in lowering the body's vital alkaline reserve causing toxaemia or autointoxication. To maintain the body's natural balance, Dr Hay recommended:

- Vegetables, salads and fruits should form the major part of your diet.
- Do not mix starch (food containing flour and sugar, except the natural sugar found in fruit) and protein (meat, game, fish, eggs and cheese) meals. They should be eaten more than four hours apart and in small quantities.
- Milk does not combine well with food and should be kept to a minimum.

The Grape Diet

Going on the Grape Diet for up to one month, together with a normal healthy diet, is one of the most effective ways to detoxify yourself.

How to take the grapes:
Start drinking one pint (about 0.6 litres) of grape juice first thing in the morning by taking a couple of swallows every ten to fifteen minutes (don't drink it all at once).

Do not eat until twelve noon. Have a normal healthy diet the rest of the day, but do not consume anything after 8pm. Only drink water. Food seems to take away the healing and detoxifying agents in the grape juice, so stick to the fast between 8pm and noon the following day (16 hours). Keep this up everyday for two to four weeks. It is particularly helpful to detoxify yourself in this way if you are on or have recently had chemotherapy or radiotherapy.

Even better, would be to liquidise whole grapes, as you absorb the goodness from the skin and seeds, but you may not like to drink the seeds. Do not use a 'juicer', as it discards the skin and the seeds and you get very little juice left over. My 45 year old Kenwood liquidiser does an excellent job. If you just cannot drink the seeds, even though they are the healthiest part, you can push the grapes through a sieve or buy seedless. 400g of grapes and a little water makes one pint (about 0.6 litres) of juice.

Dr Johanna Brant of South Africa wrote the 'Grape Cure' book over 70 years ago giving details on how she had fought bowel cancer for many years, until she cured herself and many others with her Grape Cure.

In the 30s Fred Wortman of Abbany, Georgia, USA developed an inoperable malignancy of the intestine, but could not afford the advised radiotherapy. He read Dr Brant's book, but found her grape diet too involved and cumbersome to follow, so he reduced it to its essentials – as described above – he took his own grape diet and was completely cancer-free within a month. He had his 'cure' published in a local paper. This resulted in over 600 people reporting to him that his grape diet had treated their cancer successfully.

Before you get too excited, you must not rely on this as a cancer cure.
Maybe we do not have the same type of grapes anymore as they did 60 years ago in the USA. They are sprayed with new chemicals. Pollution has become greater, as has both Geopathic Stress and Electromagnetic Stress (50 times over the last 50 years). Today thousands of chemicals are put into your food, drinks, and household products, make up etc. Maybe the Grape Diet was able to kill the weaker parasites that were around 60 years ago?
However as a detoxifier the Grape Diet is excellent combined with other detoxification methods, such as detoxifying pads and Devil's Claw tea.

I personally feel strongly that a normal healthy diet, dealing with the BIG FOUR and taking the previously described supplements, are far better for you, than some of the often soul destroying diets mentioned. If, however, you need more details on special diets, I suggest you buy a book on them or look them up on the internet.

GREEN and WHITE TEA
Eastern culture has long recommended green and white tea as beneficial to one's health and for their anti-cancer properties.

Both green and black tea, come from the leaves of the same plant, the tea plant (camellia sinensis). To produce black tea, the leaves are left outdoors to oxidise. Green tea is produced by lightly steaming the fresh cut young leaves, thereby ensuring it is high in polyphenol compounds with potent antioxidants and anticancer properties. Polyphenols are destroyed in black tea during the oxidising process.

The polyphenols in green tea block the formation of cancer-causing compounds as well as effectively detoxifying or trapping cancer causing chemicals. Green tea has also been shown to increase the activity of your body's own antioxidant system. Research has shown that the polyphenol ingredients in green tea have greater antioxidant properties than Vitamins C & E. Green tea can reduce enlarged lymph nodes.
(See in CLL (leukaemia).
Green tea seems to have an effect in reducing the onset of all types of cancer. The popular custom of drinking green tea with meals is claimed to be one of the reasons Japanese people have a lower rate of cancer then in the UK, yet they smoke far more cigarettes!

A cup of green tea contains between 100 to 200mg of the anti-tumour ingredient epigallocatechin gallate (EGCG).

It is suggested four cups of green tea per day should be sufficient to have a varied and wide ranging positive effect on your body. If this is too much for you, then take green tea as a convenient supplement.

Green tea has also been shown to help to reduce cholesterol and blood pressure. Also to reduce blood sugar in the case of diabetes.

White tea comes from the unopened buds of the tea plant. Again like green tea, it is lightly steamed. White tea is about 25% more beneficial than green tea with a smoother taste.

For the perfect cup of white tea, infuse one tea bag per person (in teapot with extra water if too strong) for 30 seconds to 2 minutes in freshly boiled water (not boiling water). Boiling water can scald white tea and impair the flavour.
Serve without milk.

Green and white teas are very good at encouraging a healthy pH (Acid/alkaline balance). (See PART ONE).

MANUKA HONEY

Manuka honey has a reputation as the best honey in the world to help with a range of diseases together with cancer.

Manuka honey comes from New Zealand, where beekeepers set up their hives in wild, pollution free areas in which manuka bushes grow. Manuka honey is unique, as it possesses remarkable anti- bacterial properties over and above other types of honey. It remains active even under the most adverse conditions.

Manuka honey will soothe, calm, protect and destroy disease producing microbes in the digestion system and help with heartburn, inflammation of the oesophagus, upset stomach, various ulcers, irritable bowel syndrome (IBS) and ulcerative colitis.
The extraordinary properties of Manuka honey were discovered by Professor Peter Molan MD. of New Zealand's University of Waikato. The properties are termed UMF® (unique manuka factor). The higher the UMF®, the more anti-bacterial activity it has. This should not be below 10 and best between 16 and 19. UK honey have some manuka properties.

SALT

Over many years, we have been told that salt is bad for us, resulting in many people being very short of salt. The salt we are warned about, giving us high blood pressure etc., is obtained from salt mines. As a result of washing with hydrochloric acid and being recrystallized, this purified salt is almost 100% sodium chloride. But sea salt, obtained by evaporating sea water, contains calcium, potassium and most notable, large amounts of magnesium, in addition to sodium. Ten grams of sea salt a day contains about 1500mg of magnesium. Magnesium has proved to be very good to prevent heart problems. In 1972 Japan changed over from sea salt to mined salt containing pure sodium chloride.
Interestingly, the death rate from heart disease almost doubled in Japan between 1975 and 1985. If you are low (check with the muscle test), take half to one teaspoon of granulated sea salt (drink water afterwards) per day for a few days. If you are sensitive to salt, take a few grains with water many times a day, gradually increasing the quantity of salt until your body can take ¼ to ½ a teaspoon at a time.
You can also add extra sea salt to cucumber and tomato slices or take one to four salt tablets obtained from your pharmacist.
It is estimated over 20% of people are low in salt. Recently, I have had several reports from people with long standing headaches who have found that their headaches have gone after taking extra sea salt. One lady, with continuous pain down one leg, had tried numerous medical drugs and therapist treatments, with no results. Her pain disappeared within days of taking extra sea salt.

WATER

It is most important that cancer patients drink enough water, as water stimulates the immune system; helps increase the body's white blood cells, flushes out accumulated toxins and enables your brain to function properly.

Our cells literally owe their lives to an adequate supply of water. It is debatable whether you must drink 8 glasses (2.5 litres/4 pints) per day because large quantities of water are contained in food. Most uncooked vegetables and fruit contain 90% water.

It helps to stagger your water intake throughout the day, rather than going for hours without anything and then drinking half a litre (about a pint). This can cause your kidneys to struggle and you may have to dash to the toilet.

If you have difficulty in swallowing water, try drinking through a straw.

Britain's leading nutritionist, Jane Clarke, claims you can count tea and coffee as part of your water intake. Previously it was thought they acted as diuretics, encouraging your body to get rid of fluid. So you can drink tea and coffee as part of your 2.5 litres. Strong alcohol is diuretic.

An indication of dehydration is if your urine is thick, dark yellow and rank in smell. Due to shortage of water your body cuts back on water usage throughout its various systems. Note that extra Vitamin B intake can also darken urine.

Water travels very quickly through the body, so be prepared to go to the toilet soon after drinking. If you have to go out soon after drinking water, eat a banana, which will prevent you having to get to a toilet urgently later.

There is no need to waste hundreds of pounds a year on bottled water. 25% of all bottled water is filtered tap water. Bottled water is only tested once a year by the Food Standard Agency and there have been some drastic failures lately. On the other hand, the Drinking Water Inspectors test tap water on average 3 million times a year and no UK water company has failed to deliver water to the laid down standard. Tap water is alive, not like dead bottled water.

Whether or not you use a carbon filter for drinking tap water is really a matter of personal preference. Chlorine in water can injure red blood cells and damage their ability to carry vital oxygen where it is needed. Putting in a tiny amount of Vitamin C powder can neutralise chlorine and will cut out the taste and odour of the chlorine. A carbon filter is adequate for producing chlorine-free tap water. Chlorine evaporates quickly in the open, so after leaving your tap water for 20 minutes in a glass, the chlorine will have evaporated.

Water from plastic bottles should be avoided as it can be contaminated with chemicals from the plastic or the chemicals they clean the bottles with before use. According to Dr. Hulda Clark, micro parasites feed on some of these chemicals. Water in glass bottles is fine; choose a 'natural mineral water', ensure it does not contain artificial sweeteners (see page 229).

Don't drink too much ice cold water; your body uses energy to heat this.

Ensure children drink four to six glasses of 'good' liquid a day.

Interesting note
In the UK, £2 billion is spent on bottled water per year. The carbon footprint on one 500 ml plastic bottle of water is equal to 1,000 pints of tap water.

OZONATED WATER

Ozone is the second most powerful disinfectant known and can rapidly destroy viruses, bacteria, fungi, micro-parasites and revitalise your whole body. Ozone will reduce side effects when having chemotherapy and radiotherapy and when recovering from surgery. You can now produce it yourself very economically and quickly on a daily basis from tap water. Nearly all of the body's activities, from brain function to elimination, are regulated by oxygen. Ozone, often referred to as 'activated oxygen' and represented chemically as 0, is pure elemental oxygen, but with three atoms instead of the usual two found in the oxygen that we breathe.

Ozone disinfects over 3,000 times faster than chlorine and without the carcinogenic effects. It has been used to disinfect water at waterworks for over 100 years. Ozone also destroys spores, moulds, cysts, yeasts, viruses and bacteria such as E.coli.
Ozone is approximately ten times more soluble in water than oxygen, so drinking ozonated water is a very powerful way to detox your body and remove those toxins through a simple chemical reaction which allows your liver and kidneys to process the waste water much more efficiently.
It is now possible to produce ozonated water very quickly with an Ozone Generator (2).

- You can drink up to 2½ pints of ozonated water per day (1½ litre).
- Apart from water, no other product is used.
- Ozonated water is very good for animals too.
- If you cannot drink cold water, put a small plate on top of the glass, with the cold ozonated water, until it is warmer.

DAIRY PRODUCTS

Dairy products have a strong link to breast and prostate cancer. Giving them up is not all that difficult and is unlikely to cause health problems.

The incidence of breast cancer in China is 1 in 10,000 women. In the West it is as high as 1 in 10 women. Prostate cancer in men in China is even lower than 1 in 10,000. In the West it is about 1 in 7 men.

Why is there such a difference? **The Chinese do not eat or drink dairy products.** (See note at end of chapter). As soon as people from China move to western countries and adopt western diets with a very high dairy product content, they soon suffer breast and prostate cancer in the same proportion as local people.

The average USA diet contains over 40% dairy products.

(2) **An OZX 3000 Ozone Generator can be purchased from Commercial Science and Good Vitality. Tel/Fax 01293 446244 www.comsci.org.uk.**

In Denmark, people on average eat more dairy products than in the U.K. and Danish women have the highest percentage of breast cancer in the world.

The higher percentage of breast cancer in Scottish women than in English women is almost in direct proportion to the higher rate of dairy products consumed in Scotland than in England.
Chinese, Japanese, Korean and Thai cook books do not mention dairy products.

Milk is only for babies.

All milk from mammals – humans, cows, goats, sheep and other species – is a powerful bio-chemical solution of great complexity uniquely designed to provide for the individual needs of young mammals of the same species. Cow's milk is great food for young calves, not for humans.

One problem is the growth factor and hormones in dairy animals, which research has shown promotes growth in breast and prostate cancer tumours. Young calves and kids need milk containing this high growth factor to make them grow at a colossal rate compared to humans. Calves slaughtered for veal are mainly fed on milk. Human babies normally take 180 days to double their birth weight; calves only take 47 days and kids just 19 days, calves gain about 1kg per day for the first 6 to 10 weeks. Cows are continually milked into their next pregnancy, when they are producing extra quantities of growth factors.

The milk sugar lactose is broken down by the body into another sugar called galactose, which is then broken down by the body's enzymes. If your digestive system is under par, there may not be enough enzymes in your body to break down galactose. Galactose may then build up in your blood, which could damage your body and lead to cancer. Don't forget if your body is in Geopathic Stress during sleep, when your body is doing its 'housekeeping', it has to put something on the back burner (delay dealing with it) mainly your digestive system, to enable it to fight the Geopathic Stress. Your body must deal with the most essential things first, like forming new cells, looking after your heart, kidneys, liver etc.

Dairy milk contains oestrogen and testosterone. Exposure to oestrogen is considered a risk factor in causing breast cancer. Similarly, testosterone is thought to affect prostate cancer. Even in small doses they can cause hormonal imbalance and biological damage.
Cows are given certain hormones (including oxytocin) to increase milk production, which cannot be destroyed even during pasteurisation of the milk. Additionally, modern methods of processing milk to prevent the cream separating by homogenisation may prevent the cancer-promoting chemicals from breaking down in our digestive system, so large quantities are absorbed into our bloodstream.

Dairy products are not only in milk, butter, cheese and yoghurt, but also in biscuits, cakes and are sneaked into soya, sunflower and olive oil spreads as buttermilk. **The problem is milk sugar, not milk fat,** so it is not resolved by using low-fat dairy products, such as yoghurt and low fat cheeses, because the bacteria used in the production of galactose from lactose make these products particularly dangerous.

The increased chances of breast and prostate cancer as we get older, may also be due to having consumed dairy products for a longer period.

Milk is an excellent culture medium that micro parasites just love. Elsewhere I explain how most people, who develop cancer, are high in micro parasites.

Professor Jane Plant CBE is a highly qualified scientist (not medical). She fully explains in her international bestselling book on breast cancer 'Your Life In Your Hands' [3] and 'Prostate Cancer – understand, prevent and overcome,'[4] why dairy products are one of the main causes of breast and prostate cancer and their effect on other cancers. Plant had many operations, radiotherapies and chemotherapies after she was diagnosed with breast cancer, but still her tumour came back. The fifth time round was cancer in the lymph nodes in her neck. She had the same type of chemotherapy treatment as she had on her previous unsuccessful treatments, for similar cancerous lymph nodes and so her doctor only gave her a few months to live.

In her extensive research for a cure, Plant discovered the relationship between dairy products and cancer. She stopped eating dairy products immediately and her tumour shrunk very quickly and was gone within five weeks. This is now over 10 years ago.
Plant is as busy as ever today and explains fully the vast research she has performed which entirely convinced her that consuming dairy products is a major contributory factor in developing cancer. Neither is it necessarily a good source of calcium for your bones.

Plant also explains while you have active cancer, your nutritional intake should be based on a diet of vegetables and fruits rather than on animal products, at least until you have recovered. Together with Gill Tidey, Jane Plant has also written 'The Plant Programme'[5] on how to make delicious food without dairy products. Two other excellent books on dairy-free diets are 'Super Soya' by Tanya Carr and Joanna Farrow and 'Health Dairy-free Eating' by Mini C and Tanya Carr. Apart from vegetables and fruit the main ingredients used in these books are soya beans, which are one of the most nutritious foods known and have been the main source of protein in oriental countries for over 4000 years. I personally have found it very easy to substitute dairy products with soya products, such as soya milk, soya cheeses and soya spreads and I am not a vegetarian.

You can make your own fresh, organic, GMO-free soya milk for just pennies per litre in a special soya milk maker taking about 15 minutes. An excellent automatic soya milk maker, in stainless steel, is 'SoyQuick' supplied by Wholistic Health Direct Telephone 017632 84910 www.wholistichealthdirect.co.uk. One family of four is now saving over £600 a year by making their own organic soya milk. (Most good health shops stock organic soya beans).

Some people claim soya milk is unhealthy, but this mainly relates to the ready-made long life soya in cartons to which stabilisers and other chemicals are added to keep the soya fresh for up to one year. Soya milk you make yourself does not have this disadvantage. Some people are allergic to soya so try rice milk or even coconut milk, which is very nutritious.

Plant gave the Plant Programme Diet to 6 women, who initially had cancer. All of them have remained cancer-free. Five other women, who refused to use her diet or who 'cheated', have had cancer return again or have died.

(3), (4) & (5) By Virgin Publishing Ltd.

Tip: Do not pour soya milk into very hot coffee or tea etc as it will curdle.

Milk sales have gone up 4% over the last few years, mainly due to the increase in sales of coffee, e.g. cappuccino and latté, which is another contributing factor in the steady increase in breast and prostate cancer.

Other Interesting Factors about Dairy Products

The only two mammals that drink milk long after the breastfeeding period are humans and cats. Cats often die young of kidney failure (cats which originally come from the East like Siamese and other oriental cats do not drink milk!)

Most cats are lactose intolerant therefore cannot digest the sugars in milk. Milk has very little to no nutritional value for cats. Good milk substitutes have been created for cats which also have some nutritional value. Always have fresh cool water available. (See chapter on Animal Cancer).

Lactating (breast feeding) mothers often have babies suffering from colic if the mother is consuming dairy products, since the antibiotics in cow's milk can pass through the mother into the baby causing digestive and many other problems. You absorb far more calcium from vegetables, which is the same source cows and goats obtain their calcium from.

Over 70% of the world's adult population are unable to digest the milk sugar lactose, which can cause abdominal pain, diarrhoea etc. Many dairy-free products are advertised as 'lactose-free'.

Cow's milk is tested for cell count of somatic pus, which comes from infections on the cows udders. If the cell count is too high the farmer is paid less for his milk (or cannot sell it), so the cows are given high doses of antibiotics. This then enters the human body, via the milk, which makes it more difficult for us to be treated with antibiotics, if our doctor finds it necessary. The antibiotics given to some cows also make us allergic to dairy products.

Mainly due to pressure from supermarkets on milk prices, cows are becoming simple milk production machines - maximum production for as little cost as possible, so milk now costs less than many bottled waters. Milking cows are filled with growth factors and hormones, so they can produce over twice as much milk as they did a few years ago (used to be 4,500-5,000 litres per cow each year, now it is up to 15,000 litres). During milking, cows used to be given rations (cow cakes) containing 12-14% protein, now they contain 22-24%.

Milking cows are sent for slaughter exhausted and at a far younger age than their natural life span. This is the meat generally sold in supermarkets. Now you can see why large consumption of beef hamburgers is so unhealthy.

Aberdeen Angus and Highland Cattle's milk is not used for dairy products, so the cows are not given extra hormones to increase milk production. That is why beef from these two breeds of cattle are among the healthiest of beef meat.

Most bull calves are killed at birth, except the ones reared and slaughtered at about 6 months for veal meat. Unfortunately, they are mostly fed on cow's milk.

Often asthma can be cured by simply eliminating dairy and sugar products from our diet

Apparently, changing from dairy to soya milk may also eliminate hot flushes during menopause.
Note:
About 8,000 years ago, when humans discovered they could drink cow's milk, their bodies could not tolerate the lactose in cow's milk. But gradually the digestive system in most humans, who drank milk, changed so it could tolerate lactose. But cows were not introduced to the East so those peoples' digestive system did not change, so generally they cannot tolerate the lactose in milk. Yet India has now become the biggest milk producer in the world.

FOOD SWEETENERS

High levels of **Aspartame** have been found in brain tumours and now a major research study has connected this sweetener with cancer. **Aspartame** has been shown to have a bad effect on your immune system and many health conditions, so it should be avoided at all costs. Also parasites love to feed on formic acid, one of the compounds **Aspartame** splits into in the digestive system (See PART ONE).

Aspartame is now found in sugar-free yoghurt, diet drinks, low calorie desserts and an estimated 5000 other products under such names as, **NutraSweet, Spoonful, Canderel, Equal, Equal Measure** etc. Aspartame is popular on two counts. First Aspartame is ten times sweeter than sugar by weight therefore a much cheaper option. Secondly low fat sugar free food with Aspartame sweetener is made popular by the myth that it is good if you are on a slimming diet, so under no circumstance should you eat 'low fat food'.

According to Dr Robert C Atkins, carbohydrates create insulin and insulin creates long term fat. Cut carbohydrates and the body burns the fat very quickly. Aspartame is put into low fat food to make it palatable to eat but it will upset the insulin balance and prevent you burning off the fat in your body. Low fat yoghurt for children is particularly unhealthy. Not only do children under 10 years old need extra fat but the Aspartame can in many cases make them hyperactive and put on unnecessary weight.

Diet Coke, Diet Pepsi, Diet Snapple, Sugar-Free Kool-Aid, Robinson's Fruit Shoot and most flavoured bottled waters contain Aspartame.

When one of my grandsons was under 6 years old, he would become unbelievably hyperactive a few minutes after he had a drink with Aspartame sweetener in it. (He was normally an exceptionally quiet and well behaved boy). I have seen the same thing happen to other small children in restaurants and on public transport.

In the digestive tract Aspartame is split into its two component amino acids and a methyl group. During metabolism, the methyl group is converted to the toxin methanol (wood alcohol) and then to a highly toxic substance formaldehyde, which can cause severe damage to the nervous and immune systems and permanent genetic damage, even at extremely low doses. Formaldehyde in turn is broken down to another toxin, formic acid. These facts are undisputed by the manufacturers.

In view of the many illnesses reported as a result of Aspartame consumption – illness which is resolved when the consumption ceases - many consumers want to know why it was ever allowed on the market. The stumbling block appears to be whether it can be scientifically proven that Aspartame consumption produces enough methanol and formic acid to cause seizures, headaches, blindness and other problems reported. The manufacturers claim that the product has been thoroughly tested, but under current law, manufacturers are allowed to do their own testing. They can carry on testing until they obtain a satisfactory result. No independent laboratories need be involved. The irony is Canderel has joined forces with Pink Ribbon Breast Cancer Campaign. Already 7% of UK households use Canderel and it is marketed in 85% of countries throughout the world. The USA Food & Drug Administration wanted to ban the manufacture of Aspartame, but was overruled by enormous pressure.

Research connecting Aspartame with Cancer

Dr Movando Soffritti, a cancer researcher in Bologna, Italy, found by carrying out a seven year study with his team, **Aspartame** was associated with unusually high rates of lymphomas, leukaemia and other cancers in rats which had been given the equivalent doses to four to five half litre bottles of diet soda a day for a 68kg person. The study involved 1900 laboratory rats and cost $1 million, was conducted at the European Romazzini Foundation of Oncology and Environmental Sciences, a non-profit organisation that studies cancer-causing substances.

The Alternative to Aspartame

Unrefined cane sugar is a natural product made by simply pressing out, cleaning and crystallising the juice from sugar cane. It is not subjected to further refining that is required to manufacture white sugar. Fruit juices as a sweetener in food and drinks are fine. The best sweetener is honey, which has powerful antioxidant qualities. Honey is also sweeter than sugar, so we use less of it. Its sugars are mainly fructose and glucose, which your body digests and absorbs more easily than sucrose.

Detoxing Yourself

It is most important while detoxing yourself that before starting certain health programmes, that you stop taking artificial sweeteners, such as Aspartame on its own and in food and drinks.

Vitamins and Minerals for Children

Nearly all children's chewable Multi-Vitamins and Mineral Supplements contain Aspartame, which does more harm than the Vitamins and Minerals do good.
The only product I have come across without Aspartame which incorporates fruit juices as a sweetener is Animal by Nature's Plus USA, well worth the extra cost and stocked by most good Health Shops

Check Yourself

Use the Muscle Test to check if a product contains Aspartame and if it is bad for you.

The Ambassador of Uganda told a conference their sugar industry added Aspartame to make the sugar taste sweeter!!!

Over $600 million worth of **Aspartame** is sold per year.

PART FIVE

EXERCISE

POWERFUL MAGNETIC THERAPY

EXERCISE

> If you have cancer, it is very important that you exercise to increase your body's oxygen supply as you fight cancer. Exercise will also increase the flow of lymph through its channels, to improve your immune system by detoxifying and eliminating the toxins from your body. Your lymphatic system has no pump unlike your heart.

One of the mistakes cancer patients make, is to wait until they feel better to exercise. Even if you have pain and are undergoing strong cancer treatment, you have to somehow rise above it and force yourself to exercise. The only time you have to be careful with exercise, is when the cancer has spread to your bones as this can make you more susceptible to spontaneous fractures.

Ideally, you should build up to a brisk walk of 30 to 40 minutes, three to four times a week.

However the best way to exercise daily is on a rebounder in your own home. A rebounder is smaller and stiffer than a trampoline and increases your gravity by 25% both on the down and up movement. A rebounder is much more efficient and cheaper than a cycling, running or rowing machine and you are less likely to get bored. I have tried them all, but for the last ten years have only been rebounding. Ensure you get a good quality rebounder, which will give you the best exercise and last for years.

You can listen to music, radio or watch TV while rebounding, so there is no excuse not to exercise. Rebounding at night may interfere with your sleep. A support bar can help if you have difficulty in standing, are elderly, handicapped or have impaired sight. If you cannot stand, sit on the rebounder while somebody creates a rebounding action behind you on the rebounder.

It is claimed that the number of white blood cells, which help fight cancer, can be doubled for one hour by rebounding for two minutes.

Exercising for ten minutes on a rebounder is the same as walking briskly for over half an hour. Exercise will also build up your energy, stimulate your metabolism and reduce any pain.

POWERFUL MAGNETIC HEALING

Magnetic Therapy has long been proved to be a simple, powerful and entirely painless method of dealing with most illnesses, injuries, other ailments and to boost the immune system. Having studied the effect magnetic therapy has on cancer tumours in numerous experiments on animals and humans, I decided to develop the most powerful magnet therapy apparatus possible.

Paracelsus (1493-1541) the famous Doctor of Medicine in the Middle Ages, informed us "The magnet is very useful in treating internal as well as external diseases".

Professor Olav Lindahl, former Chief Medical Officer in Sweden, said many years ago "Only a fanatical sceptic, totally ignorant of the published research, could today deny the powerful biological effect of magnetic therapy. **I personally would not hesitate to try magnetic therapy if I had cancer.** I would be considerably less suspicious of that than of normal treatment used in cancer hospitals".

Lindahl reported the following experiments carried out at highly respected research establishments:

Barnothy inoculated two groups of mice with cancer. In the control group, all the animals died. In the group treated with magnetic therapy, 80% survived. In another set of experiments, Barnothy inoculated mice with three different types of cancer. The tumours in the animals treated with magnetic therapy disappeared, while the untreated mice died.

Mulay worked with cancer cells in tissue culture. In repeated experiments, he treated every other culture with magnetic therapy and the rest were left untreated as a control group. The untreated culture all showed normal growth, while those treated with magnetic therapy not only failed to develop, but showed complete degeneration (tissue death).

The above experiments show magnetic therapy increased the oxygen <u>pressure</u> inside the tumours and caused a reduction in oxygen <u>absorption</u>.

Each cell in a biological organism is surrounded by a cell wall and the cell is dependent for its nourishment on food entering and waste products being expelled through the cell membrane. Any alteration in the cell wall's permeability weakens those processes. One explanation of the effect of these fields is that a magnetic field improves the passage through the cell membrane.

Another basic mechanism is the magnetic field's effect on the genetic material in the cells DNA and RNA. By marking certain basic substances (raw material) for the synthesis of DNA and RBA with radioactive trace elements (tritium), it is possible by means of animal experiments to show that certain magnetic fields stimulate the production of this genetic material.

These two mechanisms, the effect of the magnetic field on the permeability of the cell wall and the effect on the cell's genetic material, represent the two main explanations of how magnetotherapy might affect biological material and so are effective in all kinds of disorders (diseases) as well as normal (healthy) people.

It has been shown that magnetic therapy revitalises the universal biological motor, which provides each cell with chemical energy, ensuring the motor runs the correct way, otherwise tissues perish.

The North Pole calms the body and the South Pole revitalises it, which makes it difficult to use stationary magnets for healing various health problems at the same time. We then discovered a magnetic field not only becomes 20 times stronger when rotated, but by changing the poles over 260 times a second, it is too fast for the body to recognise the poles, so there is a 'pure' magnetic field which can be used anywhere on the body for any health problem or injury.

Having used lateral thinking and taking financial risks in inventing, developing and manufacturing industrial products over many years, I was determined to manufacture the most powerful magnetic therapy apparatus.

By incorporating sophisticated high speed Swiss DC micro motors and the strongest commercially available permanent magnets and installing industrial bearings, the lightweight MagneTech was developed which can be used by health practitioners and individuals.

The MagneTech has now been used by over half a million people all over the world in the last 17 years, without any side-effects being reported. It is still the most powerful magnetic therapy apparatus and the only one that has passed The Medical Device Agency European Standard certificate for medical use (CE0120). The manufacture and distribution of the MagneTech has been one of my crusades. By keeping the profit margin very low, it has made it more affordable.

A rotating magnetic field study carried out by N.G. Bakhmutskii of Russia before the MagneTech was developed, resulted in inhibiting Walker's carcinoma tumour growth as much as 90% in some cases.

In another Russian study, the effect of a rotating magnetic field on a group of 51 breast cancer patients, showed a significant positive response in 27 cases.

CASE HISTORIES

No claims are made that the MagneTech will reduce tumours, as hospitals have not yet been willing to carry out clinical trials. I am only reporting what cancer sufferers have told me. The MagneTech is not successful in all cases of cancer. However, the MagneTech can be used during other treatments to give more energy and a better quality of life. We would always advise people to contact their doctor first. In most of cases, the people also became free of Geopathic Stress.

Caz C (Devon) was diagnosed as having **cancer in several places,** *when she was four months pregnant. As no orthodox treatments like chemotherapy or radiotherapy could be given, Caz's only option was to use the MagneTech direct on her lung and neck cancer. X-rays showed the cancer did not spread during the pregnancy and Caz gave birth to a very healthy 10lb (4.5kg) baby boy.*

Elsa W (Germany) was told by her hospital doctor that there was no more they could do for her **lung cancer.** *Chemotherapy would only make her expected short life more uncomfortable. She used the MagneTech on her lungs for about half an hour each day to enable her to cough up any impurities and breathe more easily. This also enabled her to get up stairs. Her daughter also gave her half an hour's treatment with the MagneTech on her back each day to take away the pain and to make her sleep more easily. Elsa lived for another 18 months without any orthodox treatment. This was over fifteen years ago. Since then the MagneTech has been made* **4 times** *stronger.*

David K (Bournemouth) had a **tumour as big as a golf ball under his chin.** *Not wishing to have an operation as this would leave a big scar on his neck, or any other orthodox treatment, he used the MagneTech directly on the tumour for 20 minutes each day for six weeks, by which time the tumour had shrunk to the size of a pea.*

Brenda S (Hants) not only had a **large tumour on her breast, but the skin was very discoloured above the tumour.** *Brenda used the MagneTech daily and reported that the tumour shrunk to the size of a pea within 14 days and that the skin colour had almost returned to normal. No orthodox treatment was given.*

Iain P (Cheshire) A scan diagnosed a **brain tumour.** *He has used the MagneTech directly on the area for 15 minutes each day and a later scan showed no increase in the size of the brain tumour. Iain says he wouldn't dream of stopping the treatment with the MagneTech.*

Dr Karen Stevens reports "I used the MagneTech to shrink a cancerous tumour that was so big in a friend's stomach, that when he came to me 2 weeks prior to going into hospital in Liverpool to have all of his stomach removed, he had little hope of recovery. I used the MagneTech on him 9 hours per week for two weeks. When the surgeons operated two weeks later, they found that the huge tumour had shrunk to the size of his thumbnail and they took out less than a third of his stomach.

A world champion rally driver was given three weeks to live, with an inoperable brain tumour. Two MagneTechs were used for 20 minutes, direct on his brain, each day for three weeks. We do not know how long he would have lived, as he was killed in a helicopter crash two years afterwards.

See other case histories under individual cancers.

Reducing the after effects from Radiotherapy

*My wife Lena had **throat cancer** (before I knew the importance of the BIG FOUR) and was given the strongest radiotherapy possible - 10 times over two weeks. Each night when Lena came home from hospital , she felt as if her head was exploding. Ten minutes with the MagneTech at the back of Lena's head made her head feel normal again. St. Thomas's hospital said they had never come across a patient who could take strong radiation so well. They even gave her two extra days radiotherapy. Lena was the only patient smiling in the waiting room.*

Other uses of the MagneTech

The MagneTech can be used anywhere on the body for any problem and has been successful in treating bones (heal 40% faster); leg ulcers, circulatory problems, wounds, burns, PMT and period pain, infections, gangrene, ear and eye problems, frozen shoulder and whiplash, sports injuries, sinuses, dental problems, lung congestion, repetitive strain injury and to revitalise organs and the immune system.

We have thousands of case histories, but the following recent case is typical:

Sylvia W. London came into our office and showed us her left foot, where her big toe was very badly affected by gangrene. Her doctor had suggested removing by surgery the big toe and cut well into her foot. Sylvia used the MagneTech on her big toe each day and put 100% stabilising Allicin gel on her toe and took the liquid internally to kill her micro parasites.

Sylvia came back again after about 6 weeks and proudly showed her left foot, where the big toe had completely healed and needed no surgery.

I am not ashamed to admit that after personally seeing the above result, I felt proud that I had developed the MagneTech.

Important

It is very important you take account of the BIG FOUR, together with the vital supplements and exercise to obtain the maximum benefits from magnetic therapy.

PART SIX

THERAPIES TO HELP YOU FEEL BETTER

Do it yourself
There are many therapies you can use yourself on a daily basis to help you feel better such as:
- Bach Flower remedies
- Exercise (see Part Five)
- Powerful magnetic therapy (See Part Five)
- Laughter
- Meditation
- Yoga

Complementary Therapies
It would be improper and illegal for any responsible complementary therapy practitioner to offer a cure for cancer. However, used in conjunction with orthodox treatments, they can help you relax, reduce pain and tolerate any orthodox treatments far better.

Ask your doctor to recommend a complementary therapist suitable for your particular cancer or contact the relevant professional organisation (see under specific therapies) to recommend a local member. Ask at your local health shop. Often the best way is by 'word of mouth'. However a therapist who suits one person, may not suit another. It is also a question of having confidence and feeling relaxed with your therapist. **Always ensure** that the therapist is fully qualified (after professional training and not just acquired at a weekend course). Also check they are fully insured.

Remember
A. Consult your doctor before embarking on any complementary therapy, to ensure it can be carried out alongside your current orthodox cancer treatment.
B. Do not stop taking any drugs prescribed by your doctor.
C. Tell your complementary practitioner about any prescribed medication you are taking and any other treatment you are receiving.

There are over 200 types of complementary therapies. The main ones are described here:

- Acupuncture
- Aromatherapy
- Chiropractor/Osteopathy
- Healing
- Homeopathy
- Kinesiology
- Massage
- Reflexology

BACH FLOWER REMEDIES

These remedies are all prepared from the flowers of wild plants, bushes and trees for healing negative emotional states.

Doctor Edward Bach (1880-1936) discovered 38 flowers which he prepared in pure spring water, to treat emotional problems and so restore health and harmony to mind and body.

The main use is for - negative emotional states such as fearfulness, uncertainty, disinterest, loneliness, over-sensitivity, despair and excessive concern for other people. Also for physical symptoms arising from emotional problems.

The Bach flower remedies have no harmful side-effects, are non toxic and do not influence or are influenced by drugs. If the wrong Bach flower remedy is given, it has no side-effects.

The Rescue Remedy for emergencies and crisis situations including before and during cancer treatment, is a combination of 5 of the 38 remedies selected by Dr Bach. Doctors, therapists and individuals highly recommend The Rescue Remedy, so keep some in stock for emergencies.

The Bach Flower remedies can be bought over the counter, but if you want remedies containing 'mother' tinctures prepared under the supervision of the Bach Centre, look for Dr. Bach's signature on the bottle.

If your local therapist is not acquainted with the Bach Flower remedies, you can obtain information and advice re dosage and remedy indication direct from The Dr. Edward Bach Centre, Mount Vernon, Sotwell, Wallingford, Oxon, OX14 5JX Tel: 01491 832878 or to arrange a personal consultation Telephone: 01491 832877. Both numbers between 10.00 am - 3.30 pm.

LAUGHTER

You could feel a significant improvement in your life within a week and it only takes half a minute a day

Laughter has been called the greatest preventative medicine. When you laugh, you release extra hormones from your various endocrine glands into your bloodstream which can be as powerful as morphine. A really good laugh can affect your immune system for hours, bring more oxygen to your brain and create better thoughts. Laughter boosts your thymus, so it can mature more T-cells, which fight your body's enemies.

Research shows laughter can exercise muscles and nerves in your solar plexus where 70% of your immune system is stored. It causes the heart to beat faster, increases blood flow and raises blood pressure which then drops to a point that is lower than where it started. When the blood vessels dilate by laughing, protective chemicals are released which are believed to reduce the hardening of the arteries.

Research has also found that patients who cannot do physical activity to normalise or enhance their appetite, can increase the levels of the two appetite hormones, leptin and ghrelin, by using 'laughercise' to help them regain their appetite.

Try this
    A. Think of something positive
    B. Laugh a good 'belly laugh' for 15 seconds (can be silent) every morning and every afternoon.
    C. Don't skip a session.

There is the famous case of a man with terminal cancer, who decided to spend most of his time watching lots of hilariously funny videos and cured himself of cancer.

However I feel he did one or two other good things we are not told about, so laughing is only one excellent habit you should get into to make you healthier.

MEDITATION

Meditation (or mindfulness as it is often called) is cheap, 'portable' and has been shown to reverse the effects of stress by giving you inner peace, thereby benefiting you mentally, physically and spiritually.

Meditation is a useful self-help technique which can be practised without adhering to any religion or philosophy.

Research has shown meditation reduces stress, anxiety, mild depression, insomnia, tension headaches, migraines and other stress-related illnesses.

Meditation works best when you do it regularly, say for 10 minutes at the start of each day. Find a place where you are not disturbed. I suggest you sit on a chair with your back straight but relaxed, feet on the floor and your hands resting on your stomach.

To calm you down, breathe in through your nose. Hold your breath for a count of 10. This will help you to regain some extra carbon dioxide gas which will help you to calm down. Exhale through your mouth for a count of 10. Ensure you inhale enough air into your diaphragm ('belly' breathing) rather than shallow 'chest' breathing. Again hold your breath for a count of 10 and exhale for a count of 10. Do these three or four times.

Now become aware of your senses, the feeling of your body, the sounds and smells around you. Do not think about them, just notice them.

Various schools of meditation favour particular techniques. All emphasise the initial need for a focus of attention to which the mind can return if distracted. This may be the rising and falling sensation of your breathing, a mantra, a physical object such as a religious icon or a repetitive movement to improve the 'life energy' around the body.

If you have lots of thoughts racing around your mind, take a couple of minutes to write them down. This will give you a feeling of extra space in your mind.

You can meditate any time of the day, at work, when travelling to or from work, whilst walking or on transport.

You may initially need a practitioner to show you how to meditate.

YOGA

Yoga represents a holistic approach to self development which originated in India and the rest of Asia thousands of years ago. Yoga embraces many static and dynamic exercises both gentle and strong, breathing procedures from the very basic to the highly subtle and meditation arts from both a worldly and spiritual standpoint.

Yoga has been found by many to be the healing force in the treatment of anxiety, depression and can help in treating illnesses.

The main type of yoga taught in the West is Hatha yoga and under this umbrella there are three main schools:-

Sivanada, Iyenga and Ashtanga

Finding a good teacher is more important than the type of yoga you do.

Professional body: British Wheel of Yoga (BWY) has a network of 3,000 teachers.

Contact www.bwy.org.uk

ACUPUNCTURE

This is a technique which has been developed over the past 3,000 years mainly in China, whereby needles are used to puncture the skin at defined points along the body to restore and unblock the flow of 'chi' energy which acupuncturists believe is essential to good health.

There are around 800 points on your body which join up to form 12 major meridians that are named after the organs to which they are attached. These are: large intestine, stomach, heart, spleen, small intestine, bladder, kidneys, gallbladder, lung, liver plus circulation, triple warmer and the 2 central and governing meridians.

Many cancer patients have reported a reduction in pain and other health benefits before, during and after orthodox treatment by having acupuncture. This is a branch of medicine founded upon the principle that health is dependent upon a proper balance of vital energy forces within your body.

Professional body British Acupuncture Council has 3,000 members. Qualifications consist of over 360 hours of training. Contact www.acupuncture.org.uk.

British Medical Acupuncture Society has 2,500 members. Qualifications - all members are medical professionals - doctors, nurses, physiotherapists and osteopaths. Minimum training 100 hours. Contact www.medical-acupuncture.co.uk,

AROMATHERAPY

Aromatherapy is the use of essential oils or aromatic essences of plants to rub onto your skin, inhale or use in a bath or footbath.

Aromatherapy is a soothing way to relax, particularly if you are stressed. The essential oils penetrate the skin via the skin pore openings and sweat glands and is then carried round the body in the lymph system and blood. Ask your health shop which essential oil is suitable for you. This should help if you are suffering from insomnia and stress.

If you wish to have a professional aromatherapy massage, **The Aromatherapy Consortium** has over 10,000 members. To be recognised as a professional member, you must train and meet The National Occupational Standard. Contact www.aromatherapy-regulation.org.uk.

CHIROPRACTIC/OSTEOPATHY

Both therapies involve manipulating and mobilising the body structure by various hands-on techniques, thereby helping it to heal itself.

Osteopathy lays equal emphasise on the joints and surrounding soft tissues such as muscles and ligaments.

Chiropractors focus mainly on the joints of the spine and the nervous system.

Both therapies will ease neck and back pain rather than the use of painkillers. Do discuss the above therapies with your doctor and tell the therapist about your cancer treatment.

Professional bodies Both osteopaths and chiropractors must by law be registered by their appropriate council after lengthy courses at an accredited college. A list of members nearest you is available as follows:

The British Osteopathy Association at www.osteopathy.org.uk

British Chiropractic Association at www.chiropractic.co.uk

HEALING

Healing by touch or holistic healing has been known for centuries. It is all about changing the person not the illness, for it is the person that heals not the therapy.

Healing removes blockages within your system, restores the balance of energies and allows the body to move its natural state of wholeness. Many patients report feeling heat emanating from the healer's hands and a feeling of profound relaxation and peace.

Healing is sometimes called spiritual or faith healing, but healing requires no shared religion between healer and patient.

Professsional body of National Federation of Spiritual Healers has about 6,000 members. Full members must have undertaken a two year NFSH licensed healing development course. Contact www.nationalfederationofspiritualhealers.

HOMEOPATHY

Cancer patients have been able to tolerate their harsh chemotherapy and/or radiotherapy treatment better by taking homeopathic remedies. Homeopathy is one of the most well recognised complementary therapies and is available on the NHS. The remedies have no side-effects and are not addictive.

Homeopathy (Greek *homoios* (same) and *pathos* (suffering) was founded in 1796 by Samuel Hahnemann, a German doctor, on the principle that 'like cures like'. That is, a substance or preparation which can cause groups of symptoms of illness, whether physical, emotional or behavioural, in the healthy can cure similar groups of symptoms when they appear in the sick. Hahnemann further stated that the potency of a curative agent increases as the substance is diluted. Homeopathy treatment seeks to stimulate the self-healing process rather than suppress symptoms.

Homeopathy uses over 2,000 different remedies which are chosen to suit the patient's characteristics as well as treating the symptoms. The therapist will spend some time during the first session to find out about the medical history and what particular constitutional type the patient is.

Homeopathic remedies are prepared from tinctures by a number of methods depending on the nature of the source of the remedy. These tinctures are then successively diluted by a special process called succession. Each stage of succession increases the potency which is given a number and a letter. Potencies with an X affix are diluted 1:9 and those with a C affix are diluted 1:99 at each successive stage. The most 'potent' remedies of all are 200c, 1000c or even higher, at which point not even a molecule of the original substance is likely to be left. The substance can be used once it becomes soluble in a strong alcohol/water solvent.

Homeopathic remedies need to be protected from contamination. They should not be touched, exposed to sunlight or taken near meals or drinks, as their energy can easily be nullified. **Nor must the remedies be kept in a place where there is Geopathic Stress.**

It is worthwhile asking the therapist to double check with the muscle test, if the one or several remedies prescribed are suitable for you.

Professional bodies British Homeopathic Association runs postgraduate training courses for doctors, dentists, nurses, pharmacists and other statutory registered health care professionals. Medically qualified homeopathic doctors offer the additional reassurance of conventional medicine. With a GP referral, you can attend one of five NHS homeopathy hospitals or claim private health insurance.
www.britishhomeopathic.org

The Society of Homeopaths is the largest professional body for non-medical homeopaths, with over 1,000 registered members who have completed a six month registered process on top of training (three years full time, four years part time) at accredited colleges where the curriculum includes physiology and anatomy.
www.homeopathy-soh.org

KINESIOLOGY

Kinesiology (pronounced kin-easy-ology) uses manual muscle testing to diagnose imbalances in the body and its sensitivity to food, drugs and toxic substances and also to check how beneficial specific medical drugs and supplements are.

The theory is based on 'your body does not lie'. Once the body's imbalance has been identified, a variety of treatments and techniques can be recommended. Even people with similar symptoms may need an entirely different treatment plan, as each person is unique.

Kinesiology's truly holistic approach of addressing both physical and mental/emotional issues make it especially powerful in identifying the most suitable therapy for cancer patients. The therapy is often carried out by most therapists as a prelude to any treatment.

Professional body: **Academy of Systematic Kinesiology Limited**

Contact www.kinesiology.co.uk

MASSAGE

The majority of hospices in the UK offer massage for cancer patients to promote a general feeling of comfort and to boost the circulation and immune systems.

Massage may be the oldest and simplest form of medical care. Greek and Roman physicians valued it as a principal method of relieving pain. Gentle massage or stroking can trigger the release of endorphins, the body's natural pain killers. Massage is now being included in nurses' degree programs.

In trials at The Royal Marsden Hospital, London in 1995, massage was shown to reduce anxiety and improve quality of life in cancer patients. Massage has also been shown to produce more natural killer cells that destroy invading microbes.

The basic techniques

Stroking aids circulation and relaxes tense muscles. The therapist's hands glide smoothly and rhythmically over the skin either alternately or in a slow fanning or circular motion.
Kneading stretches and relaxes muscles and is particularly useful for fleshy areas such as thighs. The action is like kneading dough, using alternate hands to squeeze and release flesh rhythmically between fingers and thumbs.
Friction is deep, direct pressure to release tension in the muscles around the spine and shoulders. Even pressure or small circles is applied with the thumbs.
Hacking is applied by the side of the hands in alternate short, sharp taps.

Therapist

Your doctor may be able to recommend a massage therapist. Private practitioners will often visit you at home. Members of professional bodies have attended an accredited college and have received training in anatomy and physiology.
Contact **The British Massage Therapy Council** at www.bmtc.co.uk

REFLEXOLOGY

Reflexology is based on the principle that there are areas or reflexology points on the feet and hands that correspond to each organ, gland and structure in the body.

By working on these reflexes mainly with thumbs and fingers, the reflexologist reduces tension and relieves congestion all over the body. As circulation in the feet slows down - through illness, wearing badly fitted shoes or lack of exercise - then crystalline deposits form at the nerve ends. By deep compression foot massage, the deposits are broken up, encouraging the whole body to keep working at peak efficiency. Reflex areas that are tender to the touch signal malfunction, disease or deterioration of the corresponding organ or function.

There are reflex points in the feet for all parts of the body and these are arranged in such a way to form a map of the body in the feet. See diagram.

Professional body: Association of Reflexologists has more than 7,000 members. Members must have trained on courses accredited by the association.
Contact www.aor.org.uk

REFLEXOLOGY CHART

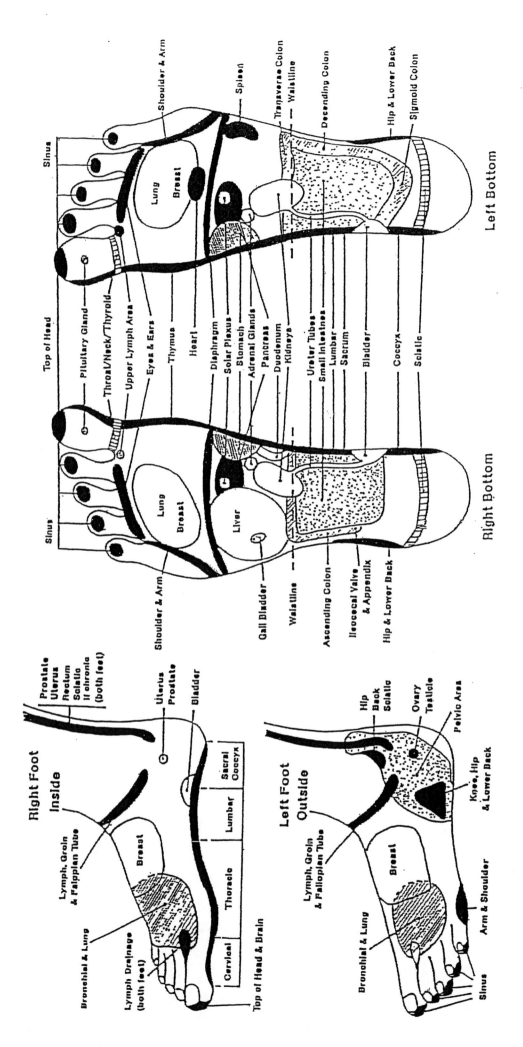

PART SEVEN

INSIDE YOUR BODY

CONTENTS

- Your immune system and how to strengthen it

- Functions of your organs and glands

- Inside your body diagrams

YOUR IMMUNE SYSTEM - and how to strengthen it.

> If you get cancer it is because your immune system has been weakened. The success of any orthodox cancer treatment will depend on you improving your immune system. Remember cancer is not a contagious disease from outside, it develops in your body due to an inefficient immune system, which you can have even if you feel fit and reasonably well.

I have heard of many cases where a cancer patient after orthodox treatment, has been in remission, but died soon afterwards of pneumonia, septicemia, heart problems etc. due to treatment which has further weakened their immune system. It is, therefore important to build up your immune system before you have surgery, chemotherapy and/or radiotherapy.

I remember well, after each of our son's tough chemotherapy treatments, he was sent home very weak with no advice on how to strengthen his immune system. That was 25 years ago when even less information was given.

A strong immune system can stop cancer in its tracks by identifying cancer cells and can mount an effective attack against tumours and groups of renegade cells that may have spread from a primary tumour.

Lymph System

The lymph system is your main immune system. It consists of a network of vessels throughout your body which link together the spleen, tonsils, thymus gland and a multitude of lymph nodes. These nodes generally occur in clusters mainly around the neck, armpits and groin. The lymph system contains a watery or milky fluid which comes from the white blood cells. This fluid flows into innumerable tiny ducts and capillaries. Eventually the lymph fluid makes its way back into the bloodstream via the thoracic duct and the right lymphatic duct through to the two subclavian veins near the neck. These veins unite to form the inferior vena cava through which the blood flows back to the heart.

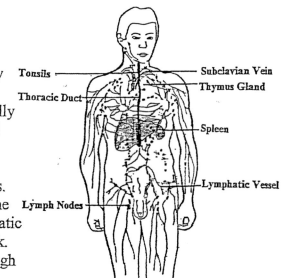

The role of the lymph system is:
- to maintain tissue fluid and protein balance throughout the body by removing and re-circulating excessive amounts from any part of the body.
- to produce and circulate lymphocytes all round the body in order to protect it from infection, cancer and other alien matter thereby providing immunity.
- to assist with the circulation of nutrients (proteins, fats, sugar etc) vitamins, minerals, trace elements and hormones to all cells in the body.
- to remove waste products and other toxic matter from the body tissues, thereby maintaining its inner healthy environment.

Lymphocytes are produced in the bone marrow and come in two forms. **T-cells** travel to the thymus (behind the breast bone) which produce hormones that help to mature the T-cells which have many functions in the body's immune system. **B-cells** produce antibodies to neutralise foreign matter in the blood and tissues and are matured by passing through the bursal equivalent in the Peyer's patches surrounding the intestines.

Certain types of T-cells signal to other white blood cells, that cancer cells are present. Some lymphocytes can produce various anti-cancer chemicals, known as cytokines, which include tumour necrosis factor, interleukin and interferon. These are the body's own 'chemotherapy', but they do not harm healthy cells as administered chemotherapy does.

Antibodies scurry around your entire body from one molecule to another checking all identification badges, known as epiliop which consists of about ten letters made up of amino acids. If the molecule is a foreigner, the antibody immediately attaches itself to the invader or cancer cell and calls on other antibodies, T-cells, neutrophils and macrophage cells that proceed to the site of the antibody to arrest and destroy the foreigner.

Macrophages are the vacuum cleaners of the immune system swallowing everything that is not normal healthy tissue, including old dead cells. They can digest over 100 bacteria in seconds and still continue.

Monocytes are immature white blood cells circulating in the bloodstream. Once they leave the bloodstream and come into the lymph system, they 'puff-up' to five times their original size and become deadly macrophages.

Neutrophils are five times smaller than macrophage cells. They are also summoned by the antibodies to destroy foreign bodies.

Killer T-Cells are a special form of lymphocyte capable of migrating to the site of a cancer and destroying the malignant cells before they can divide. In a normal strong immune system, killer T-cells will descend directly into a minuscule tumour and begin devouring and disintegrating it. As a consequence, many tumours never make it beyond this asymptomatic stage. Unfortunately, killer T-cells have little effect against large tumours. Their main value is in protecting against the spread of micrometastases, those tiny blood and lymph accumulation of cancer cells that would otherwise seed a new tumour growth, by using almost 100 different biochemical poisons to kill foreign proteins.

If your lymphatic system is strong, healthy, circulating properly and is kept well informed by antibodies, your lymphocytes get in there and clean up in no time at all. But if the crack armies of your immune defence force are weakened by malnutrition, lack of proper exercise, microbes - mainly parasites - too acidic blood, emotional upset, the presence of too much toxic waste in your body and weakened by a bad environment (mainly Geopathic Stress), the balance of power can swing in favour of the mutant (cancer) cells, which can soon build a cancer colony that will try and destroy your entire body.

At least 95% of all cancer patients are 'immunosuppressed', meaning that they have a total lymphocyte count of less than 1200 cells/mm³. The low lymphocyte number can be detected by a Complete Blood Count (CBC) a routine and inexpensive medical test.

Chemotherapy destroys up to 30% of your immune system. You will most likely die if you lose more than 40%. Chemotherapy and radiotherapy are often ineffective in the long run, because the elimination of the tumour does nothing to change the causes that allowed the tumour to grow in the first place.

Geopathic Stress

As fully described elsewhere, Geopathic Stress is the most important issue to deal with in order to strengthen your immune system and if dealt with in the first place, can nearly always prevent cancer. If you already have cancer, dealing with Geopathic Stress will ensure that any treatment will be 100% more successful. Many people with cancer have told me they sleep and feel so much better after sleeping in a good place. Often people with brain tumours have said they stopped waking up with headaches. Your immune system just cannot operate fully when Geopathic Stress is present and, as mentioned before, cancer always starts where the body is most Geopathic Stressed. So check your bed and 'favourite' chair for Geopathic Stress and move then into Geopathic Stress-free places in your home, however inconvenient it is. Don't forget to check your workplace.

Healthy Diet

More than 4,000 different food additives are currently in use in processed food. On average we swallow 2.3kg (5lbs) of additives each year. Most are alien particles. Our immune system has to deal with each one and this places an extra burden it so try and stick to unprocessed foods - fruit, vegetables (best green leafy and uncooked if possible), fresh fish, meat, chicken, milk, butter, eggs, nuts etc. and make a point of looking at the labels for ready made soups, sauces, meals, butter substitutes etc.etc.

TOP (I feel this is so important that I am repeating it)
Remember the following when you are eating:
T is for time. Give yourself time to eat. The French are not necessarily healthier because they drink wine, but it relaxes them, so they spend longer eating. The Scandinavians light candles with their meals, which helps them relax and therefore they have fewer digestive problems.
If you eat under stress, your stomach can close down for up to two hours, so you take no benefit from your food.
O is for oxygen. Eat slowly so you can breathe more whilst eating so more oxygen enters your stomach, making your calories burn more efficiently and thereby your body obtains the maximum benefit from your food. If you do not burn your calories properly, they will be stored as fat.
It is of major importance to your overall wellbeing to replace your "friendly" bacteria (probiotics), destroyed by many medical drugs including antibiotics. Often probiotic products (including yoghurts and fermented food) fail to reach the intestines, because they are destroyed by the acid environment of the stomach.
Bio-Culture capsules by Pharma Nord contain up to 4 billion in each capsule of the most important "friendly" bacteria lactobacillus acidophilus and bifidobacterium lactis. The capsules need not be kept in the fridge and contain live bacteria at the time they are taken. The capsules are guaranteed not to dissolve before they reach your small intestines where they are needed.
P is for pleasure. Take pleasure in everything you eat, then your stomach will digest it, even if you are eating something you know is a little bit 'naughty'! Have that cream cake or what you long for, now and again. Your stomach will cope as long as you take pleasure in eating it.
You must feed your soul.

Water

Drink plenty of water to stimulate your immune system, because water increases the body's white blood cells and flushes out accumulated toxins (see Part Four).

Parasites

They must be eliminated as micro parasites are continuously attacking and weakening your immune system (see Part One).

Thymus

More than 25% of your immune system, the T-cells, are matured by the thymus. The thymus is the one organ you can influence and strengthen yourself very quickly, by pleasant music, laughter, meditation, relaxation and activities that create pleasure and happiness. Also by light tapping directly a few times with your flat hand. See magnetic therapy below.

Exercise

Your lymph system does not have a pump, unlike your heart. Exercise greatly assists the circulation of your lymph system. Harvard University studied 5,000 women who graduated from 10 USA colleges between 1925 and 1981. They found that the less active women were 2½ times more at risk of developing cancer, than the former athletes among them. Remember, 2 minutes on a Rebounder doubles your white blood cells. (See Part Five).

Magnetic Therapy

Place a powerful high spinning magnetic apparatus on your thymus for one or two minutes to strengthen it. Magnetise your kidneys and liver to give them strength to filter out toxins and alien bodies from your immune system. Also use for say 20 minutes on your solar plexus, where 70% of your immune system is located and under your feet to strengthen your whole body through to your reflexology points.

Acid Alkaline Balance

It is vital your blood is slightly alkalised (see Part One).

INSIDE YOUR BODY

FUNCTIONS OF YOUR ORGANS & GLANDS

I am surprised how often I meet people, who have little idea where their various organs and glands are and how they function.

ADRENAL GLANDS produce a number of hormones such as adrenaline, cortisone and sex hormones.

BRAIN STEM controls heart beat and breathing

CEREBELLUM controls balance, muscle tone and co-ordination of movement.

COLON mainly removes considerable quantities of water from digested food.

DIAPHRAGM moves up and down to help lungs inhale and expel air.

DUODENUM & SMALL INTESTINE
the major part of digestion and absorption takes place here. Hormones are released into the blood from food.

ENDOCRINE GLANDS are the major glands of the body. They secrete hormones and release them into the blood.

GALL BLADDER stores and concentrates bile, this is released into intestines when needed.

HYPOTHALAMUS regulates body temperature, appetite and releases some hormones.

ILEOCAECAL VALVE prevents residue of food passing back into the small intestine.

KIDNEYS eliminate the toxic waste products from the body's metabolism and maintains stable fluid and electrolyte levels.

LARGE INTESTINE is the combined name for colon and rectum.

LARYNX is the voice box.

LIVER removes toxic substances produced in the small intestine and produces proteins. Stores and processes vitamins and excretes bile as waste product, which also aids the digestion of fats.

LUNGS extract oxygen from the air and remove carbon dioxide and water from the blood.

LYMPH NODE is a small mass of tissue which filters lymph and produces lymphocytes.
Important group of nodes are found in the groin, around lungs, in the armpit (24%) and behind the ears.

PANCREAS produces enzymes for digestion, bicarbonates to neutralise the acid coming into the small intestine from the stomach and also some gut hormones, such as insulin to control sugar and fat metabolism.

PARATHYROID GLANDS secrete the parathormone hormone which controls the distribution of calcium and phosphate.

PITUITARY GLAND controls the release of many hormones.

SIGMOID COLON forms faeces.

SOLAR PLEXUS is a region of the lower abdomen (above the navel) which contains 70% of your immune system.

SPLEEN filters out old red and white blood cells from the circulation and destroys them. It contains many cells of the immune system and defends the bloodstream against invading micro organisms such as bacteria and viruses.

STOMACH mixes food with gastric juice to partially break down proteins. Contents move into the duodenum over several hours.

THYMUS GLAND matures T-cells, which recognise and fight viruses and bacteria. It also produces hormones to regulate the development of peripheral lymphoid tissues. (A much under-rated gland, affected by stress).

THYROID GLANDS under the control of the brain and pituitary gland, release iodine containing hormones, which control metabolism and growth.

INSIDE YOUR BODY

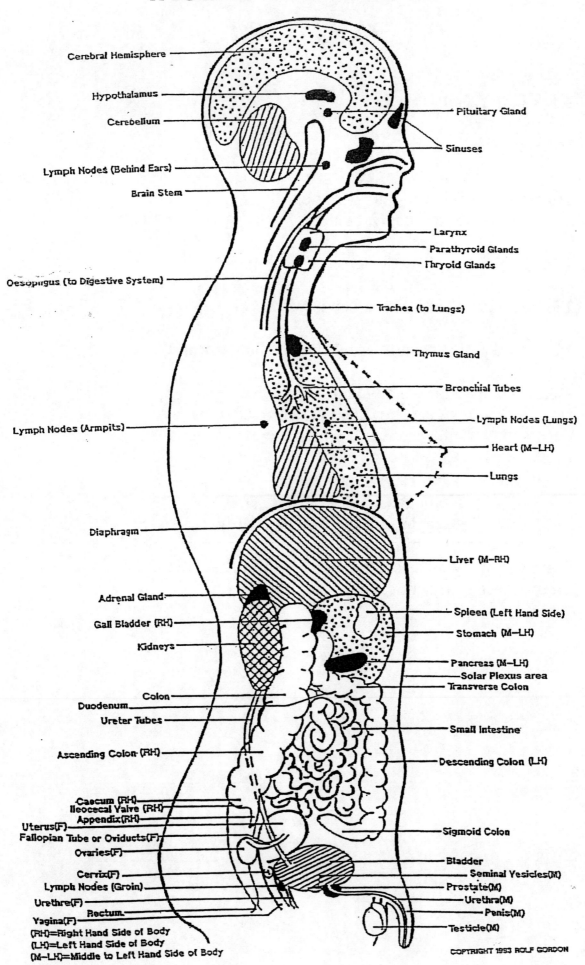

Cerebral Hemisphere

Hypothalamus

Cerebellum

Pituitary Gland

Sinuses

Lymph Nodes (Behind Ears)

Brain Stem

Larynx

Parathyroid Glands

Thyroid Glands

Oesophagus (to Digestive System)

Trachea (to Lungs)

Thymus Gland

Bronchial Tubes

Lymph Nodes (Lungs)

Lymph Nodes (Armpits)

Heart (M–LH)

Lungs

Diaphragm

Liver (M–RH)

Adrenal Gland

Gall Bladder (RH)

Kidneys

Spleen (Left Hand Side)

Stomach (M–LH)

Pancreas (M–LH)

Solar Plexus area

Transverse Colon

Colon

Duodenum

Ureter Tubes

Small Intestine

Ascending Colon (RH)

Descending Colon (LH)

Caecum (RH)
Ileocecal Valve (RH)
Appendix (RH)

Uterus(F)
Fallopian Tube or Oviducts(F)

Ovaries(F)

Sigmoid Colon

Bladder

Cervix(F)

Seminal Vesicles(M)

Lymph Nodes (Groin)

Prostate(M)

Urethre(F)

Urethra(M)

Rectum

Penis(M)

Vagina(F)

Testicle(M)

(RH)=Right Hand Side of Body
(LH)=Left Hand Side of Body
(M–LH)=Middle to Left Hand Side of Body

COPYRIGHT 1953 ROLF GORDON

CANCER - the full menu

251

PART EIGHT

ADVICE AND HELP

CONTENT

- Hospital - What to take with you
  - Your survival guide

- How to help people with cancer

- Financial problems - when you have cancer

- Insurance and vaccinations when travelling abroad

- Charities - MacMillan Cancer Support
  - Marie Curie Cancer Care
  - Look Good - Feel Better
  - Hospices
  - Children's Charities
  - Teenage Charities Trust
  - Maggie's Cancer Caring Centres

There are many other cancer charities, but these are the main ones I know of who deal with cancer patients direct.

HOSPITAL

- **What to take with you**
- **Your survival guide**

> You are no doubt worried about going to hospital for your cancer treatment, but perhaps also about what to take with you and any infections you may pick up in hospital. Here is a check list of what to take and how to protect yourself against hospital acquired infections (HAI) and how to treat yourself if you get infected.

SUGGESTED LIST OF WHAT TO TAKE WITH YOU

You may only need some of these things if you are only expected to stay in hospital for one or two nights, but pack the rest in a bag at home for someone to bring if you should have to stay in longer.

- Two pairs of pyjamas or two nightgowns
- Dressing gown
- Slippers
- Clean underwear, socks, tights/stockings for when you are going home
- Toilet bag to include:
  - Hair brush/comb
  - Toothbrush and toothpaste
  - Shampoo
  - Bar or liquid antibacterial soap
  - Body lotion and other creams you normally use (not containing petroleum products if possible).
  - Natural body deodorant (free from perfumes and chemicals)
  - Oregano Germ Spray (make yourself by putting 3 drops of super strength Oregano Oil in a spray bottle with water) or use Germ-A-Clenz
  - Air freshener
  - Razor for shaving
  - Address book, paper, envelopes, stamps
  - Wax earplugs to cut out most of the noise of other people snoring etc.
  - Eye shades in case you wish to sleep when lights are on, or during the day.
  - A bottle of cordial such as elderflower, pink ginger or drops of 'Jif' lemon juice does wonders for the taste of hospital water
  - crystallized stem ginger in case you should feel nauseous
- Vitamins and minerals you normally take - see under surgery and chemotherapy (Part Two) i.e. what you should <u>not</u> take. You may not like to show these to hospital staff in case they do not know how beneficial they are and they may take them away. I know from personal experience how weak my mother became in hospital because she was not allowed her usual supplements. (She was only in hospital for investigations, not for an operation. She picked up again in days, when I 'smuggled in' her usual supplements which she took in secret).

- Plenty of washed fruit to keep your energy reserves up. Do not assume that others will bring these in for you.

The most essential supplements to take each day are:
- Q10 minimum 100 mg in soya oil capsules (not tablets)
- Vitamin D minimum 40 mcg (1600 IU) in capsules containing oil (not tablets)
- Seaweed (good quality) - to boost your intake of vitamins, minerals etc.

Also recommended:
- Vitamin E minimum 350 mg
- Vitamin C minimum 1000 mg
- Selenium and Zinc minimum 200 mcg
- Fish Oil minimum 1000 mg

- Oxygen enriched capsules if you get a tummy upset, are constipated or if you are already taking it. This will give you extra oxygen to fight microbes and give you energy.
- For hospital acquired infections and to boost your immune system, use 100% stabilised Allisure® allicin liquid, capsules or gel.
- MagneTech if you dare! This will help to heal any surgery scars faster, fight HAI, revitalise your immune system, deal with bed sores and reduce pain etc.
- Loose change for magazines/newspapers (or bring your own).
- Mobile phone (ask hospital staff if you can use your mobile phone by your bed in case it interferes with any hospital equipment).

YOUR SURVIVAL GUIDE

Hospital Acquired Infections (HAI)

Unfortunately since hospitals in the UK have contracted out cleaning to private companies, we have some of the dirtiest hospitals in Europe. Within hours of admission, you will most likely have various strains of bacteria on your skin as well as in your respiratory and digestive system.

If you are healthy, most bacteria will not do you any harm, but if your immune system is low or you have an injury/broken skin, catheters or drips may be inserted, bacteria are then able to enter your body, multiply and can then be life-threatening.

Quite rightly, NHS hospitals focus on MRSA and C-difficile, but they are only responsible for about 15% of HAI. The far more common infection is E-coli which now accounts for about 33% of HAI, around 22,000 cases in hospitals a year. Other deadly HAI are surgical site infections, HAI caused by infected tubes etc. inserted into the body and pneumonia and other respiratory infections.

Unfortunately 25% of people carry the superbugs with them into hospitals either as a patient or as a visitor.

What to do if you get MRSA , E-coli etc.

Most antibiotics, including *methicillin,* can no longer destroy superbugs. Luckily, if your immune system is strong (unfortunately it will not stay strong for long on hospital food alone), the superbug will eventually go away. As described in Part Four, 100% stabilised

Allisure® allicin was shown to successfully destroy all 52 cases of MRSA in a study at the University Hospital, East London. It is recommended you take 4 x 450 mg allicin capsules each day, starting one week before going to hospital and carry on while in hospital to lessen the chance of getting HAI, stop any microbes multiplying and boost your immune system. If you should still get for example MRSA, take 2 x 5 ml of allicin liquid twice a day with food; later reduce to 1 x 5 ml twice a day.

Deep Vein Thrombosis (DVT) or pulmonary embolism
Anyone who is immobile for any length of time is at risk of blood thickening and forming clots in the lower limbs. These clots can start to travel around the body. If they lodge in the pulmonary blood vessels of the lung, they can kill instantly by cutting off the blood supply to the heart and brain.

Even young fit people who have no blood disorders can die from clotting in hospital. DVT is blamed for more than 60,000 deaths of hospital patients each year, which is half as many as the 120,000 who die from cancer. Many of the deaths caused by DVT are not properly recorded, but often shown as heart attacks or strokes as a cause of death, as fewer post-mortem examinations are carried out today.

Even if you are only in hospital for a few days and not having surgery, you should be assessed for anti-clotting drugs. If you are not given anti-clotting drugs, take 100 mg of Q10 every 4 hours (200 mg before you go to sleep). Wear surgical stockings and move your legs every 4 hours or get somebody to exercise your legs for you. Better still get out of bed for a walk if you can.

Malnutrition
About 10,000 hospital patients a year in the UK are more malnourished leaving hospital than when they went in, which can cause 30% more complications and a 40% higher mortality rate. When you are seriously ill your body needs more energy in the form of calories, vitamins etc. to recover than a healthy person. Aim for carbohydrate rich food such as pasta also full-fat milk, butter and always have a pudding.

Unfortunately several things can prevent you getting enough to eat:
* You don't feel hungry when you see the hospital food.
* You are asleep when your food is placed next to you and it is cold and inedible by the time you wake up.
* Nobody helps you with food if you have difficulty feeding yourself or reaching the food.
* Even when you are well, some people find it difficult to open a packet of sandwiches.

How to help overcome the above:
* Get family and friends on a rota to bring your favourite food to you each day. Also ask them to bring some energy drinks (with a straw).
* If you are having sandwiches, ask the food trolley staff or a fellow patient if no hospital staff are willing, to open and cut the sandwiches into small pieces.
* Ask fellow patients to help feed you.
* Do no forget to take all your supplements.
* If you find the main course a bit dry, order soup and pour it onto the main meal.

Cleanliness

Wash your hands regularly throughout the day particularly, after every visit to the toilet, with an antibacterial liquid. Often microbes that cause infection come from you. Also ask any hospital staff that come into contact with you, including doctors and any visitors, to wash their hands with antibacterial liquid beforehand.

Do not forget that bacteria etc. are easily transferred to toys, magazines and books etc., so use an antiseptic spray like Oregano, Germ-A-Clenz.

Fluids

Try and drink two litres (over three pints) of liquid a day. Not only water, but juices, tea and coffee count towards the two litres. This will help your body to heal and prevent infection, pressure sores, electrolyte imbalance in your blood, nausea, weakening of your immune system, heart irregularities and other complications especially if you are older.

Surgical operations

Before any operation, clip all your nails short to minimise bacteria hiding underneath. Have a long hot shower using plenty of antibacterial soap.

You may also consider

- taking a mobile phone picture of each doctor (ask first)who examines you, in case you have to explain to others which doctors came to see you.
- asking doctors to clean their stethoscope before using it on you.

HOW TO HELP PEOPLE WITH CANCER

> **I want to help one of my best friends who has just been diagnosed with cancer. What can I do?**

When you first meet your friend after he or she has received the bad news try not to break down in tears. Treat your friend as you always have. No special pitying voice, no special treatment. Your friend's personality has not changed. Hug your friend if you always do, otherwise don't. Later carry on talking and argue about daily life and subjects as before. Don't come unannounced nor ask endless intruding questions or give loads of advice.
If you bring flowers, make sure they come in their own vase or pot, so they do not entail a lot of work to display them.

It has been observed that cancer patients only recall 10% to 25% of what is said by the doctors during consultations, so offer to go along with your friend and make as many notes as possible. Consider taking a tape recorder and ask if you can record the consultation. Some specialists tape themselves and hand it to the patient. The tape can then be replayed when your friend is in a better position to absorb the information.

Before the next consultation, help your friend to write down all their worries and questions he or she want answers to. Ensure the doctor is asked everything about the proposed treatment and its side effects and ask for a second opinion if not happy with the answers. A final decision can always wait a few days. Your friend may consider changing to another GP or consultant if unhappy with the way they are being treated or the treatment suggested.

Consider helping your friend to set up a Facebook page on the internet and post regular reports on how he or she is feeling and how treatment is going. This can save hours of repetitive updating for everyone. Some people may also be too embarrassed to phone or visit.

If your friend is worried about how to tell any of his or her children, advise them to talk in an open and honest way, depending naturally upon the age and understanding of the children. It is usually best to tell them individually if there is more than one child, so the child can show emotion and ask questions without interference from any sisters or brothers. Also, it is difficult to cuddle more than one child at a time. Tell them cancer is a serious but treatable illness and that you may feel very sick if the treatment involves chemotherapy and radiotherapy.

Try to help as much as possible with laundry, ironing, cleaning, preparing and dishing up daily meals. Maybe organise a rota of friends, who can make and bring along ready-made meals each day, if your friend is alone and feeling very low during treatments.

Help with looking after pets e.g. dog walks etc.

If your friend has children, help transporting them to and from nursery, school, Scouts, sport, parties etc. Again organise a rota with friends.

Don't forget to help and/or get others to help with transport, as your friend may be involved in over 50 trips for check-ups, treatment and follow-up appointments.

Sometimes your friend will just need you to be with them to lessen their loneliness or perhaps to simply listen quietly to any worries they may have.

Don't always ask if your friend needs help, just do it.

On visiting somebody in hospital, don't start with "how are you"? If they look better, tell them so. If not, talk about something else, like pretty flowers, cards etc. Wait for the patient to volunteer to talk about how they feel, latest treatment etc. Make your stay short, no matter how long your journey has taken.
You may, of course, be a close family member or a friend who the patients just wants you 'to be there', talking now and again, helping with eating etc. or just to hold their hand.

I highly recommend you read the late Deborah Hallan's book 'What can I do to help?' published by Short Books.

FINANCIAL PROBLEMS - when you have cancer

Financial hardship is often second to the physical pain of cancer as a cause of stress.

75% of the 270,000 new cancer patients each year suffer financial difficulty. People don't realise how expensive having cancer can be. The cost can vary depending on the type of cancer you have and how the treatment affects you, such as chemotherapy or radiotherapy which can leave you physically exhausted and nauseous (see Part Two).

Transport
The cost of going back and forth to hospital day-in, day-out, can be very considerable. You might have to make many journeys for diagnostic checks, surgery, chemotherapy, radiotherapy and follow-up appointments. Some specialist treatments like radiotherapy, may be located hundreds of miles away.

Public transport is not always an option. You may fear that pain and fatigue will make you too ill to stand if you don't get a seat or that nausea will force you to get off several times before finishing your journey. Contact with the public will also increase the risk of infection, so if you cannot drive yourself, you have to rely on expensive taxis or the generosity of friends and family - only to be stung by parking charges on arrival. Which? magazine found that nearly one in three English hospitals do not provide information in their car park about parking discounts, which can range from weekly or monthly permits, to multiple entry passes and even free parking, especially if you are going to hospital for treatment such as chemotherapy or radiotherapy - do enquire at the hospital reception.

Also ask for help with transport to and from clinic appointments. If you drive yourself, you may be entitled to road tax exemption and a disabled (blue) badge. The congestion charge is waived for anyone (not just people with cancer) undertaking a long course of treatment in a central London hospital.

Other expenses
You may lose weight and need to buy new clothes; you may need extra heating if staying at home more and the added expense of special diets.

Benefits
The Government benefit system for cancer patients is very complicated and it involves much form filling. Hundreds of millions of pounds worth of benefits go unclaimed each year. People living on their own may be under even more financial pressure. Over 90,000 people of working age are diagnosed with cancer each year. Most cannot work during cancer treatment and nearly one third cannot hold down a job after treatment.

Most large hospitals with cancer centres have people who can give expert advice about financial entitlements to welfare and employment rights. Ask your clinical nurse to make an appointment. Macmillan Cancer Support can also help (see Page 261).

Depending on the stage of your cancer, you may be eligible for many of the following Government benefits:

- **Statutory Sick Pay** (SSP) for a maximum of 28 weeks if you have earned enough to pay National Insurance (NI). If you are still unable to work after 28 weeks you may be able to claim Incapacity Benefit via Form SSP1 from the Department of Work and Pensions.
- **Incapacity Benefits** if you are self employed and make regular NI contributions.
- **Occupational Sick Pay** this is usually paid as a top up to SSP - you will not get both but SSP becomes part of Occupational Benefit.
- **Income Support** if you are not entitled to SSP or Incapacity Benefit. This includes disability and care premiums.
- **Disability Living Allowance** this can usually be back-dated to the time of your diagnosis, is not means tested and is worth up to £100 per week.
- **Housing and Council Tax Benefit and Rebate.**
- **Carers Allowance**
- **Attendance Allowance**
- **Working Tax Credit**
- **Help from the Social Fund**
- **Child Tax Credit**

Deferring payments Most banks, building societies, landlords, councils and utility companies are nearly always willing to defer payments. Get a letter from your hospital consultant or social worker. Ask your hospital clinical nurse to arrange this. Make several photocopies.

Mortgage Contact the manager of your mortgage provider, as arrangements can usually be made to suspend payments for a few months. Alternatively, it may be possible to pay interest only or extend the term of the mortgage. The Department of Work and Pensions may help with interest payments.

A helpful friend who will not take 'no' for an answer may be needed to assist you to manage your finances and obtain all the benefits you are entitled to.

INSURANCE AND VACCINATIONS WHEN TRAVELLING ABROAD

> **If you have had or are having cancer treatment, what better tonic than to travel abroad to a sunny climate for a short break.**
> **However you have to take into account travel insurance and vaccinations.**

Travel Insurance

The lack of available travel insurance has, until recently, been a source of great frustration to cancer patients seeking to take a therapeutic holiday break abroad. Many tried up to ten insurance companies and over half went on holiday without travel insurance.

In 2002, Dr Kirsh Shastri launched what is now called **InsureCancer**. After personal experience of cancer, he was horrified at the lack of reasonably priced and accessible travel cover for those suffering from or in remission from cancer. InsureCancer has developed a pioneering insurance risk assessment and underwriting methodology providing travel insurance for individuals. This includes patients with active, metastatic, relapsed or terminal cancer travelling to all destinations worldwide, including the USA. Children with cancer can also get travel insurance. Insurance is only available for people living in the UK.

It is important, however, for your oncologist to confirm in writing that you can travel with little or no risk to your health.

In 2007 InsureCancer was given The Queen's Award for 'Enterprise in recognition of pioneering insurance underwriting innovation for those affected by cancer'.

InsureCancer is authorised and regulated by the Financial Services Authority.
Contact: Dr Krish Shastri, Director, InsureCancer, 76 Crooksbury Road, Farnham, Surrey, GU10 1QD
Tel: 01252 780192 Fax: 01252 783698 Email: Krish.Shastri@InsureCancer.com

Unique also provide travel insurance for cancer patients Tel: 01603 828210

Vaccines

You should not travel to certain holiday destinations if you require live-virus vaccines, if you have a weak immune system or if you have had chemotherapy or total body radiotherapy during the previous six months. Steroid therapy can weaken your immune system for three months. A diagnosis of, lymphoma, leukemia or a cancer related to HIV infection may also mean that you need to avoid live-virus vaccines.

It is safe to have inactivated vaccines after cancer treatment. However, they may be less effective if you have weakened immunity, so you will need to discuss this with your doctor.

Macmillan Cancer Support will send you a copy of *Travel and Cancer* which includes a list of active and inactivated vaccines. This information is also available on their website - www.macmillan.org.uk.
Tel: 0808 808 0121

CHARITIES

MACMILLAN CANCER SUPPORT

MacMillan Cancer Relief offers excellent help in many ways and can also assist if you are supporting a relative or friend.

Macmillan nurses provide expert care in hospital and at home, are up-to-date with new treatments and are concerned with emotional as well as physical health. They use their specialist skills to provide emotional support, pain relief, symptom control, information and advice to people living with cancer from diagnosis onward.

Macmillan specialists, consultants and doctors deliver cancer treatment and care, undertake research and advise and teach other health professionals.

Macmillan health and social care professionals work across a range of disciplines, many delivering cancer treatment to patients (e.g. radiotherapy) or helping to improve the quality of life following treatment (e.g. occupational therapy). They help people who need social, practical and emotional support. All these professionals have expert knowledge to help people affected by cancer.

Macmillan cancer care centres provide a healing environment for patients at all stages of their illness. Designed and created by Macmillan specialists, they use architectural and design principles, which have been shown to improve people's response to treatment and help them recover faster. Over 100 projects have now been completed.

Macmillan information and support services when you, or the person you are caring for, are upset or frightened, it can be hard to absorb information - or remember to ask the doctor the questions you want answers to - perhaps about treatment or caring for someone at home. Macmillan can help provide up-to-date information about all aspects of cancer including different cancer treatments and individual drugs and any possible side-effects.

Financial help and advice Macmillan can help people struggling with the additional costs associated with having cancer - such as hospital parking or fares. Some people also face extra heating and clothing bills. If working, having cancer or caring for someone, may also mean a break from work and a significant loss of income, small grants can sometimes be given to help meet specific costs, for example, a short break or a washing machine.

Macmillan CancerLine provides free information and emotional support for people affected by cancer, both patients and their family and friends. You can reach the service via freephone 0808 808 2020 Monday to Friday 9am to 6pm, via a telephone service for the deaf and hard of hearing (0808 808 0121), by email (cancerline@macmillan.org.uk) or by writing to CancerLine, Macmillan Cancer Relief, 89 Albert Embankment, London, SE1 7UQ. A link to Language Line Interpreting Service allows callers to be converse in 150 languages. If you leave a message out of hours, they will call you back.

'Help with the Cost of Cancer' is a very useful booklet which tells you more about benefits, grants and financial help generally and can be requested free through CancerLine.

MARIE CURIE CANCER CARE

Research has shown that 64% of people would choose to die at home. In reality only 25% achieve this.

Marie Curie Nurses now make that wish possible for thousands of cancer patients throughout the UK and now care for 50% of all cancer patients who die at home. The nurses work day and night to provide care for patients in the comfortable and familiar surroundings of their own home.

The Marie Curie Nurses are also there for families and carers, providing practical and emotional support at what can be an exhausting time. All services are free of charge to patients and carers.

Nine Marie Curie hospices across the UK provide free specialist support in a relaxed, friendly and comfortable environment.

Marie Curie employs more than 2,700 nurses, doctors and other healthcare professionals and provide care to around 29,000 terminally ill patients each year.

www.mariecurie.org.uk

LOOK GOOD - FEEL BETTER - for women with cancer

Cancer treatment can have a demoralising effect on a women's appearance affecting self-esteem and confidence at a time when a positive attitude is very important.

The charity holds free skincare and make-up workshops regularly at over 50 locations throughout the UK in hospitals and care centres, for up to 12 people at a time. Volunteer beauty consultants take everyone through a specially designed 12-step skincare and make-up regime. At the end of two hours of learning, fun and laughter, women leave feeling relaxed and full of renewed confidence in their appearance. They are all given a gift bag filled with 17 different products donated by major companies throughout the beauty industry.

To make a booking contact www.lookgoodfeelbetter

HOSPICE

Hospice Care aims to improve the lives of people whose illness may not be curable. They care for a quarter of million patients in the UK each year.

Hospices offer the following service:
- medical and nursing care
- pain and symptom control
- rehabilitation
- taking care of peoples' emotional, spiritual and social needs
- therapies, including physiotherapy and complementary therapies
- practical and financial advice
- support to families and close friends both during illness and in bereavement

Palliative care is the name for the type of care provided by Hospices and is also provided in other places such as hospitals and care homes.

People may be referred for Hospice Care as soon as a cancer diagnosis is made, not just at the very end of their life. **Respite care** is also available for short stays at regular intervals to give carers at home a break.

Hospices are also available for people with other life-limiting illnesses such as neurological conditions (e.g. Motor Neurone Disease), HIV and heart and lung diseases.

Some Hospices have a Christian foundation, but Hospice Care aims to meet the needs of people from all cultures and religions and those with no faith.

St. Christopher's Hospice in Sydenham, South London, was the first Hospice to be opened in 1967. There are now 217 Hospices and palliative care inpatient units in the UK with 3,194 care beds. There are 41 children's Hospices with 311 beds in the UK. There are now Hospices all over the world.

Funding

Hospice Care in the UK costs over £½ billion a year, of which only 32% comes from the Government, leaving the Hospice Care charity to raise about £350 million.

Over 100,000 people are volunteers in local Hospices in the UK. It is estimated that the value of volunteers to independent charitable Hospices in the UK is over £112 million per year.

The service to the individual Hospice Care patient is free.

Hospice nurses can also arrange home visits especially to help with pain control.

CHILDREN'S CANCER CHARITIES

CHRISTIAN LEWIS TRUST CHILDREN'S CANCER CHARITY

This was started to enable Christian, who had neuroblastoma cancer, to have the trip of a lifetime to Disneyworld, Florida. The charity provides help and support to families all over the UK who are trying to cope with the unthinkable. The services include their Holiday Programme which aims to provide a unique programme of supervised holidays at special facilities where the family can get away, from the pressures of hospitals and treatment, to luxury static caravans on the coast of Wales or to resort holidays at both Walt Disney World in Florida and Disneyland in France.

The Trust has also become expert in finding specialist travel insurance cover for families with children affected by cancer. www.christianlewistrust.org.uk

CANDLELIGHTERS

Candlelighters is a cancer charity to help support children, teenagers and their families in Yorkshire.

Based at St. James's University Hospital, Leeds it was formed in 1976 and is run by parents of children who have or have had cancer, ex-patients and the medical staff who treat them.

Contact Sally Amos (Company Secretary), The Candlelighters Trusts, Childrens' Day Hospital, St. James's University Hospital, Leeds, LS9 7TF 0113 2470 373, Fax: 0133 2470248

STARLIGHT CHILDRENS' FOUNDATION

This charity brightens the lives of seriously and terminally ill children by granting their wishes and providing hospital entertainment to help take their minds off the pain, fear and isolation of their illness.
Starlight began in 1987 and now helps over 500,000 children all over the UK. Where possible, mums, dads, brothers and sisters are involved to strengthen family bonds at what is often a time of great stress and to give everyone happy memories to share, no matter what the future may hold. Starlight receives neither Government nor Lottery support.

Contact Starlight Children's Foundation, Room PRW1, P.O. Box 4267, Goring, Reading, RG8 0WY   Tel: 020 7262 2881 Fax: 020 7402 7403

OTHER CHILDREN'S CHARITIES

Cancer and Leukaemia in Childhood Trust (CLIC)	Support for childhood cancer and leukaemia.	www.clic.uk.com 0808 808 1010
Helena & Douglas House Hospice	Hospice for children offering short term and terminal care.	helenaanddouglas.org.uk 01865 794749
Family Funds	Some financial help for parents of chronically sick children. Help with bedding, clothing etc.	www.familyfund.org.uk 0845 1304542
Rainbow Trust	Support families who have children with a life threatening or terminal illness.	www.rainbowtrust.org.uk 01372 363438
Sargent	Provides practical and financial help and short breaks for families and young people specialist centres in Scotland and South London.	www.sargent.org.uk 020 8752 2800
Tenorus	Cancer charity - free helpline, financial help, free publications	www.tenorus.com 0808 808 1010

TEENAGE CANCER TRUST

This Trust believes that young people have a much better chance of fighting cancer if, they are treated by teenage cancer experts, in an environment tailored to their needs.

Teenage Cancer Trust units in NHS hospitals currently enable half of the teenagers diagnosed with cancer in the UK, to have access to dedicated specialist support. The units bring teenagers with cancer together with new friends of their own age so they can support each other.

It is hoped by 2012 that every teenager with cancer in the UK can be treated in a Teenager Cancer Trust unit. The Trust's family support network gives mums, dads, brothers and sisters the chance to meet other people, who understand their situation at every stage of the cancer journey and beyond.

An annual meeting specifically for young people with cancer is organised to give them the chance to share experiences and learn more about their disease. This allows about 400 young people from all over the country to learn and have fun together for one weekend.

The Trust holds the only World Conference focusing solely on cancer and the adolescent, where experts from all over the world share information and research helping to improve the lives of young people with cancer internationally.

Contact Teenage Cancer Trust, 93 Newman Street, London, W1T 3EZ
Tel: 020 7612 0370

MAGGIE'S CANCER CARING CENTRES

Maggie's Centres are a haven to help people to live with cancer

Before Maggie Keswick Jencks died of cancer in 1995, she laid down the foundation for the first Maggie's Centre, next to The Western General Hospital, Edinburgh.

Each Maggie's Centre offers information, psychological support, advice on nutrition, exercise and relaxation therapies. Every person visiting the centre will be helped to find his or her own best way of coping with the disease. There is no right way. The centres are a haven, where you can make yourself a cup of tea in friendly surroundings. Have a chat with other cancer patients or with an information and support specialist, browse the library or access one of the courses designed to help people live with, through and beyond the disease. All services are free and cater for all religions.

I was very impressed when I visited the Maggie's Centre in London, which like all the centres, was beautifully designed to create a feeling of warmth, full of life with a view through large windows onto a lovely garden. You just did not realise that you were next to a large busy hospital.

Maggie's Cancer Caring Centres

Edinburgh	- The Stables, Western General Hospital in Edinburgh, Crewe Road, Edinburgh, EH4 2XU	Tel: 0131 537 3131
Glasgow	- Dumbarton Road, The Gatehouse, Western Infirmary, 10 Dumbarton Road, Glasgow, G11 6PA	Tel: 0141 330 3311
Dundee	- Ninewells Hospital, Tom McDonald Avenue, Dundee, DD2 1NH	Tel: 01382 632999
Highlands	- Raigmore Hospital, Old Perth Road, Inverness, IV2 3UJ	Tel: 01463 706306
Fife	- Victoria Hospital, Hayfield Road, Kirkcaldy, KY2 5AH	Tel: 01592 643997
London	- Charing Cross Hospital, Fulham Palace Road, London, W6 8RT	Tel: 020 7386 1750
Interim Centres		
Oxford	- Churchill Hospital, Old Road, Headington, Oxford	Tel: 01865 225690
South West Wales	- North Residence, Singleton Hospital, Sketty Lane, Swansea	Tel: 01792 285868
Lanarkshire	- Flat 78, Residential Accommodation, Wishaw General Hospital, 50 Netherton Street, Wishaw, ML2 0DP	Tel: 01698 358392
Hong Kong	- Tuen Mun Hospital	

PART NINE

HOW TO DETECT GEOPATHIC STRESS (GS)

> Testing for dangerous GS places is the most important thing to do if you have been diagnosed with cancer and prevent the cancer returning after the 'all clear'.
> It is important to check for GS to prevent many other illnesses. If you have cancer, ask somebody else to test as one checking straight into GS.

The main methods of detecting GS are:

> Muscle Test
> L-Rods
> Pendulum
> VegaTest - carried out by therapists

ALLERGIES AND GALL BLADDER STONES have little to do
with cancer, but I feel they must be described as they affect millions of people each year and you can do something about it yourself.

Check for food and drink allergies
Being allergic to certain food and drinks can cause all sorts of health problems like headaches, migraines, skin rashes, sinus and digestion problems etc. Headache alone accounts for 4 million visits to the doctor, 25 million missed workdays and over £60M spent on over the counter painkillers. The main cause of migraine is being allergic to cheeses, red wine and chocolate. One in seven people are allergic to milk. See how you can check what you and your family are allergic to.

Check for environmental allergies
Sneezing and having sore eyes is not necessarily due to grass pollen. See how you can check and maybe avoid the source of the allergy.

What is good for me
Check not only what is bad for you, but also what is good or what you are in need of.

Gall Bladder Stone Flush
This flush can be carried out by yourself without pain, at little cost, in less than a week with 95% success rate. This treatment has been carried out by millions of people for over the last 25 years to prevent long term pain and surgery etc., but still not accepted by most doctors.

CHECKING FOR GEOPATHIC STRESS (GS)

The big problem is that there are no instruments which are accurate and selective enough to check for GS. Therefore one has to use the ancient art of dowsing. This is no doubt the main reason why doctors feel dowsing is parapsychic (for which no adequate scientific explanation exists) and do not want to get involved.

Dowsing has been practised for over ten thousand years and has now been approved by all major religions, as long as it is for the good of mankind.

The Chinese knew how to dowse for GS over 4,500 years ago and avoided building houses in GS places. Often people could be punished if they built on what they called dragon lines.
Sig Lonegren has dowsed hundreds of ancient sites all over the world, but has never found GS under any inhabited site of any peoples whose culture was obviously working with earth energies.

Professor Helmuth Hoffman, a Director of the Institute of Electrotechnique, has stated that the success of dowsing is so evident, that scientists can no longer afford to disregard the evidence. Even Albert Einstein believed in dowsing.

Hundreds of thousands of people use dowsing, but many keep it to themselves in case others disbelieve them. You will be surprised how many doctors and health practitioners use dowsing with pendulums to diagnose patients (often out of sight in another room).

Dowsing with L-rods are used daily by farmers and others to dig or drill water wells with 95% accuracy, used by companies to discover oil, coal etc and by council workers to pinpoint unchartered drains etc. Last year Thames Water found hundreds of water pipe leaks with 100% accuracy by dowsing. These could not be found by any other means.

The effect of harmful, high frequency earth vibrations has been called many names such as *dragon lines, black streams, cancer lines, negative green rays, harmful earth rays,* even *ley lines*. (Hartmann and Curry lines are not GS lines [1]). However, over 20 years ago I persuaded everybody to call them Geopathic Stress Lines (geo from the greek word for earth and pathic from the word Pathos = to suffer or cause disease) which they are now universally called.

Most people can learn the art of dowsing to find out if they are sleeping, sitting or working in a place free of Geopathic Stress.

You can check by dowsing the health of your body, which and what dosage to take of vitamins, minerals, Bach Flower or homeopathic remedies etc. and what drugs and treatments are good or not so good for you. You can also dowse to find out which food and drinks you are allergic to, if any. This is particularly important for babies and children.

There will always be a family member or friend who can can dowse if you find it difficult yourself.

(1) My book 'Are You Sleeping In A Safe Place' explains ley lines , Hartmann and Curry lines. It also explains how to use dials to dowse for almost anything in detail and how to map dowse from a distance.

GEOPATHIC STRESS AND SLEEP

Sleeping in a GS place is particularly stressful as a large area of your body is exposed to the GS. Also most people sleep during the night when GS is stronger. During sleep your brain is supposed to rest half the time and is busy healing your body the other half. However, if you are GS during sleep, your brain has to spend all of its' time working due to the strain of GS and you therefore wake up feeling tired.

During sleep the brain does your body's 'housekeeping' which includes creating 80% of your new cells, giving the right signals for your body to operate properly creating and absorbing the correct level of vitamins, minerals etc. together with adjusting your hormone balance. GS will interfere with this process and leave your immune system weak. All these functions will usually return to normal fairly soon after GS has cleared out of your system.

It is therefore very important, that the 1 sq. meter (10 sq. ft) you sleep on and therefore spend about one third of your life on, must be free from GS.

If you always feel restless in bed and do not feel refreshed in the morning, or have other symptoms which have resisted treatment, try moving your bed, or sleeping in a different room. If you subsequently feel better, it is very likely that your original sleeping place was in a GS place.

Many people find they sleep better on holiday, not just because of different surroundings, but because they have slept in a bed not affected by GS. Unfortunately it can also be the other way round where people sleeping in strong GS places away from home, has resulted in the onset of a long term illness.

IMPORTANT

Children who sleep in GS places will find that they react very quickly to GS later in life. People who sleep in good places as children, may take many years to be affected when in adulthood they sleep in a GS place. This is particularly noticeable when a double bed is GS all over. The person who was GS as a child, will be affected much sooner (years even), than a partner who was not GS as a child.

SURVEYING

If you are testing for GS with the muscle test, both of you should stand next to or sit on a bed or favourite chair while being tested. If you find the bed or chair is GS, test other places to find a place that GS free.

When dowsing with L-rods or a pendulum, make a plan of your complete bedroom floor and indicate where the bed/s are. Any GS lines found should follow from room to room. You will find the GS lines are exactly in the same place downstairs (unless you are in a bungalow, then any GS may extend into the living room etc). A GS line is normally anything from just under 2.5 cm (inch) to over 30 cm (1 ft) wide.

All rooms should be crossed in two directions at right angles to one another in order not to miss any GS lines by moving too close to the direction of a GS line. Each room should be crossed in one direction and then in the opposite direction. It is always a good confirmation when you find the same line on the way back.

No matter how many floors high the building is, the same pattern will be duplicated.

Have you found the right lines? If you have concentrate completely on the GS lines that are harmful to your health, you will only react to these when using the L-rods or pendulum. Double check with the muscle test if GS is found on beds, chairs etc.

If you are unlucky enough to sleep in a place **crossed** by two GS lines, one can almost be sure you will become ill, if you are not so already.
Don't forget to check your favourite chair is in front of the TV, in the kitchen and your place of work if you spend many hours in the same place. Many cases of cancer in the lower parts of the body have been detected in people who have sat for long hours daily on the same office chair, which is found in a GS place. The Metal chair legs help to concentrate GS onto the body.

Now move your beds and favorite chair or sofa outside GS lines. Some people put castors under their bed if the best place to sleep is right up against a fixed wardrobe or at an awkward angle, so they can move the bed during the day. You may even have to sleep in another room.

There was a tragic case where parents were warned that the life of their 7-year-old daughter was at risk because her bed was standing on an extremely strong GS line. The parents were sceptical and reluctant to move the child's bed because that would have involved removing a built-in wardrobe. The child died.

Your car may also be parked in a GS place making you GS every time you and your family are in the car, which may cause tiredness and even car sickness.

There are some excellent GS neutralisers on the market, but when it comes to cancer you just must sleep in a GS free place wherever that place may be in the house. You only have one life!

MUSCLE TEST

This is a versatile and accurate diagnostic technique which can be carried out by any two people based on the theory 'that your body does not lie'.

The Muscle Test can be used to check if a specific place is affected by Geopathic Stress and to double check your findings of the L rod or the pendulum. Your body can clearly tell whether a place is good or bad for you.

How to check for Geopathic Stress

Ask a willing friend (test partner) to hold out one arm at shoulder height, parallel to the ground (sitting or standing erect). Place one of your hands (palm down) on their wrist, with your other hand on their shoulder (you can be behind or in front of the person). Now ask your test partner to 'resist' with all his/her strength while you push down on their wrist quickly and firmly to assess how much pressure it takes to push the arm down. The idea is to push just hard enough to test the spring and bounce in the arm, not so hard that the muscle becomes fatigued. It is not a question of who is stronger, but of whether the muscle can lock the shoulder joint against the push. In most cases a test partner will resist the pressure and the arm will remain outstretched.

Now start checking if a bed, chair, desk etc. is in a Geopathic Stress place. When checking ask "Is there Geopathic Stress here?" If the answer is yes, your test partner's arm will go down. The weaker the arm, the stronger the Geopathic Stress. If you find Geopathic Stress, start finding places where there is no Geopathic Stress. If it is a small bedroom and the Geopathic Stress is mainly by the pillow, try sleeping the other way round.

Most people will find that they immediately sleep better when they have moved their beds from a Geopathic Stress place to a good place. It is almost magic how babies sleep better and stop crying when moved out of a Geopathic Stress place.

The Muscle Test is ideal for visually handicapped people.

The Muscle Test can also be carried out while you are both sitting down.

With experience, the Muscle Test can be done with your test partner's elbow on a table and your hand only on their wrist. You may like to test the other way round, so you can see what your arm feels like in a Geopathic Stress place. Don't test too much Geopathic Stress in one day, certainly not more than two properties a week. If you find Geopathic Stress, you should both wash your hands afterwards to get rid of the Geopathic Stress.

You will not necessarily get cancer by sleeping in a very Geopathic Stress place, but it is almost unheard of for anybody to get cancer unless they are Geopathically Stressed.

The Muscle Test can also be used to check almost anything:-
- whether specific treatments, medical drugs, supplements, Bach Flower and homeopathy remedies etc. are of benefit or not.
- also to check how allergic one is to certain foods, drinks and toxic substances.

Remember weak arm = bad

When testing, it might help to concentrate by writing the name of the specific treatment, drug, supplement etc. on a separate piece of paper. Ask the person you are testing on, to hold the paper (or actual tablet etc.) in their free hand. Alternatively, both of you should just concentrate on the question.

If the treatment, supplement etc. is good, the arm being tested will stay strong. If you wish to know how many capsules of say Vitamin D to take, test until the arm goes strong again.

Don't forget, that the answers may vary from day to day. One day tomatoes might test good for you, the next day bad. Don't get fanatical and test everything you eat.

If you wish to test a young child, your test partner should place their free hand on the child and let the child hold the names of tablets etc.

If you find the Muscle Test is obviously giving the wrong answers, you and/or your test partner may have a complication called switching. Try holding an obvious toxin (e.g. strong toilet cleaner), a 'strong' response to a toxin will indicate that you are switched. To un-switch, try a few short thumps with the palm of your hands on the thymus (on your chest just below the collarbone). You may even have to ask somebody else to test.

If checking whether a Geopathic Stress neutraliser has cleared the Geopathic Stress, it is important to ask "now my neutraliser is installed, has it cleared the Geopathic Stress in **this room/home**?" Don't just ask "has the neutraliser removed the Geopathic Stress?" because the Geopathic Stress will still be active below your home, beyond the powers of the neutraliser.

If you are on your own in a shop or pharmacy and would like to check if, say, a supplement is any good for you, try putting the tips of your thumb and first finger (or second finger) together. Put the first finger of your other hand through the 'O' you have created and pull. If the finger is **not** held back (don't pull too hard), you have got a negative answer. Some people find they blink if they get a negative answer.

L-RODS

The earliest form of dowsing for water etc. involved using a Y-shaped willow twig as a dowsing rod. Holding the twig with both hands, the single twig facing forward will turn downwards when crossing a stream of underground water, sometimes with such force it could scorch the hands.

It was discovered about 26 years ago that most people could learn to use a pair of L-shaped steel wire rods to locate GS lines fairly accurately.

How to make the L-rods

A pair of L-shaped wire dowsing rods can be easily made from two wire coat hangers:

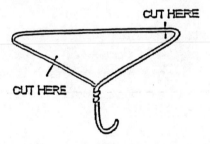

Cut where indicated and straighten the bend out so that it becomes a right angle.

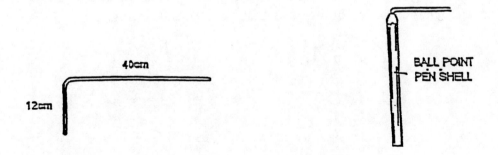

To enable the rods to swing more easily, the shells of cheap ballpoint pens can be used as sleeves on the short end (see above). To prevent the L rods swinging about too freely outdoors, you could shorten the rods or use heavy gauge wire e.g. brazing rods.

It is not important what material your dowsing tool is made out of, as long as it is reasonably balanced and you feel comfortable using it.

PRACTICE

These L rods are each held in the fist by the short length and carried in front of the chest with the longest length pointing forward.

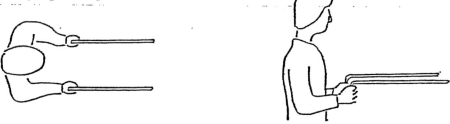

The horizontal section of the rod must not rest on the hand and the thumb must not be on top of the bend, otherwise the rod cannot swing freely.

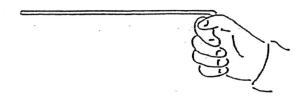

You must now learn to hold the rods completely horizontal and steady. This is achieved with a little practice. The end of the rods must not point upwards, otherwise they will fall sideways when you move and the rods must not hang down otherwise too much force is needed to swing them sideways.

So learn to keep the rods horizontal and try to hold them steady when you move slowly forward. You should adopt a sliding walk, akin to that of a cat creeping up on its prey. The most important thing is to hold the body completely steady as you move forward, thereby keeping the arm and rods unaffected by body movements. As soon as you have mastered this you can start searching for your first GS line.

THE SEARCH

The rods will react either by swinging out sideways or by crossing over one another. Curiously enough it makes no difference which way the rods swing.

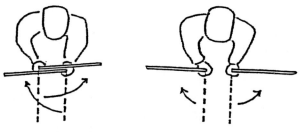

You must concentrate on exactly what you are seeking, as the rods can be used to find many other things, such as water pipes, drains, electrical cables etc. Focus your concentration on Geopathic Stress lines and you will not be attuned to other signals.

In the beginning, say to yourself "I am looking for GS lines and I want the rod to swing out when I get to one". As you are walking, it is important you keep a clear image of GS lines in your mind and that you keep focusing on them. To prevent yourself having expectations as to where the lines are, it might help to keep repeating to yourself "Geopathic Stress lines".

When you have found a GS line, walk forward and back over it a few times until you become familiar with the forces that are influencing the rods. You will soon learn to distinguish accurately between twistings which are due to your own movements, and those, which are due to GS lines.

When you find a GS line, it is as if a magnet is pulling on the rods.

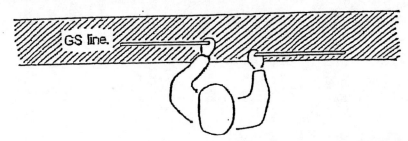

No matter whether the rods cross or swing sideways initially, they will afterwards place themselves parallel to the GS line they have located.
Therefore you should not approach the GS line at an angle of less than 45 degrees. Cross the area in various directions.
If you walk more or less in the same direction as the GS line, you run the risk that the rods will not register, as they will continue to point forward in the direction of the GS line.
When the L-rods swing back to the search position, you have reached the other edge of the GS line.
Remember, keep a loose grip on the rods, keep them horizontal and concentrate on the Geopathic Stress, not on the rods.
When this has been mastered, you can start your first survey for GS in a house.

To practice dowsing with rods for the first time, it is usually better to go out for example into some open woods, where there is no wind, you are not overlooked and where you can be completely relaxed about finding Geopathic Stress lines (and anxious e.g. when dowsing your own home). I found this the best way to start dowsing with rods.

TYPICAL BEGINNER'S MISTAKES WHEN DOWSING WITH RODS

1. The thumb locking on top of the rod.
2. The horizontal rod resting on the index finger.
3. Gripping the rod too tightly (if it has no sleeve).
   Finding the rods are spinning around in circles. Try and drop the tip of the rod down a bit then back horizontal, as you gain more experience.
5. Walking too fast.
6. Forgetting to mark the position of the GS lines!
7. Not working to a systematic plan.
8. Forgetting to go through each room in two directions at right angles to one another.
9. The reaction on the rods coming too late.
10. Relying on the rod to indicate the direction of the GS lines accurately before you have experience.
11. Not concentrating on Geopathic Stress lines.
12. Assuming that you have found a crossing just because the rods cross. To be certain you have found a crossing point, you must find two or more lines independent of each other and determine the place at which they meet, like roads at a road junction.

PENDULUM

Using a pendulum is another way to check for Geopathic Stress (GS) lines.
A pendulum can very easily be made with a thread secured to a small weighted object, such as a key or a ring, but I find a well-balanced brass pendulum with a central point, gives the clearest results. Several designs can be purchased in various materials including crystal, but an expensive pendulum in for instance silver, will not necessarily give you better results.
What is important is that you feel comfortable with your pendulum.

Hold the string or chain between
your thumb and forefinger and
allow the pendulum to swing.
Experiment using different lengths
of string or chain, starting with 3-4"
(7-10 cm).

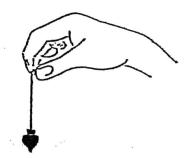

Start by swinging the pendulum gently back and forth in the initial search position while repeating to yourself "Search for GS lines" or just concentrate on GS lines. Keep moving slowly across the room you want to check until the pendulum starts to rotate either way. You now know that you have hit a GS line.

Now ask yourself the direction of the GS line is going and the pendulum should stop rotating and move back and forward in the direction of the GS line.

You can check the width of the GS line by crossing the line until the pendulum stops swinging in a circle. This indicates the other edge of the GS line.

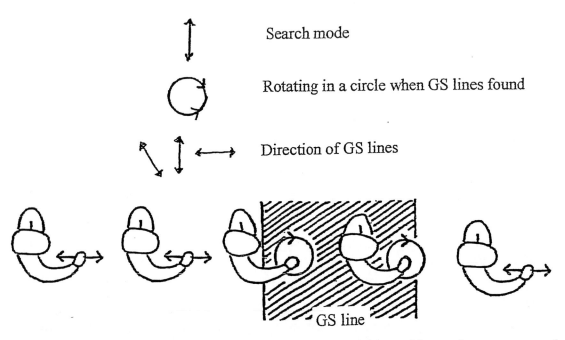

As with L-rods, one way to practise is to take your pendulum with you into open woods where there is no wind,people and homes influencing your findings. If you are in a mixed wood, you will nearly always find a GS line going straight through a big oak tree,one of the only types of tree to thrive in GS places. In a mixed wood, 80% of lightening will strike oak trees, due to the water, which creates the GS, running under the tree.

PRECAUTIONS TO BE TAKEN WHEN SEARCHING

Very often, the person searching for GS lines may feel exhausted after a little while. It is as if you have been drained of energy, but the tiredness will disappear after a rest. If you feel bad while searching - stop. This is very important. You should certainly not search for GS lines if you are already tired, ill, depressed, or have cancer, as you will only aggravate your condition. So ask someone in good health to dowse for you. Don't dowse more than two properties a week.

It is a good idea to take a shower or at least wash your hands under running water after a search.

Do not dowse during stormy weather or during full moon, as the GS will be extremely strong then.

For various reasons do not let children become involved in dowsing. Children are very sensitive to Geopathic Stress and find that they can dowse for the lines quite easily. However, they shouldn't be exposed to the influence of GS unnecessarily while they are still growing and developing. Also, young children might not always appreciate that searching for GS is a serious endeavour and might treat the whole thing as a game.

NON CANCER CASES

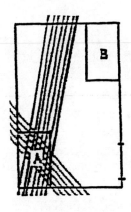

Peter (18 months old) had been in and out of Hospital all his short life with breathing problems and could not play for more than a few minutes at a time. His mother rang me up on a Friday and I advised her to move his cot from 'A' to the other side of the room 'B'.

His mother rang me up the next Monday and said jokingly, "You should never have advised me to move Peter's cot. He has now become too lively, I can hardly control him." Peter came to see me several years after with his mother, who informed me he had not seen a doctor since his cot had been moved.

"Dear Rolf,

Our 19-year-old daughter Claire has been suffering from ME for many yeas and she always slept badly. On your advice, we moved her bed as you had suggested (from 'A' to 'B'). The first night she went to sleep straight away for the first time in many years and slept like a baby all night. This has not only improved her health, but Claire can now study for about 20 minutes most days. Before she could hardly get from her bedroom to the lounge and could only study once a week for 15 minutes. Thank you for all your help. Best Wishes Ann (Mother)"

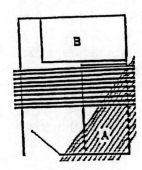

"Dear Rolf Gordon

I am writing to thank you from the bottom of my heart for the dowsing information for my house. (14/03/2005). For me this has been a breakthrough in supporting my recovery from ME. After 11 years with the condition and the last 7 years when I have been unable to work, I now feel that I am emerging into the light once more.

Yours sincerely
Paul Hancock

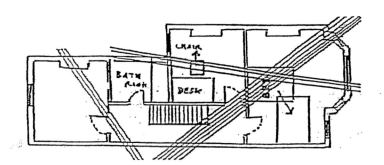

For Paul Hancock

Checked for Geopathic Stress
lines *Rolf Gordon*

Move bed and chair as indicated
by arrows

VEGATEST

This is a device for diagnosis and therapy on the basis of bio-energetics and electro-acupuncture.

The VEGATEST method has been used by doctors and health practitioners for many years all over the world. **It is an excellent method of testing to see if you are suffering from Geopathic Stress.** The VEGATEST can also be used to check the state of various parts of the body and to establish if you are intolerant to a range of different foods and drinks.

An ampoule is placed in the VEGATEST machine, or in circuit in the VEGATEST EXPERT. The patient holds an electrode while the practitioner places a probe on an acupuncture point. A minimum amount of voltage passes through the probe to provoke a response from the acupuncture meridian. The result is shown on the meter of the VEGATEST machine.

Practitioners who use VEGATEST equipment have all been professionally trained. To find your nearest practitioner contact Noma (Complex Homeopathy) Ltd., Unit 119, Solent Business Centre, Millbrook Road West, Southampton, SO15 0HW Tel: 02380 770513 Fax: 02380 702459, the UK supplier of the equipment who will give you a list of local practitioners who have VEGATEST equipment.

CHECKING FOR FOOD AND DRINK ALLERGIES

Up to 30% of adults and 50% of children are affected by the foods we eat and the environment we live in.
Food allergies can be caused by the thousands of chemicals introduced into modern foods and drinks, prescription drugs and antibiotics taken direct or indirectly due to intensive farming, where we get small daily doses of antibiotics from meat, eggs, cheese and other dairy products.

Allergies can cause:
fatigue, depression, anxiety, irritability, aggressive behaviour, nervousness, insomnia, asthma, aching joints, digestion problems, frequent infections, headaches and sinus problems. In children learning difficulties and or behavioural problems including being hyperactive. Main causes of migraines are cheese, chocolate and red wine.

Check with one of the following tests:
- The muscle test (see previous chapter).
- Get a good dowser to check you out (it is often very difficult to check yourself by dowsing).
- Go to a nutritional therapist or allergy expert who can check you out by Kinesiology or VegaTest to help devise a diet that cuts out all allergy provoking foods and introduces a suitable check list of foods and drinks that can trigger food allergies:
  - Gluten (in barley, rye, wheat, oats etc)
  - Dairy foods mainly cheeses which contain the amino acid tyramine
  - Eggs
  - Corn
  - Peanuts
  - Citrus fruits
  - Tomatoes
  - Mushrooms
  - Peppers
  - Eggplant (also known as aubergine)
  - Potatoes
  - Artificial Sweeteners such as Aspartame
  - Chocolate including drinks which contain the amino acid tyramine
  - Red wine which has a high concentration of sulphites
  - Caffeine drinks including coffee, tea and cola drinks
  - Alcohol
  - Junk food
  - Chemicals added to food
  - Food and drink with added sugar
  - Fizzy drinks
  - Gravy mixes
  - Packaged or tinned food

Headaches can also be caused by Geopathic Stress, low blood sugar, oestrogen in oral contraceptives, hormone replacement therapy and being too low in salt (see page 223), Asprin, Paracetamol etc. which can have a painful rebound effect when their intended effect wears off and smoking. They can also be caused by stress on the eyes, too much reading or computer work or wearing incorrect glasses. Resting the eyes in the palms of the hands helps. See your doctor if you have medical conditions such as fever, high blood pressure, meningitis or a brain tumour.

CHECKING FOR ENVIRONMENTAL ALLERGIES

There is a huge misconception that if you sneeze and have sore eyes a lot, it must be hay fever. It is most likely you are allergic to the allergens below. To pinpoint and avoid the source is the most crucial part of tackling any allergy. You can use the test described previously or have an allergy test for the allergies listed below at a high street chemist. It takes half an hour and involves a pin-prick to the finger.

Grass pollen, house dust mites, dogs, cats, birch pollen, hazelnut pollen, mugwart pollen, stinging nettles pollen, latex, the moulds aspergillus fumigatus, alternaria alternata and calodosportium herbarum (the last two are often found in houses with poor ventilation and in low, damp areas).

WHAT IS GOOD FOR ME

Don't forget to use the tests at the beginning of this chapter to find out what is good for you and what you are looking for, e.g. what vitamins, minerals, enzymes etc.
In case of cancer, it is vital that you also check if you need 100% stabilised allicin, Q10, Vitamin D, Bicarbonate of Soda (for your pH) etc.

GALL BLADDER FLUSH - simple, inexpensive and easy to perform

An estimated 20% of you will develop gallstones in your gall bladder at some time in your life. This could entail many months of severe pain waiting for an NHS operation, like major surgery to remove the gall bladder or remove the stones with keyhole surgery or crush them by ultrasound. It could involve a long recovery time and you may not be able to eat normally for a long time - if ever - afterwards.
Surgery may also lead to major pain and suffering for years afterwards. A private operation could cost over £4,000.
It is estimated as many as 3 million people world wide have now carried out the simple, painless and inexpensive gall bladder flush themselves, with an over 95% success rate and it only takes 6 days.

How to carry out the gall bladder flush

1. For 5 days prior to 'flush' drink 2 litres of fresh pure apple juice daily (normal juice from shops). The malic acid in the apple juice softens the gallstones and makes their passage through the bile duct smooth and easy. During the 5 days eat normal meals, but don't overeat.

2. On the sixth day
   A Have no evening meal
   B At 9 pm take 1 or 2 teaspoonsful of Epsom Salts or Andres Liver Salts dissolved in 30 to 60 ml (1 to 2 fluid ounces) of warm water. This will widen the bile ducts, thereby also making it easier for the gallstones to pass.
   C At 10 pm mix half a cup, 120 ml (4 ozs), olive oil with 60 ml (2 ozs) fresh lemon juice. Shake vigorously and drink all down.
   D IMMEDIATELY upon finishing the olive oil and juice, go to bed and lie on your right side with your right knee drawn up towards your chin. Remain in this position for 30 minutes before going to sleep. This encourages the olive oil to drain from your stomach, helping contents of the olive oil to move into the small intestine.

3. Next morning the stones will pass. They will be yellow grey or green in colour and soft as putty, varying in size of grains of sand to some as large as your thumbnail. You may have the urge to go to the toilet several times before the stones pass. You are unlikely to feel any pain, but will be amazed by the results.

4. If you are not satisfied with the results, try the flush out a few days afterwards or even double the dose of olive oil and lemon juice.

It may be advisable to have a flush out at regular intervals, say four or five years apart.

Notes
- The apple juice can be diluted with any amount of water.
- If you cannot tolerate apple juice for some reason, you can drink cranberry juice instead as it also contains malic acid.
- If you are allergic to olive oil, you can use other cold-pressed oils such as grape seed or sunflower oil. Do not use processed oils like canola or soya oil.
- People who suffer cancer, candida, diabetes, hypoglycaemia (deficiency of glucose in the bloodstream) or stomach ulcers, may have difficulty drinking apple or cranberry juice in large quantities. They can take malic acid in powdered form. Avoid malic acid capsules, especially if they contain other ingredients. Mix ½ to 1 teaspoon malic acid with a litre of water. If possible, drink 2 litres per day.
- It is best if you have enough time the morning after the night you had the flush, when you are not under any pressure and have time to rest.

Some of the letters and comments on Gall Bladder Flush I have received:

Mrs B O (London, SW7)	Using GBF, six stones came out as big as pennies. Cancelled gall bladder operation.
Mrs P M (Clonhill, Beds)	Tried GBF which resulted in many stones coming out, confirmed by scan.
Mr R D (London, SE19)	Had enormous pain. Scan confirmed many stones in gall bladder. Took the recommended GBF. Early next morning passed about a hundred small stones soft as putty. For the last fifteen years I have been able to eat fats and cream chocolate cakes without any discomfort.
Hairdresser	Bit disappointed only got 5 stones out, but they were as big as small finger nails!
Mrs E M C (Cardiff)	'Over the moon' GBF flushed out hundreds of stones.
Mrs M H (Kingston, Surrey)	Scan showed nor more stones after GBF.
Practitioner (E K, Belfast)	'I have given details about GBF to a number of my patients, one of whom was about to have his gall bladder removed. He ran out of count at 72 stones after having done the 'washout'. One of my patients flushed out stones as big as Quails Eggs!!'
Robin O'S (Kent)	'GBF worked fantastic'.

Gilda W, Practitioner (Aberdeen)	GBF flushed out 64 gall stones, some as big as finger nails.
Bob O'S (Kent)	First GBF flushed out many stones. Second flush a month afterwards flushed out two half inch stones, plus many smaller stones.
Darren Russell	'Thank you sooooo much for posting this information, the GBF worked for me and I expelled close to ¼ pint of material, one as large as a Robin's egg. I was in terrible pain. I tried the flush and feel soooooo much better, and the thought of having an operation really did NOT appeal to me. All I can say is Thank You'.

P.S. Andy Warhol, the famous modern artist, died on 22 February 1987 in a New York Hospital following a gall bladder operation.

Your gall bladder

It is a small pear-shaped sac situated underneath the liver to which it is attached by fibrous tissue. **Bile** produced by the liver, passes to the gall bladder via the cystic duct for storage and concentrated by absorption of the water content through the gall bladder walls. When food containing fat passes from the stomach to the duodenum, bile is released into the duodenum via the common bile duct, where it aids the digestion of the fats. More digestion enzyme juices are released from the pancreas through a duct, which join the bile duct just before the entrance to the duodenum. When the large amount of fat from the olive oil enters the small intestine, the gall bladder squeezes bile out with such force it pushes out any gallstones which have been softened at the same time.

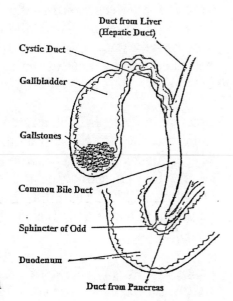

SUMMARY

Remember, 42% of people are likely to be diagnosed with cancer and one in three of all deaths in the UK are due to cancer and even more if you take into account the people who die from some of the aggressive orthodox treatments. It is, therefore, very important that you take into account the BIG FOUR which affect all cancer cases. I firmly believe that the NHS could save billions a year if we all took the BIG FOUR seriously.

It is important that you take adequate supplements, vitamins, minerals and trace elements that modern food no longer supplies. They also help to fight the thousands of chemicals incorporated in modern food. Eat a healthy diet yes, but don't forget to feed your soul by enjoying what you eat, even something a little naughty now and again, as long as you keep your blood acid alkaline balance slightly alkaline by taking Bicarbonate of Soda (see Part One).

If you have cancer, pamper yourself, treat yourself to a massage and for women perhaps enjoy a beauty treatment. Go to the theatre or cinema and try and have a good time with friends. Talk regularly about your health problems and fears with your partner, best friend, your therapist and/or other cancer patients. Ask for help in all sorts of ways from your friends. Keep your head high and convince yourself that you will recover, by believing and saying 'I will kill this cancer' and don't let anybody tell you otherwise'. A 15 year long study of breast cancer patients concluded that those who showed a fighting spirit and healthy sense of denial, had significantly better survival rates than those who held on to a hopeless and resigned attitude.

I plan to update this book on a continuous basis, so if you have any constructive criticism, interesting observations or case histories (names will not published without your permission), then please contact me in writing (keep letters brief please). The address for correspondence is:
Dulwich Health Limited, 130 Gipsy Hill, London, SE19 1PL or Fax: 44(0) 8766 6616. Kindly note that due to time constraints, I regret I am unable to accept telephone calls or e-mails.

I know it may well take as long to convince the medical profession that the BIG FOUR are some of the main reasons we get cancer, that it took Charles Darwin to convince the church about the contents of his book 'The Origin of Species'.

At least I have convinced over a million people worldwide, how harmful Geopathic Stress is to their health.

STOP PRESS   November 2012

Barnard S in Switzerland, diagnosed with severe oesophageal cancer, contacted me about six months ago. I ensured the BIG FOUR was taken care of. The doctor has just confirmed Barnard no longer has cancer. The doctor said, with tears in his eyes, that he had never had such good results in a severe cancer case before.

Many other health problems can be helped by taking care of the BIG FOUR.
Lupus This wretched disease causes joint pain, skin rashes and tiredness. Often involves hair loss, weight loss, problems with your kidneys and other organs. We have successfully treated two women. Mary, in her forties, was diagnosed with Lupus 2½ years ago, which made her feel very fatigued, had a 'butterfly' rash across the bridge of her nose, joint pains all over and felt no better after long orthodox treatment. After applying the BIG FOUR, she no longer has problems with Lupus and is now an active teacher again.

Liz, who is 72 years old, had Lupus for over 4 years. She had a heavy rash on her face, could not walk and lost most of her hair. Now, she walks up to 4 miles most days. She no longer has a rash nor joint pains and her hair has grown back. Liz's liver and kidneys are now working normally again. This was achieved by taking care of the BIG FOUR.

Lyme disease is caused by mites (mainly from deer and sheep) biting you and very soon affects almost every organ of your body, commonly involving your skin, joints, heart and nervous system. Lyme disease has been cleared in nearly all the people who have applied the BIG FOUR, after long term antibiotics had failed.

Micro parasites I believe that the main cause of Alzheimers, MS and Parkinson disease is micro parasites in the brain. Hopefully after I have carried out my research, one can prevent people with these illnesses getting worse.

INDEX - see also Contents page 4